Arthroscopy

Arthroscopy

Richard L. O'Connor, M.D.
Founding Member, International Arthroscopy Association
Consultant in Orthopaedic Surgery
West Covina Hospital
West Covina, California

With Two Contributors

J. B. Lippincott Company
Philadelphia · Toronto

ISBN 0-397-50371-7

Library of Congress Catalog Card Number 77-4908

Printed in the United States of America

3 5 4 2

Library of Congress Cataloging in Publication Data

O'Connor, Richard L
Arthroscopy.

Bibliography: p.
Includes index.
1. Knee—Examination. 2. Knee—Surgery.
3. Arthroscopy. I. Title. [DNLM: 1. Endoscopy.
2. Knee joint—Radiography. 3. Knee injuries—
Radiography. WE870 018a]
RD561.024 616.7'2 77-4908
ISBN 0-397-50371-7

This book is dedicated
with admiration and respect to my parents,
Josephine J. and Roger R. O'Connor.

Contributors

Robert C. Bechtol, M.D.
Founding Member, International Arthroscopy Association
Consultant, Department of Orthopaedic Surgery
Santa Rosa Memorial Hospital
Santa Rosa, California

Richard L. O'Connor, M.D.
Founding Member, International Arthroscopy Association
Consultant in Orthopaedic Surgery
West Covina Hospital
West Covina, California

Lou A. Wettermann
Executive Vice President
Richard Wolf Medical Instruments Corporation
Rosemont, Illinois

By the street of by and by, we arrive at the house of never.

Cervantes

Preface

My purpose in preparing this monograph is to share knowledge and experience with those interested in arthroscopy during what I believe to be its watershed period. Diagnostic arthroscopy appears to be well accepted, and the basic diagnostic equipment has been developed by many instrument makers to meet the subtle differences demanded by a great number of arthroscopists. Now, the emphasis will be on the development of therapeutic equipment and techniques.

There is no substitute for learning arthroscopy one-to-one: a physician teaching another in a clinical situation. Indeed, many arthroscopists proficient in the technique are swamped by visitors. One of the problems posed by attempting to learn the technique in this way alone is that the knowledge shared is necessarily incomplete due to limitations imposed by chance and selection of patients.

The information in this monograph is based on observation. But though I feel that my interpretation of these observances is accurate, it is not written in granite. I want to add too that many ideas have been obtained from other arthroscopists and are not acknowledged because they have rapidly entered the realm of general information. For any faulty interpretation, I assume responsibility.

Arthroscopic examination is an individual situation between patient and physician in an attempt to solve a problem. Usually, as no other orthopaedist familiar with arthroscopy is present, there is no chance for consultation or spreading of the responsibility onto a committee's shoulders. Caution and reflection are vital, particularly when one is confronted by an unusual situation; stereotyped answers are of little value; statistic analyses, used to attempt to solve a given problem, are misleading. I can only stress what has been stressed often enough about other matters: when in doubt, do nothing.

Advancement of knowledge depends upon tools—mental and physical. Prior to the advent of arthroscopic examination, considerable emphasis was placed on mental tools derived from increasing personal and collective experience with interpretation of the patient's history and physical examination. This was supplemented by radiographs with the enormous limitations of the plain roentgenogram, and, later, the blind areas of the arthrograph. The addition of a new tool opens new horizons, but allows observations without an established norm. Again, emphasis must be placed on a return to the supremacy of the mental tool to correlate facts obtained by both the conventional and the newer sophisticated methods. Hopefully, this monograph will help to find a norm against which the pathologic state may be better appreciated. That additional information is needed is suggested by the fact that 60 per cent of my arthroscopic cases were referred by a multitude of orthopaedists who recognized problems that conventional methods did not clarify. Arthroscopy will also have its limitations, but these areas must also be defined.

Many persons have contributed in great measure to this monograph. Professor James Harkess of the University of Louisville supplied the original impetus; Dr. Masaki Watanabe, Dr. Sakae Takeda, and Dr. Hiroshi Ikeuchi shared with me their technique and encouragement; Dr. Keith Walker, Dr. Paul Harmon, and Dr. William McColl of West Covina and Dr. Robert Allen of Glendora, California, provided constant encouragement during the initial difficult stages of mastering the technique. Dr. Robert Jackson of Toronto, Canada, and Dr. Ward Casscells of Wilmington, Delaware, opened the North American continent to the concepts of arthroscopy, and without their original efforts mine would have been severely curtailed. The administration of the West Covina Hospital and the operating room personnel have done everything in their power to provide an atmosphere conducive to investigation.

The Richard Wolf Company, Kittlingen, Germany, directed by Herbert Schubert, with the help of optical engineer S. Hildebrandt and electronic engineer H. Wurster, helped develop the necessary equipment. Special thanks are extended to Seymour Shubin for reviewing the manuscript, and to L. Wettermann, Vice President of the Richard Wolf Company, U.S.A., for help with the chapter on endoscopic instruments and for three years of helpful suggestions in modifying the arthroscopic equipment. Dr. Robert Bechtol of Santa Rosa, California, shared his provocative thoughts on future developments in his chapter.

Last, but not least, I want to thank my assistant, Barbara Swan, for providing loyal and dependable help throughout my arthroscopic troubles; Helen Darcel for her art work; my daughter, Mary Anne, for her grammatical corrections; Lewis Reines and Carole Baker of the J. B. Lippincott Company for their encouragement and editorial assistance; and Dolores DeHaven for managing my office.

Many have contributed to this monograph, but the sole responsibility for erroneous interpretation is mine. If one wants to have absolute evidence to support a monograph on observation, he will pass the street of by and by and reach the house of never.

RICHARD L. O'CONNOR, M.D.

Contents

1 *From Endoscopy to Arthroscopy*

Lou A. Wettermann

HISTORY

The word *endoscope* is derived from two Greek words, *endo* from the word *endon,* "within," and *scope* from the word *skopein,* "an instrument for observing or seeing."

The concept of the endoscope comprises all devices for visual examination and observation of body cavities. Owing to varying anatomical relationships, there are many very substantial differences in the construction of these individual devices. For example, entirely different requirements apply for the arthroscope, cystoscope, laryngoscope, laparoscope, and gastroscope.

Medical endoscopy had its start in the early 1800s when Bozzini devised a speculum instrument to put light into the body cavity. This instrument, called the Lichtleiter (Fig. 1-1), illuminated deep cavities by reflecting light. It consisted of a tube divided in two, with a candle inside a box. Light was reflected through half of the tube by a slightly concave mirror. The operator viewed the light field through a cuplike eyepiece attached to the other half of the tube. In 1876 Nitze designed a cystoscope that used a platinum loop for illumination. He realized that the light source had to be within the distal tip, but at that time Edison was engaged in efforts

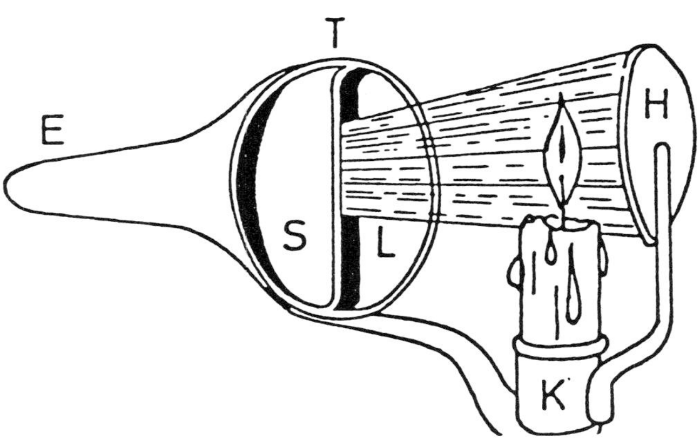

Fig. 1-1. The Lichtleiter consisted of (E) a main housing, (T) a separation wall, (S) a viewing channel, (L) a light channel, (K) a candle holder, and (H) a concave mirror.

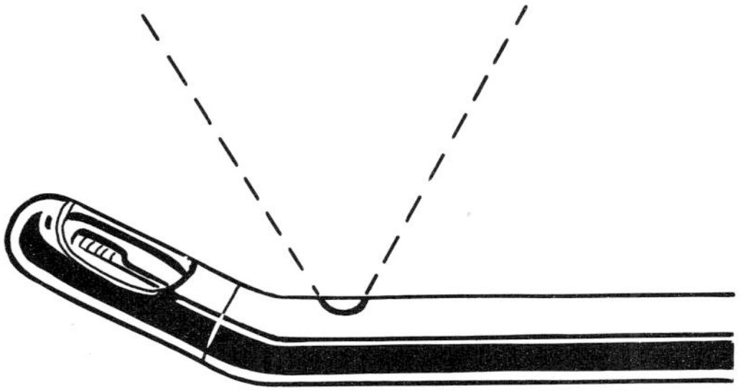

Fig. 1-2. Right-angle viewing cystoscope with incandescent lamp.

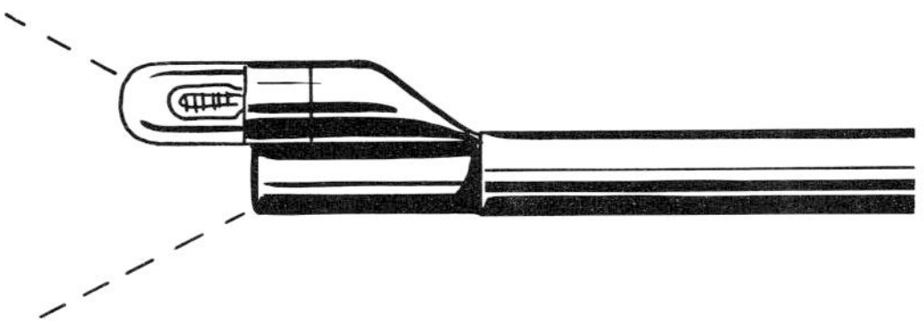

Fig. 1-3. Direct viewing endoscope with incandescent lamp.

that culminated in his invention of the light bulb, which had to be miniaturized for use in the endoscope. By 1883 the incandescent bulb had been reduced in size to fit the diameter of an endoscope, and Nitze in the following years developed one of the first true endoscopes. The lens system used in these first endoscopes was of a simple design, which had, besides a prism to reflect an image 90 degrees, only a few lenses, and which provided only limited light transmission.

FUNDAMENTALS OF ENDOSCOPES

An endoscope consists of three basic elements: mechanical parts, an illumination system, and an optical system.

Mechanical Parts

The mechanical part of an endoscope consists mainly of the instrument's rigid housing or sheath. This comes in several shapes and diameters. It must have a smooth surface, since in most cases it comes directly in contact with the mucosa of the internal organs and it is frequently inserted into narrow passages of the human body. Some endoscopes require trocar sleeves with trocars, the sleeves including stopcocks for inserting gases or fluids. The arthroscope (which is an endoscope used for examining the interior of a joint) requires a trocar for piercing the fibrous capsule. The trocar is removed and replaced with an obturator for the safe passage of the scope through the synovium or for difficult maneuvers through the joint. The trocar or obturator is then replaced with the telescope. A 15 gauge 1½ inch stainless steel needle is used for a counterdrain. The material originally used for the rigid sheaths was either brass or nickel-silver, and it was coated with nickel or chrome. Today most endoscope sheaths have incorporated the illumination as well as the optical system into their main housing so the need for thin walls with dependable rigidity becomes obvious. Thus, the use of stainless steel for sheaths has become widespread.

Illumination System

The incandescent lamp, once subminiaturized, was eventually embedded into the distal portion of the endoscope. (Fig. 1-2). Several different versions were used, depending on the viewing direction. If a 180-degree angle of vision was needed, lamps would be placed on a separate lamp carrier that positioned the illumination next to the endoscope shaft so that a straight viewing direction was achieved (Fig. 1-3).

The Optical System

It was Nitze who first incorporated a lens system into early endoscopes. It consisted mainly of an ocular transmission system and an objective lens, which, depending on its application, provided the different viewing angles needed. The con-

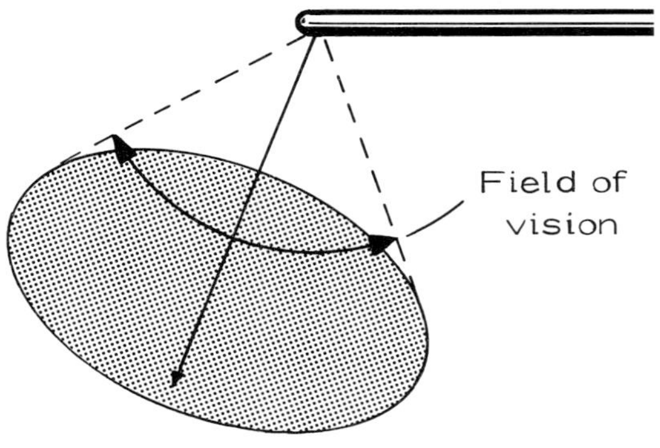

Fig. 1-4. Note the distinction between the field of vision and the complete visual field obtained with an encoscope.

struction of a modern endoscopic lens system is of special design, and therefore is not comparable to that of a microscope, binoculars, or standard astronomical telescopes. All lens systems for endoscopes are adjusted to infinity, thus allowing the examining physician to view the internal parts of the human body without increased magnification, but still within a considerable field of vision. The endoscopic lens system is therefore nothing more than a magnifying glass following the principles of Galileo, except that the objective lens is separated from the ocular by means of a lens system designed to transfer the image. The lens system consists of several lenses that reverse the image. A reverse prism is then used to achieve a noninverted image.

CLASSIFICATION OF ENDOSCOPES

Endoscopes are classified according to their viewing angle, field of vision (Fig. 1-4), method of illumination, site of illumination, type of optics, and method of introduction, and whether they are designed to be used in air or liquid. The great variety of viewing angles is illustrated in Fig. 1-5. The most common ones are sometimes referred to as follows:

Direct Vision: 180° to 170° angle of vision
Fore Oblique: 135° to 165° angle of vision
Right Angle: 110° to 90° angle of vision

MODERN TELESCOPES

Manufacturers of endoscopes* in the United States and in Europe have recently made several major innovations in their instruments, largely as a result of the introduction of fiber optics and of greatly improved lens systems. This conversion

* The telescope contains the lens system of the endoscope. The arthroscope, a specialized type of endoscope, contains the telescope and the mechanical parts necessary to provide joint irrigation.

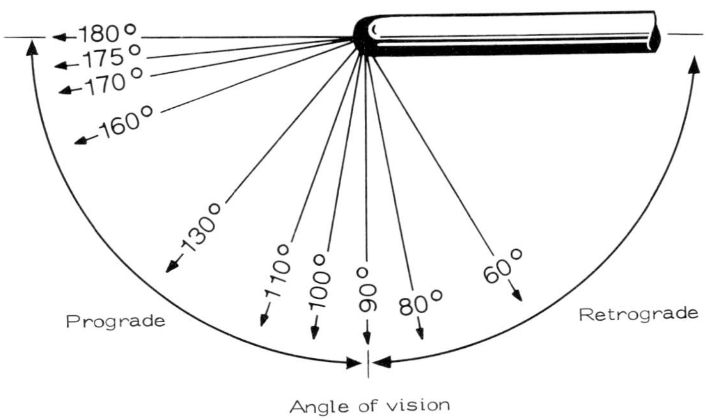

Fig. 1-5. Different angles of vision may be obtained with an endoscope.

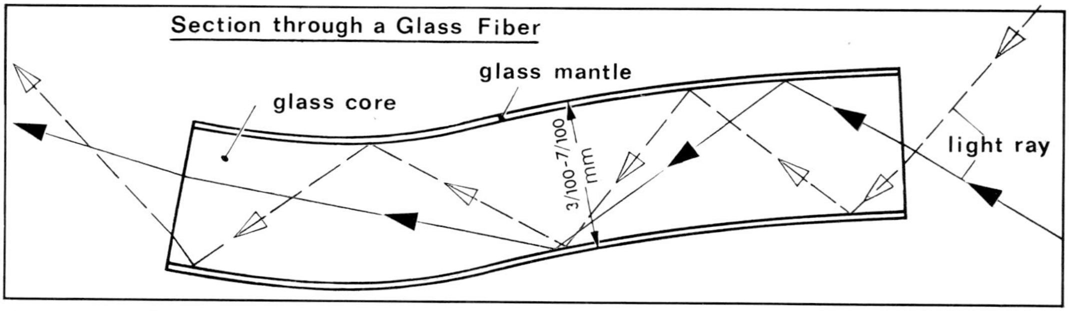

Fig. 1-6. The basic process of light transmission through optical glass fiber. The inner glass core must be coated with a thin film of glass of a lower refraction index in order to prevent light from leaking through its sides.

has greatly benefited practitioners of endoscopy.

Fiber Illumination

The development of endoscopy has always been greatly influenced by the availability of illumination. Light is a necessity for all visual examinations (especially documentation), such as 35-mm. still photography, cinema photography, and television.

The principle of using fiber optics to transmit light, or images, from one place to another through a flexible fiber bundle is not new. Early in 1950, A.C.S. Van Heel of the Netherlands began to improve the optical coating of fiber bundles in order to make them usable for illumination (Fig. 1-6), but until 1958 industry was unable to produce fiber optic bundles for transmission of either images or light at a reasonable cost. However, the resolution of such financial difficulties has rendered endoscopes with incandescent lights obsolete.

The current generation of endoscopes utilizes fiber optic illumination whenever possible. By omitting the distal incandescent lamp (Fig. 1-7), the so-called dead length of the objective is reduced to a minimum (Fig. 1-8). The incandescent lamp was a necessary extension at the distal tip of the telescope, and this extension prevented close-up examination. With a fiber illumination system, the space between the distal tip and the objective window was reduced considerably, allowing examination at a much closer distance.

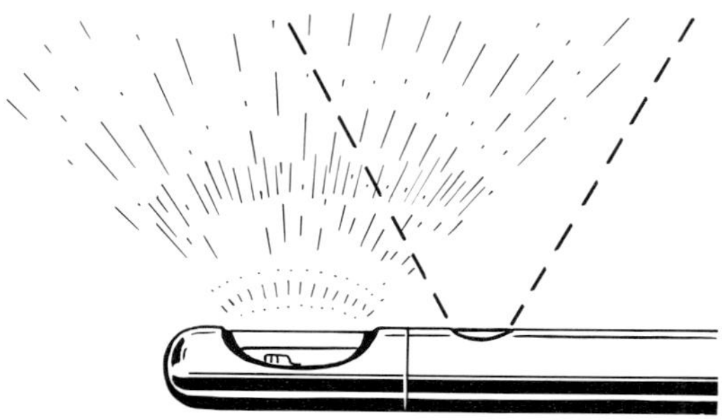

Fig. 1-7. Distal tip of an endoscope with incandescent illumination and *extended* space between tip and objective window.

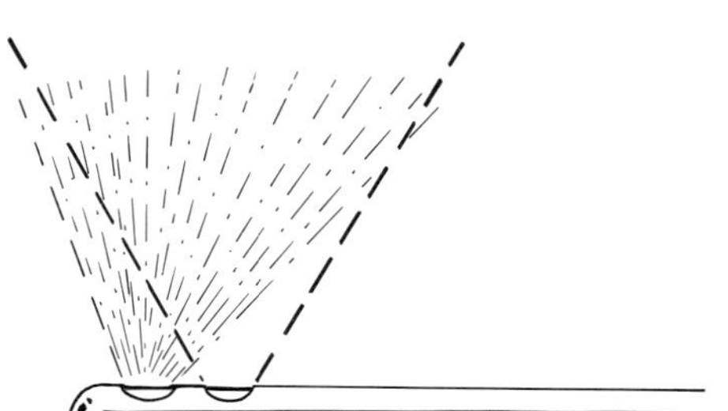

Fig. 1-8. Distal tip of an endoscope with fiber illumination and *reduced* space between tip and objective window.

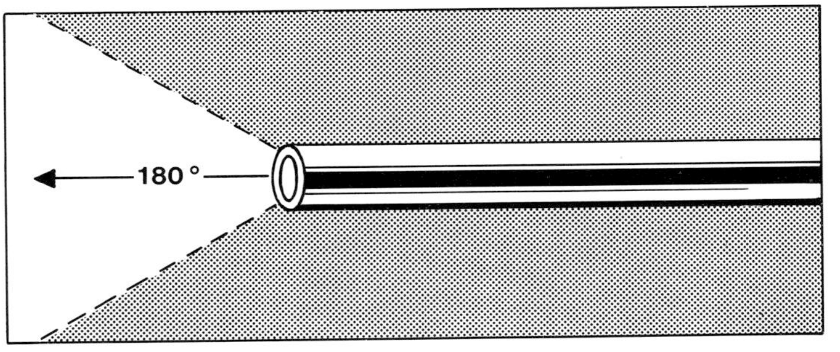

Fig. 1-9. Direct-viewing endoscope with fiber illumination (ring of light).

The light carrier with the offset lamp, which had been used prior to the availability of fiber optics (and which had caused difficulties when inserting or rotating the instrument), is rendered completely unnecessary, since it is now possible to place the fiber-illuminated bundle around the circumference of the objective window (Fig. 1-9).

An endoscope with fiber illumination (Fig. 1-10) consists of the fiber light projector with its cooling facilities, the fiber light cable connected to the projector and endoscope, and the scope with fiber illumination. The light source is now separated from the endoscope, and it is possible to produce a cold and powerful light without having to take into consideration the heat or weight factor. The advantages of a self-contained light source are as follows:

1. The size of the source is immaterial. It can therefore be of a very high intensity, and can be provided with a powerful cooling system.
2. In case of a defect, it is easy to repair or replace the light source.
3. A single light source can feed various instruments simultaneously.
4. Reliability and life of the light source are enhanced in comparison with internal illumination systems.
5. Replacement of the lamp is possible during examination.
6. The necessity to store many types of small lamps is eliminated.

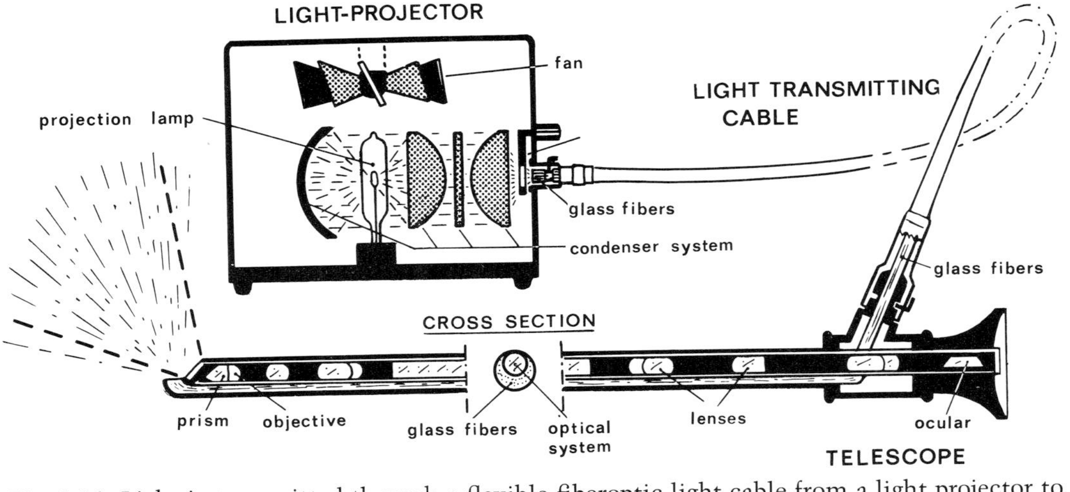

Fig. 1-10. Light is transmitted through a flexible fiberoptic light cable from a light projector to the tip of an endoscope where it provides illumination for visual examination and observation of body cavities.

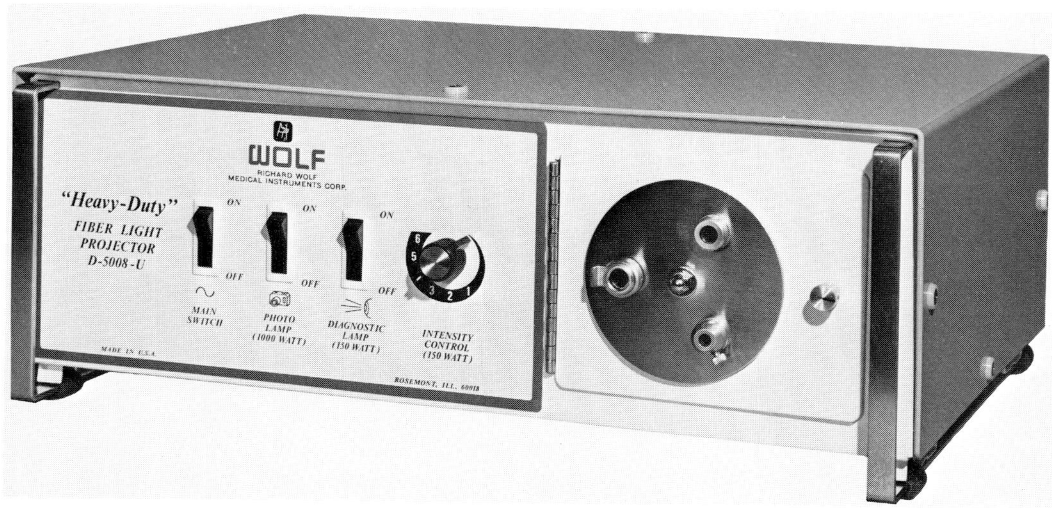

Fig. 1-11. Photographic fiber light projector with two alternating light sources.

The advantages of light transmission through a fiber light cable are as follows:

1. The light emanating from the light transmission bundle is cold.
2. The light transmission cable is flexible and elastic, and its length can be selected according to clinical requirements.
3. The light transmission cable can be sterilized with a cold solution in a steam autoclave or a gas sterilizer.
4. Safety is increased during examinations by eliminating any electrical hazards.
5. Endoscope construction has been simplified by eliminating electrical wires and connecting cords.

With newer and more powerful lamps available, it is possible to utilize the newer endoscopes for most documentation systems. One model, the Marc 300/16A lamp and its power pack, is incorporated into a heavy-duty light projector (Fig. 1-11), and is designed for both still and cinema photography.

Rod Lens System

With the availability of fiber illumination and improved lens systems, the entire concept of endoscopy was revolutionized. Within the last few years all major endoscope manufacturers have introduced new lens systems. In 1960, Hopkins, an English scientist, introduced a new design for a lens system that is known today as a rod lens system, which achieved a remarkable increase in light transmission and expansion of the field of view. Instead of the conventional system in which small lenses are separated by large air spaces, it contains long rod lenses with short air intervals. The rod lens system established a milestone in the development of the conventional lens system and, with the help of computers, it was now possible to redesign the conventional lens system using newer types of optical glass and coatings, and also to perform an exact computation of lens specifications. The basic difference between the computerized conventional lens system Lumina-S and the Hopkins rod lens system is illustrated in Fig. 1-12. Both of these systems offered improved definition of details due to increased resolution, maximum brightness without loss of contrast, natural reproduction of all colors, and a large field of vision with greater magnification.

Factors Influencing the Development of Optic Systems. The evolution of lens systems in endoscopes has resulted from an ongoing adjustment between the phy-

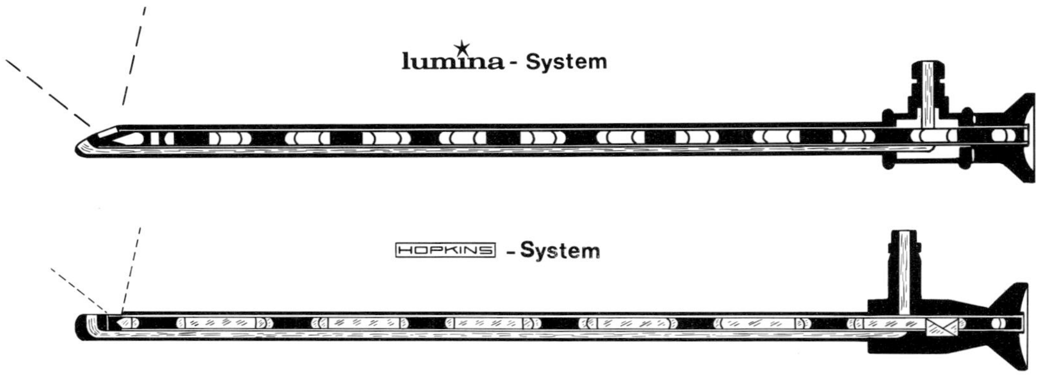

Fig. 1-12. The basic difference between these two systems is in the use of air space and the sizes of lenses applied.

sician, with his special clinical requirements, and the technician, with his knowledge of the exigencies of materials and the laws of optics. With the use of computers and with continued discussion between industry and the medical profession, endoscope design strives for wide-angle optics without increased barrel distortion, stronger magnification, perfect color reproduction with good contrast, and high resolution capabilities without loss of field depth.

THE STANDARD ARTHROSCOPE

The first attempt at observing the inside of the knee joint with a cystoscope dates back to the early 1900s. It was through the efforts of Takagi and later Watanabe that arthroscopy equipment was first developed. In 1957 the No. 19 and No. 21 arthroscopes were introduced. The No. 19 scope was for routine examination and the No. 21 was for purposes of photography.

Important Features

Because of the difficult anatomical situation, endoscopes for examination of the knee joint must meet very strict requirements. The following features of the arthroscope (to name only a few) are of great importance:

1. Field of vision (the greatest angle between two light rays going through the lens, at which image definition is acceptable)
2. Angle of vision (the angle between the axis of the telescope and the centerline of the field of vision)
3. Depth of field (the distance over which satisfactory definition is obtained when the lens is in focus for a certain distance)
4. Field stop or aperture (an opening, usually circular, in an opaque screen, whose diameter determines the field of view of an optical instrument)
5. Magnifying power (the ratio of the apparent size of a plane image to the apparent size of the object, as the latter would be seen without the magnifying instrument)
6. Resolving power (the ability of an optical system to resolve, i.e., separate two entities)
7. Illumination
8. Diameter of instruments
9. Irrigation flow
10. Photographic capability
11. Ability to be sterilized

Improvements in Design

Numerous instruments have been used for knee arthroscopy in the past, but all have needed improvement. Within the last year, major manufacturers of endoscopes have introduced several models of

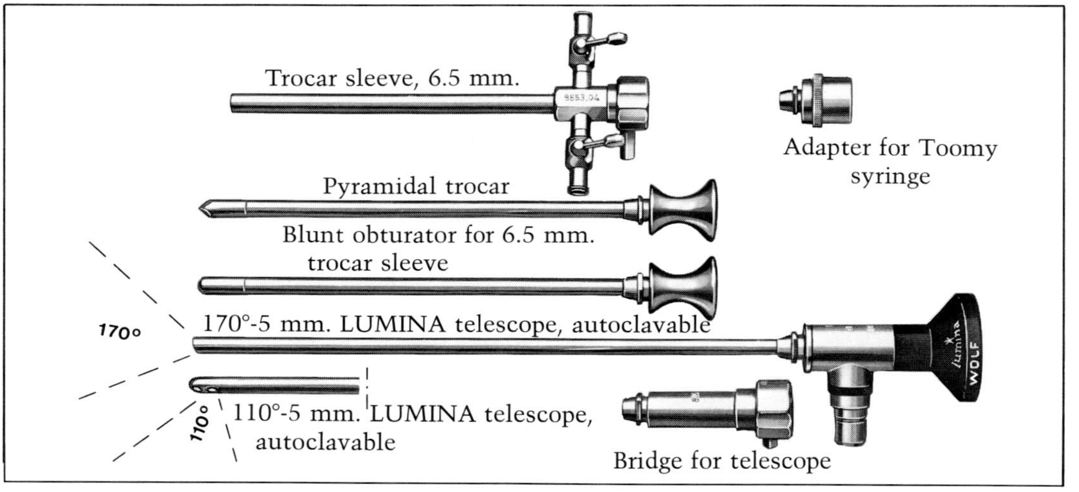

Fig. 1-13. A standard arthroscope.

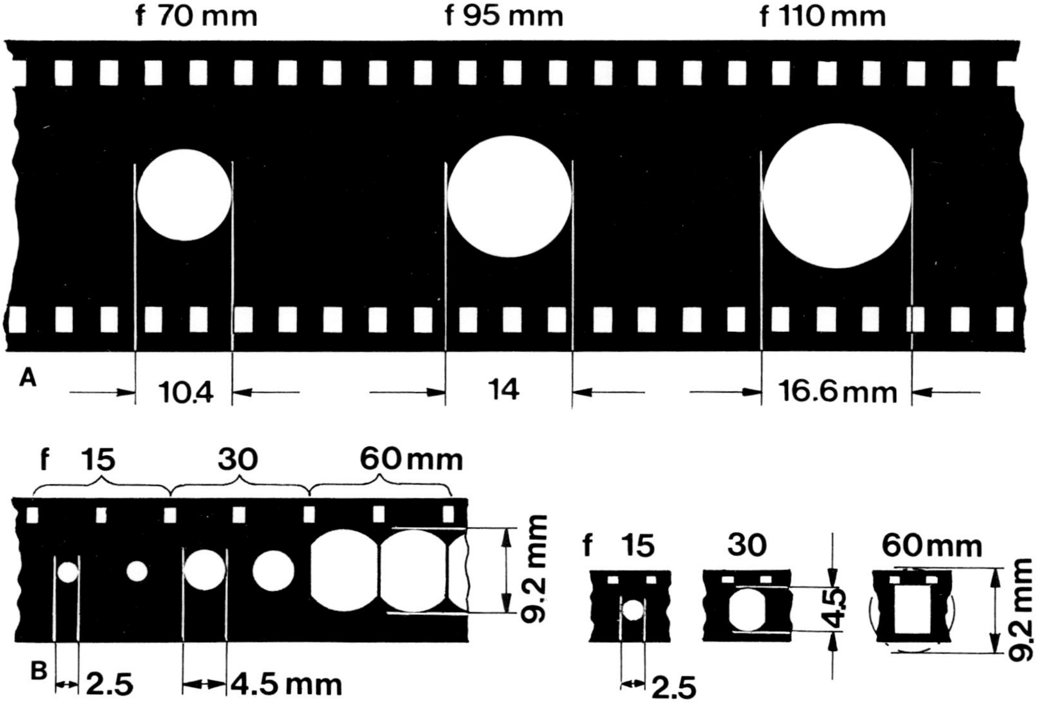

Fig. 1-14. Lenses of different focal lengths used with either movie or SLR cameras determine the size of the exposed picture. Recommended for 35 mm. film are F 70, F 95, and F 110 mm. lenses, and for motion pictures F 15, F 30, and F 60 lenses.

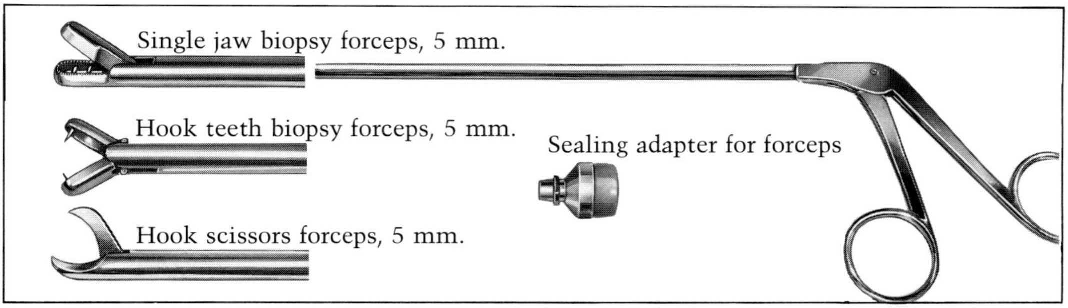

Fig. 1-15. Operating instruments.

arthroscopes with different design features, and in 1974 Dr. Richard O'Connor and the Richard Wolf Corporation introduced a completely new design of arthroscope, known as Type 8853 (Fig. 1-13). For years Dr. O'Connor had used different models of arthroscopes, but he felt that all had needed some improvement. This new design succeeded in circumventing most of the difficulties inherent in the old models, by means of the following features:

1. The space between telescope and sheath is increased without enlarging the total diameter, resulting in an increase in irrigation flow.
2. The number of fiber light transmitting bundles inside the telescope is increased to permit greater light transmission for greater photographic capabilities.
3. Fiber-illuminated bundles are placed in a complete circle around the objective window (ring of light) to assure an even distribution of light. This avoids under- or overexposed pictures in both still and motion photography.
4. Easy and reliable connections between camera and arthroscope can be made, to obtain documentation by viewing through camera and telescope simultaneously.
5. The system can easily be adapted to any standard photo fiber light projector, without attaching or using additional equipment.
6. The sharpness of the telescope tip is minimized, to avoid the scuffing and scraping sometimes caused by panning with endoscopes.
7. Telescopes with diameters of 2.5 and 5 mm. can be interchanged, thereby permitting the use of biopsy forceps under direct vision.
8. The entire arthroscopic system can be steam sterilized at 272 degrees F. for 10 minutes.
9. Properly fitting operating forceps and other accessories can be added to the system.
10. Rigid or flexible teaching devices can be attached to the telescope.
11. Standard single lens reflex cameras can be used.

Photographic Capability

In light of these design features, it is now possible to obtain full-frame color slides and exposed pictures measuring up to 25 mm. in diameter. For adapting the arthroscope to the camera, there are choices of different lenses with different focal lengths. These give different size images and scales of enlargement (Fig. 1-14). By increasing the size of the exposed picture, however, one must also increase the available light and sacrifice the depth of field. It is now possible to produce 16-mm. motion picture films in which the complete frame is exposed; the same rules apply as with 35 mm. still photography.

The design of current standard arthroscopy equipment also allows the use of standard reflex cameras for documentation.

The adaptability of the arthroscope to color television systems was demonstrated at the American Academy instruc-

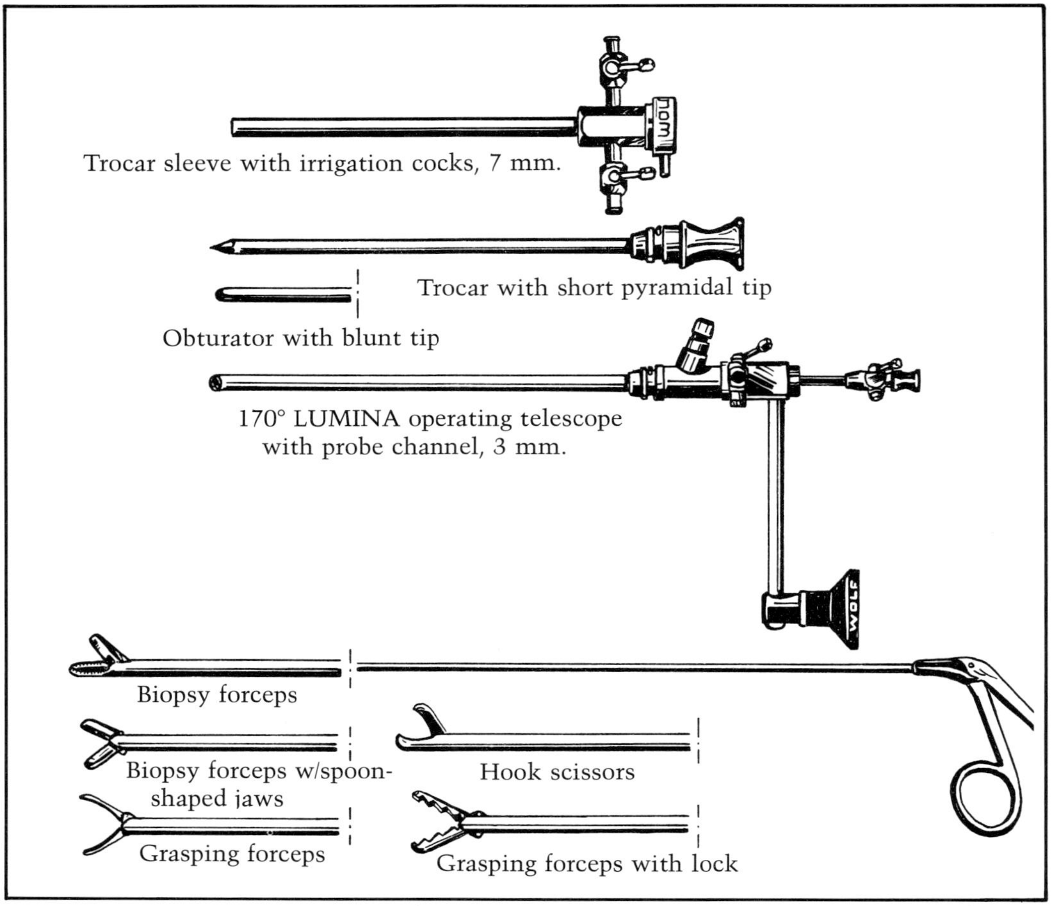

Fig. 1-16. The operating arthroscope.

tional course on arthroscopy in Anaheim, California in March, 1976, and it is now possible to make color videotapes for educational purposes.

Operating Accessories

Operating accessories for the Type 8853 arthroscope include, besides a basket-type biopsy forceps, a hook-type scissors, and a retractor forceps, which can be used for the removal of loose bodies by adding a hook tooth on the opposite end of each jaw (Fig. 1-15). Adapters were selected to connect the trocar sheath with the Toomey syringe or Ellik evacuator for faster irrigation with the largest lumen possible.

THE OPERATING ARTHROSCOPE

A completely new arthroscope design (Type 4857, Fig. 1-16) was introduced by Dr. O'Connor early in 1976. The optical system, fiber illumination, irrigation channels, and a channel for operating instruments were built into one single shaft, allowing the surgeon to view his operating instruments at all times.

CLEANING AND STERILIZATION OF ARTHROSCOPES

Cleaning

Without question, these new endoscopes require special handling and care.

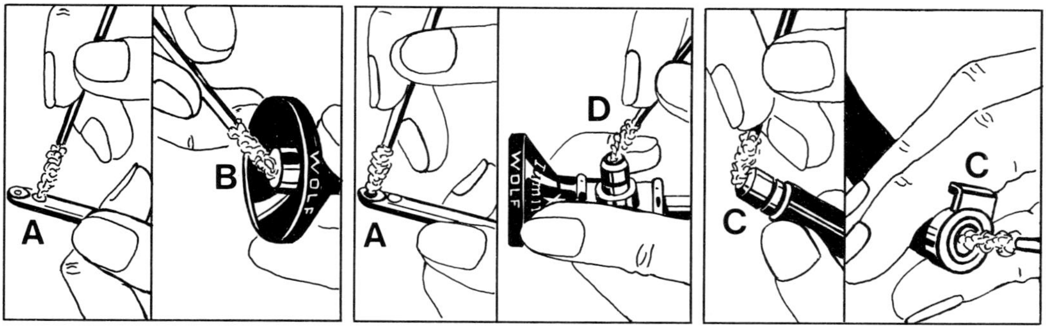

Fig. 1-17. It is vitally important to clean all transmission surfaces as illustrated.

The lens systems, incorporated with fiber illumination into small sheaths, are fragile, and must be handled like the precision instruments they are. Extreme care should be taken when the scope is to be cleaned and sterilized. The procedure for general cleaning is as follows:

1. Clean thoroughly with a soft brush, mild soap, and warm water.
2. Use a cleaning rod with cotton for inside of sheaths.
3. Rinse in warm water.
4. All distal objective lenses (*A*) and ocular windows (*B*) must be cleaned individually with a cotton swab dipped in alcohol to assure clear viewing. Be careful not to scratch the objective of the scope (Fig. 1-17).
5. All fiber end surfaces on light cables (*C*) and telescopes (*D*) must also be cleaned periodically as in Step 4 to guarantee maximum light transmission.

Oiling. Stopcocks, locks, and other mechanical parts should be lubricated with oil periodically (Fig. 1-18). Lubricating oil is used for the trocar sleeve, forceps, and L.L. connector.

Sterilization

Proper care and maintenance is important for the efficient and safe operation of sophisticated surgical equipment. To obtain maximum service life, it is recommended that the autoclavable telescopes be routinely gas sterilized, and steam sterilized in emergency situations. Even though instruments are designed to withstand the heat and pressure of a steam autoclave cycle, one cannot expect a lifetime equal to that of instruments that are gas sterilized. Only equipment that is specially marked can be steam autoclaved; the manufacturer's instructions must be closely followed. When sterilizing arthroscopic equipment the following points should be kept in mind:

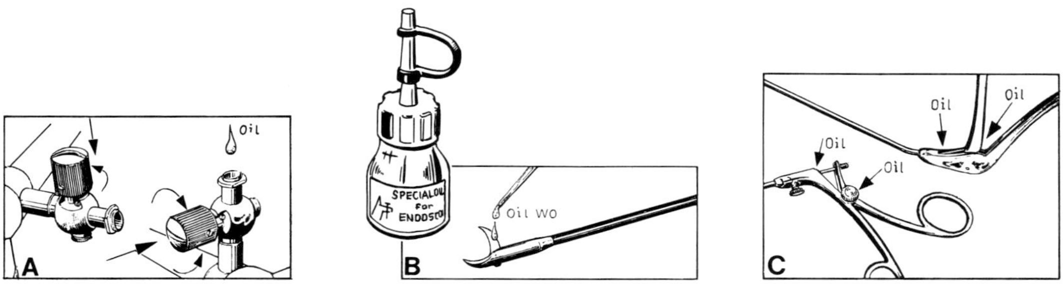

Fig. 1-18. It is necessary to lubricate mechanical parts periodically as illustrated.

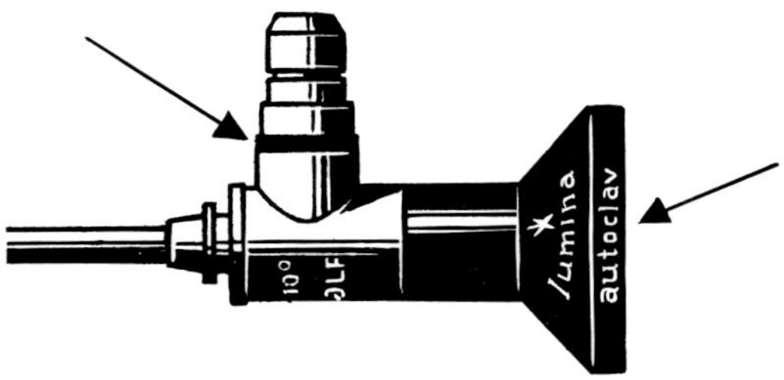

Fig. 1-19. Richard Wolf steam autoclavable telescopes are identified by a permanent red band around the fiber light cable connector and the word *autoclave* is engraved on the eyepiece.

1. Don't use any solvent (except alcohol or acetone) on the instruments.
2. Don't sterilize in carbolic acid.
3. Don't steam autoclave *standard* fiber-illuminated telescopes.
4. Don't allow instruments to remain immersed in *any* solution beyond the time recommended by the manufacturer of the solution.
5. Don't use bichloride of mercury or other corrosive solutions as a germicide.
6. Don't use clamps or forceps when handling instruments.
7. Don't pick up or handle instruments in bunches.
8. Don't handle telescopes at the distal end. Grasp them at the eyepiece end.
9. Don't pile instruments or cables on top of one another. Heavy instruments can cause fiber breakage.

Soaking—Cold Sterilization (Disinfection). For all telescopes and accessories an activated glutaraldehyde solution (Cidex) may be used. This solution destroys within a short time most microorganisms, including *M. tuberculosis* and viruses. It does not affect rubber, plastics, and lens cements; however, instruments of stainless steel should not be immersed for excessive periods. In addition, metal and rubber items should not be immersed simultaneously; remove all rubber sealing caps and disinfect them separately. After sterilization, the instruments should be rinsed twice with distilled water. Minimum soaking time is 20 minutes. For maximum time, see the instructions on the bottle.

Gas Sterilization. For all telescopes and accessories, gas sterilization may be used. Telescopes must be placed separately in a perforated metal container with gauze or cloth inserts folded loosely about each telescope. Other instruments should also be placed in gauze or cloth inserts in fixed position to avoid wobbling or damage. Do not autoclave instruments in a plastic bag or container. Follow the manufacturer's instructions of the autoclave for adjusting and servicing. Ethylene oxide gas is recommended. The temperature should not exceed 60 degrees C. (140°F). The pressure should not exceed 8 pounds. Preferably, the pressure should be between 6 and 7 pounds. The length of time is not important as long as the temperature and pressure are stabilized at the points mentioned.

Steam Autoclaving. For Richard Wolf steam autoclavable telescopes, this method may be used. Proper care and maintenance is important for the efficient and safe operation of sophisticated medical/surgical equipment. Even under ideal conditions heat and pressure during a steam autoclave cycle will reduce the life of any optical system (Fig. 1-19). It is our recommendation that all telescopes be gas sterilized or cold soaked to achieve maximum life expectancy, unless otherwise required. The sterilization method should be selected and accepted keeping this information in mind. Instructions for steam autoclavable telescopes are as follows:

1. Do not use autoclaves that incorporate a fast vacuum system to initiate faster heating and/or cooling.
2. Telescopes must be placed *separately* in a perforated metal container with gauze or cloth inserts folded loosely about each telescope (Fig. 1-20). Since autoclave equipment is subject to temperature variances, we suggest the autoclav-

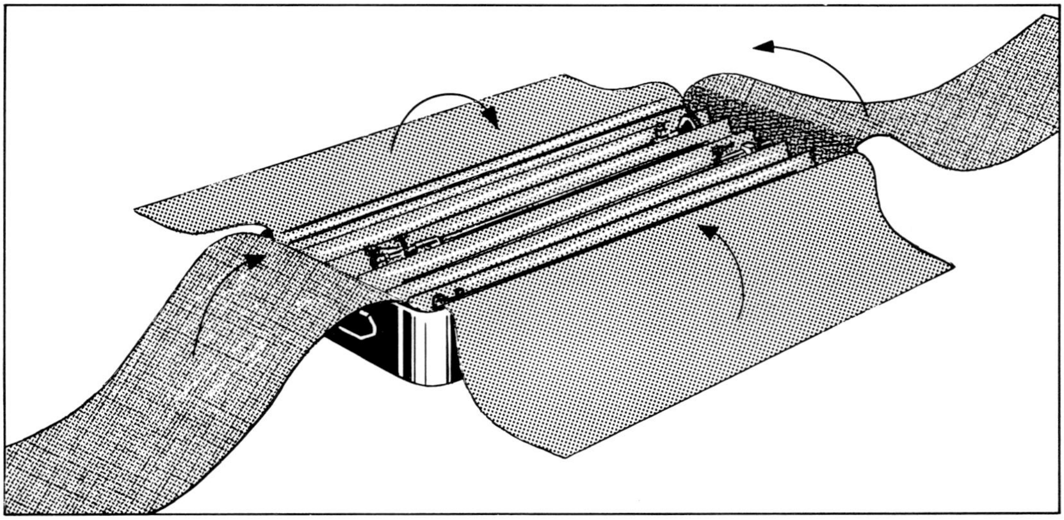

Fig. 1-20. It is mandatory to place each steam autoclavable telescope separately in a container as illustrated.

able telescope be placed in the coolest part of the sterilizer if proper calibration of that equipment has been established.

3. The maximum sterilization cycle must not exceed 10 minutes at 134 degrees C (272°F) at 2.2 atmospheric pressure.

4. After removal of the telescopes from the autoclave, they should be cooled slowly to room temperature.

DO NOT IMMERSE OR RINSE IN COLD WATER OR ANY OTHER LIQUID.

REFERENCES

1. Draeger, V. H.: Das Endoskop. Medizinal-Markt/Acta Medicotechnica, *23,* Jahring, Nr. 5/1975.
2. Franke, G.: Endoscopes—Principles and Problems of their Optics. Medical Market; Acta Medical-Technical [Special excerpt from sixteenth year (1968); notebook 3], pp. 372–374. Berlin, Helios Publishing House, 1968.
3. Quint, R.: Endoscope Instrumentation. Clin. Obstet. Gynecol., *12:*463–483, 1969.
4. Zeman, E. and Pavlinec, M.: Fibre Optics in Medical Engineering, Acta Technica CSAV, No. 2, 1969.

2 Indications, Techniques, and Complications of Arthroscopy

INDICATIONS FOR ARTHROSCOPY

Applications

The primary reason for performing arthroscopy is to obtain as much useful information as possible in planning treatment; however, it should be stressed that arthroscopy is only one technique that may be used in the assessment of a knee problem. Considerable helpful information is gained by conventional methods of clinical examination, roentgenograms, arthrograms and, occasionally, bone scanning techniques. If, at a particular point, the clinical assessment and other ancillary tests still leave the problem unsolved, arthroscopy is indicated.

The arthroscope is particularly useful when the clinical situation suggests the possibility of internal derangement of the knee and the roentgenogram and arthrogram do not substantiate this. Certain tears of the meniscus, particularly early tears transverse to the long axis of the meniscus, are not demonstrated by the arthrogram. When there is a conflict between compartment localization clinically and arthrographically, the arthroscope is the final arbitrator.

Closed synovial biopsies may be obtained under direct vision. The synovium does not respond uniformly to the disease process; instead some areas show more advanced pathology while other areas appear relatively normal, so selection of diseased areas for biopsy is facilitated by arthroscopy.

Any knee on which surgery is to be performed might first be examined with the arthroscope. This gives the beginning arthroscopist an opportunity to improve his technique and develop confidence in his interpretative abilities. Quite frequently, as he gains experience, the arthroscopic findings will alter or obviate the operative procedure.

Precise recording of pathologic states can be obtained during arthroscopy by either still or motion photography. Such documentation has been found to be useful in resolving medicolegal matters.

Specific Indications

A definite indication for arthroscopy, associated with a high yield of information, is hemarthrosis following a twisting injury that produces no clinical signs of instability. In this situation numerous unanticipated abnormalities may be detected and quite frequently early diagnosis of meniscal tears or a tear of the anterior cruciate ligament may be made.

Arthroscopic evaluation of the patient

with a torn meniscus allows at least a tentative prognosis. The question Is the meniscus torn? leads to the next question, How is the meniscus torn? Does it interfere with the mechanical function of the knee? Must it be totally excised or will partial excision relieve the localized pain and instability? Of greater significance are the questions, Are the femoral condyles, tibial plateaus, and patella covered with glistening, physically unaltered hyaline cartilage, and if not, what is the degree of alteration? Subtle changes in the matrix of the condyles are better observed with the magnification possible with the arthroscope than with the naked eye. As the physical alteration progresses to fibrillation and fragmentation the outlook for normal knee function diminishes. Obviously learning this information *before* the arthrotomy incision permits a more critical determination by the surgeon.

The presence of loose bodies within the joint is an excellent reason to perform arthroscopy, because quite often these bodies can be removed under arthroscopic control.

Certain metabolic conditions, such as acute or chronic crystalline synovitis resulting from gout or calcium pyrophosphate deposition, may improve after arthroscopic examination and thorough joint lavage.

The status of osteochondritis dissecans may be followed and information obtained regarding potential viability of the osteochondritic fragment. Postoperative healing of the defect may be assessed by ballottement with the obturator, and on occasion Smillie nails can be removed under arthoscopic control.

The presence of a popliteal cyst in an adult whose clinical examination and arthrogram do not reveal the source of the intra-articular pathology may be confirmed by arthroscopy.

Arthroscopy may be useful in treating the patient with partial fibrous ankylosis of the knee not yielding to manipulation under anaesthesia. Adhesive bands in the suprapatellar pouch may be cut under direct vision, allowing increased motion not previously obtainable by manipulation.

Arthroscopy is useful in analyzing the knee of the adolescent female, as originally suggested by Casscells.[1] In the presence of continuing complaints and negative findings it is reassuring to both the physician and the patient's family that no pathology requiring operation is present and a more positive attitude may be taken by the advising physician.

Arthroscopy may be useful in evaluating postoperative results of meniscectomy and ligamentous repairs and in following the progress of degenerative changes within the joint. Assessment and continued observation by arthroscopy of the rheumatoid knee has been suggested by Dr. Watanabe.[2]

THE AUTHOR'S TECHNIQUE OF ARTHROSCOPY (AFTER WATANABE)

Insertion of the Arthroscope

A tourniquet, though rarely inflated, is placed high on the thigh of the involved leg either before or after the patient has been anesthetized, and the leg is scrubbed for 5 minutes with a povidone-iodine (Betadine) solution. Draping is then completed with the knee region free. The knee is flexed approximately 40 degrees, and an area a thumb's breadth above the lateral tibial plateau and just lateral to the patellar tendon is selected for the insertion of a 15 needle, 1½ inches long.

The needle is directed towards the intercondylar notch, which makes an angle of 45 degrees to the patient's leg and 45 degrees to the plane of the floor. As the leg is gradually extended, the needle slips through the fibrous capsule, fat pad, and synovium and passes beneath the patella lying on the trochlear groove of the femur. The needle is then slid back and forth to make sure it lies free within the joint cavity and the joint is then distended with sterile normal saline solution until the quadriceps bursa is firmly distended. Care must be taken not to rupture the quadriceps bursa at this point. The inferior site of the insertion of the needle serves two purposes: (1) it gives a visual landmark for the proper insertion of the arthroscope, and (2) retrosynovial injection of the normal saline solution is avoided. This latter complication of the technique is seen following distention of the joint using the classical lateral suprapatellar approach, which may well obscure vision of the suprapatellar recess until the saline is reabsorbed and may also cause unnecessary delay in examination. When the quadriceps bursa is full, the needle is removed.

The Incision. The leg is then flexed approximately 40 degrees and a quarter-inch stab wound is made in the same location one thumbs breadth above the lateral tibial plateau and at the lateral edge of the patellar tendon. (When a lateral meniscectomy is contemplated, this incision is best made in a direction that may be incorporated into the skin incision.) The surgeon now firmly grasps the water sleeve and trocar as a unit, his index finger resting against the skin to prevent overpenetration of the trocar against the femoral condyles during its insertion. The fibrous capsule is pierced by the gradual twisting motion of the trocar and water sleeve. When resistance is no longer felt from the fibrous capsule, the trocar is then removed and the blunt-tipped obturator inserted. (After acquiring considerable experience you usually do not need the obturator.) The knee is then gradually extended and the obturator and water sleeve pass through the synovium and beneath the patella over the trochlear groove of the femur to rest in the suprapatellar recess. During this maneuver, little fluid is lost from the joint.

Insertion of the Counterdrain. A Veres needle or other large-bore needle (15 gauge) is inserted medially and slightly superior to the patella and is aimed at the middle of the patella. The Veres needle is specially constructed so that when its sharp tip no longer meets with resistance as it is inserted, the blunt tip is released. Using this needle minimizes the scuffing of the patellofemoral joint during manipulation of the knee. The medial suprapatellar location for this counterdrain insertion is felt to have an advantage over the lateral insertion employed by many arthroscopists because flow is cut off more often during examination of the lateral compartment when the needle is inserted through the superior lateral approach.

Completion of the Assembly. When the Veres needle is in place and good outflow is established, the obturator is removed and the telescope with the bridge attached is inserted. The tubing that is used to deliver the normal saline solution is then connected to the water sleeve. The containers are usually elevated 3 feet above the level of the knee to give sufficient hydrostatic pressure to provide good irrigating flow throughout the joint. Attaching the fiber optic cable to the arthroscope and the light source completes the assembly, and you are now ready to view the knee.

Examination of the Knee

Early in my experience I wore the usual sterile cap and mask to prevent possible contamination, but I soon found it unnecessary. Examination of the knee is done in a methodical manner, always following the same steps.

Examination of the Suprapatellar Pouch. The quadriceps bursa and suprapatellar recess are examined first. As the telescope is moved side to side and partially withdrawn, the side walls, roof, and floor of the quadriceps bursa are examined. The instrument is partially and gradually withdrawn from the joint until

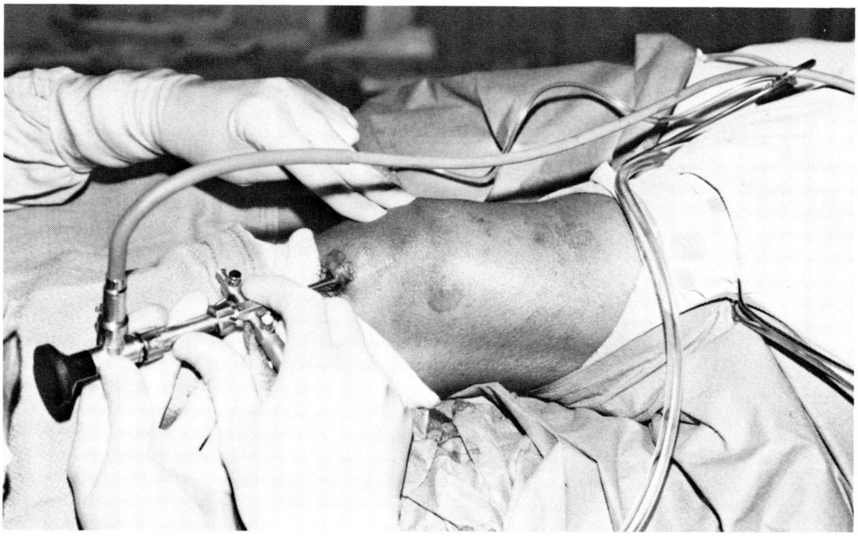

Fig. 2-1. Examination of patellofemoral joint and quadriceps bursa of the left knee. Gentle movement of the patella exposes its many surfaces. To study this region adequately, the arthroscope should be moved from side to side and advanced and retracted.

the undersurface of the patella comes into view. The examiner moves or tilts the patella medially and laterally with his hand, exposing various portions of the patella's undersurface (Fig. 2-1).

Examination of the Medial Compartment. After the quadriceps bursa and patellofemoral articulation are examined, the instrument is brought into the medial compartment.

To accomplish this maneuver, an assistant partially flexes the knee while the examiner rotates the arthroscope, keeping its tip pressed against the synovium medially and the body of the water sleeve against the surface of the medial femoral condyle. Flexion of the knee necessary to accomplish this is approximately 40 degrees. The illumination on the skin over the medial portion of the knee gives striking evidence of the position of the arthroscope if the examiner loses his orientation. The instrument is then brought into the medial compartment, slipping between the medial femoral condyle and medial tibial plateau over the middle half of the medial meniscus by withdrawing the telescope approximately one inch. The anterior half of the medial meniscus is examined in external rotation with mild valgus stress and 40 degrees of flexion. To obtain visualization of the posterior half of the meniscus, however, the foot must be externally rotated and the leg extended to all but the terminal 10 degrees and a valgus stress applied (Fig. 2-2). There is variation from knee to knee. The amount of flexion necessary to examine the posterior half of the meniscus is variable, but its position is between 20 degrees of flexion and complete extension. Occasionally it is helpful if the examiner presses his finger over the joint line. Meanwhile, the position of the leg is controlled at all times by the assistant.

Examination of the Intercondylar Notch. Following visualization of the medial compartment, the knee is bent to approximately 60 to 70 degrees and the instrument is brought into the intercondylar notch region. This may be obscured by the presence of the ligamentum mucosum and (as it particularly seems to the beginner) the omnipresent fat pad. The

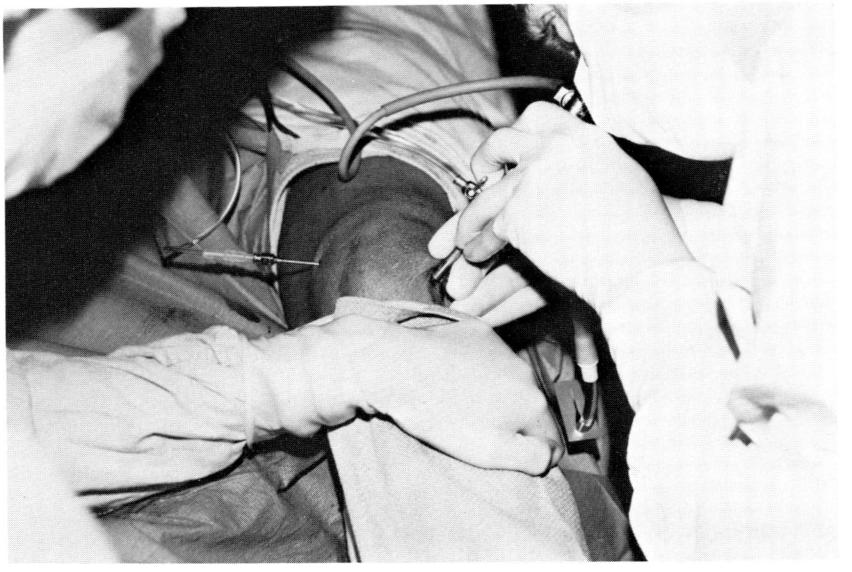

Fig. 2-2. Examination of the posterior half of the medial meniscus of the left knee. Note the irrigating needle superior and medial to the patella. A valgus stress is applied by the assistant's left hand; his right hand holds the foot and applies an external rotary force to the leg.

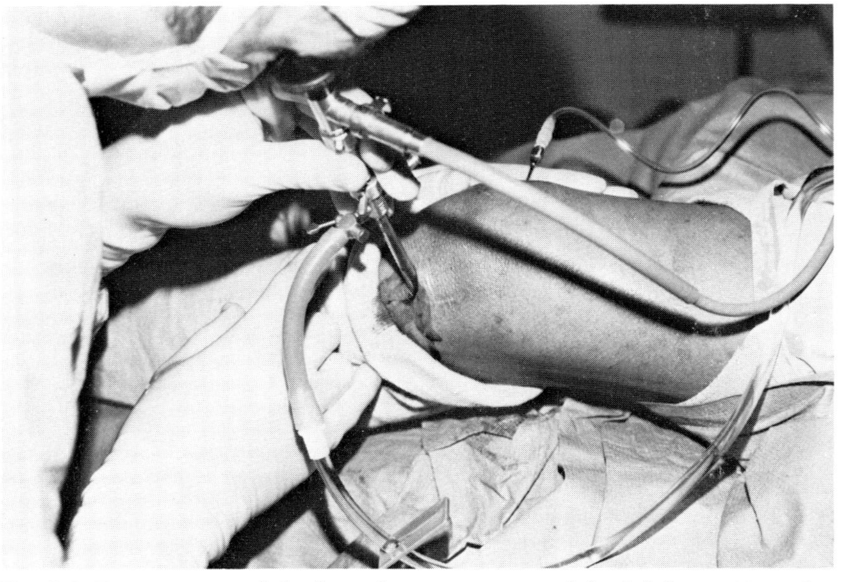

Fig. 2-3. Examination of the lateral compartment of the left knee. Note the assistant's left hand applying a varus stress; the right hand is holding the foot in internal rotation, and the amount of flexion is varied. A good look at the anterior cruciate ligament can be obtained in this position, as the ligamentum mucosum is separated from the anterior cruciate ligament.

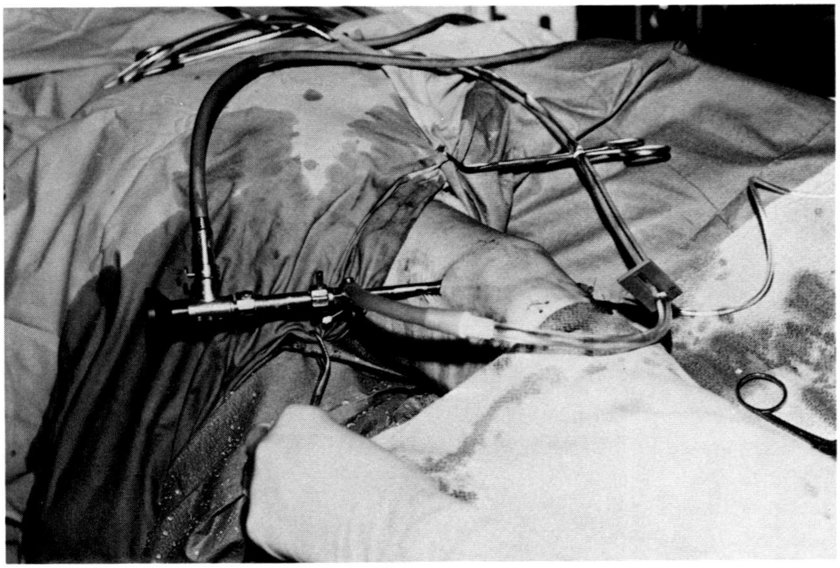

Fig. 2-4. The lateral suprapatellar approach to the right knee. The arthroscope is resting in the quadriceps bursa superior to the patella. The retropatellar surface is best studied from this approach.

ligamentum mucosum is a thin, or sometimes thick, ligamentous-appearing structure extending from the intercondylar notch anterior and slightly central to the origin of the anterior cruciate ligament, inserting centrally on the fat pad. It may consist of a septum dividing the medial and lateral halfs of the joint. Routinely, the femoral origin of the posterior cruciate ligament is observed medially, and the distal two-thirds of the anterior cruciate ligament may be seen as well.

Examination of the Lateral Compartment. The lateral compartment is entered by positioning the patient so that the leg is brought upon the operating table with the hip in external rotation; the knee is flexed at 20 to 30 degrees and a varus stress is applied, which causes internal rotation of the tibia (Fig. 2-3). The arthroscope is passed along the lateral femoral condyle. It may be necessary to vary the amount of flexion to bring the instrument into the joint line. Routinely, the posterior tibial attachment of the lateral meniscus is observed first, then the inner rim is followed laterally and advanced anteriorly by partially withdrawing the arthroscope. From this position, the anterior cruciate ligament can be seen and the instrument may be passed across the joint line beneath the ligamentum mucosum into the medial compartment to study the anterior attachment of the medial meniscus as well. In the majority of patients, a nearly complete assessment of the joint may be obtained by observation through this lateral infrapatellar approach.

On occasion—particularly when one wishes to examine the peripheral margin of the anterior half of the lateral meniscus or a degenerated knee with 10 or more degrees of varus deformity—the lateral compartment is best visualized by the medial infrapatellar approach. The counterdrain is then closed and the knee distended again. A quarter-inch stab wound is made one thumb's breadth above the medial tibial plateau and just medial to the patellar tendon, and the instrument inserted. The trocar and water sleeve are pointed again at the intercondylar notch region, and a twisting motion is used to penetrate the fibrous capsule. The same technique is repeated with the obturator while the leg is extended. The lateral femoral condyle is then followed posteriorly to gain access to the joint line.

In addition to the medial and lateral approach, the suprapatellar approach may often be used (Fig. 2-4). The knee is distended and a quarter-inch incision is made about 1 inch above the superior pole of the patella, either on the medial or lateral aspect of the knee. The previously described method of insertion is used, by aiming the instrument towards the center of the patella. This view has been found to be extremely useful in observing the patellofemoral articulation in varying degrees of flexion and extension. It also facilitates a more nearly complete study of the undersurface of the patella. Loose bodies in the quadriceps bursa are easily identified and removed.

Termination of the Arthroscopic Procedure

At the termination of the arthroscopic procedure, the irrigation system and fiber-optic cable are removed. The telescope is removed from the joint, with the water sleeve left in place. The joint is then irrigated of clots or debris. The wound is then loosely closed with a suture at each incision site. The joint is again fully distended, and if the tourniquet has been inflated this is now released. After a few minutes the counterdrain is opened to observe the outflow. When this is clear, the needle is removed and a light pressure dressing is applied.

If bleeding continues, the knee is again distended with 50 to 100 ml of saline and held for 5 minutes. If the patient has required multiple arthroscopic approaches, saline solution may dissect along soft tissue fascial planes, distending the leg and the thigh. This has not proven troublesome, as the solution is quickly reabsorbed in the postarthroscopic period. When arthrotomy is performed following arthroscopy, the patient is reprepped and redraped.

Discharge of the Patient. If the patient does not require arthrotomy, he is allowed to walk as soon as he is fully awake and is discharged from the hospital that same evening. The sutures are removed 4 days after the operation. Activity level is dictated by the patient's pain response to the procedure, which varies. I have had several patients who have even played football the following day, as well as several who have complained of discomfort for about 7 days. Many patients state that their knee feels numb following arthroscopy. Analgesics stronger than aspirin are rarely necessary.

CONTRAINDICATIONS AND COMPLICATIONS

I feel that there are only two contraindications to arthroscopy:(1) skin abrasion, a laceration or abscess in the vicinity of the knee; and (2) fibrous ankylosis of the knee with flexion less than 50 degrees.

Complications following arthroscopy, while rarely encountered, can occur and they must be recognized. They are listed below. The quadriceps inhibition found following arthrotomy of the knee has not occurred in my experience, except when hemarthrosis develops.

Scuffing of the Articular Cartilage

This complication is secondary to the passing of the instrument from compartment to compartment and can be partially avoided with the use of the obturator for inserting the arthroscope into the joint. Increased experience with the technique also lessens the chance of this complication developing.

Infection

In my experience, there has been no infection recognized following arthroscopy of the knee. However, four infections occurred in patients who had arthroscopy followed by arthrotomy. Intense orthopaedic interest has been raised by the potential for joint infection; therefore, details of these four infections will be described.

Case 2-1. Infection After Medial Ligamentous Reconstruction

Immediately following arthroscopy, a medial ligamentous reconstruction was performed. Infection was suspected on the fifth postoperative day and proven on the fifteenth postoperative day. Exploration of the operative site revealed necrotic material on only the medial side of the joint. The patient was treated by wide incision of the joint capsule medially and laterally. The culture grew out a *Staphylococcus aureus* coagulase positive. Superinfection occurred with a pseudomonas. The patient's follow-up at one year revealed a full range of motion and moderate joint instability necessitating the use of knee brace for work.

Case 2-2. Infection After Lateral Meniscectomy

Three weeks following arthroscopy, a lateral meniscectomy was performed. The patient's subsequent course was uneventful. Two weeks following surgery, a hemarthrosis of the knee was aspirated. The patient gave no history of fever or chills, and the range of motion was improving. Two weeks following this, the patient complained of malaise and stated that she had run a temperature for a day or two of 100 degrees and had a chilling sensation. Study of the aspirated joint revealed a 70 ml. effusion with cloudy synovial fluid with a markedly elevated white count, but no organisms grew. Several more cultures were obtained, which also failed to confirm the diagnosis of an infection. Arthroscopy was then performed, which revealed whitish plaques studding the synovium; culture of biopsy material from these areas grew out a *Staphylococcus aureus* hemolytic coagulase-positive. The patient responded immediately to irrigation of the joint with a cephalothin (Keflin) solution. She has good quadriceps strength and no apparent permanent changes within her knee. Her range of motion is full.

Case 2-3. Infection After Realignment of the Quadriceps

Six months following arthroscopy in a 39-year-old obese female, a medial realignment of the quadriceps mechanism was performed. Infection was noted on the fourth postoperative day, and the wound opened. The infection was brought under control rapidly and secondary closure of the wound performed.

Case 2-4. Infection After Medial Meniscectomy

One month following arthroscopy, a medial meniscectomy was performed. The patient's postoperative course was marred by excessive pain, but he had no fever. Six days following surgery, after discharge from the hospital, he developed fever and chills, and a bloody specimen of synovial fluid grew out a *Staphylococcus aureus* coagulase-positive. Arthroscopy was performed and irrigating tubes inserted into the knee through the arthroscope, and the patient was maintained on closed-circuit irrigation for a period of 7 days. He has regained full range of motion. Three months following the diagnosis of this infection the knee again became swollen and warm, but synovial fluid cultures and white blood count were normal. Arthroscopy was again performed and numerous necrotic synovial tips found. The necrotic debris was washed from the joint. The effusion and synovitis responded very rapidly to this, and the patient has regained a full range of motion and good quadriceps strength.

Swelling

Occasionally persistent swelling over the site of the insertion of the arthroscope occurs; usually the swelling is in the lateral fat pad. This complication has been noted numerous times, but gradually, with time, the fat pad becomes less swollen and the discomfort decreases.

Instrument Breakage

Early in my experience with the Watanabe No. 21 arthroscope, a light carrier was broken from the tip and lodged in the joint, but retrieval was not attempted inasmuch as surgery was contemplated. This complication has not occurred with fiber-optic arthroscopes, and it can be avoided with the Watanabe No. 21 by moving the instrument with the light carrier as the leading edge, forcing it against the telescope. Reversal of this direction causes the protruding bulb to be stressed at its most vulnerable point—the junction of the light bulb at the stem—and weakened.

Hemarthrosis

Hemarthrosis requiring aspiration has been seen in three of my patients following arthroscopy.

Thrombophlebitis

A 34-year-old patient developed swelling in his leg 10 days after arthroscopy. This necessitated hospitalization and anticoagulation therapy. No pulmonary embolus has occurred following arthroscopy.

Synovial Rupture

Occasionally when the joint is overdistended with saline solution, a definite pop is heard within the knee, and a defect is noted in the quadriceps bursa superiorly by arthroscopy. This, however, has not been associated with clinical problems.

REFERENCES

1. Casscells, S. W.: Arthroscopy of the knee joint, a review of 150 cases. J. Bone Joint Surg., *53A*:287, 1971.
2. Watanabe, M., Takeda, S., and Ikeuchi, H: Atlas of Arthroscopy, ed. 2. Tokyo, Igaku Shoin, 1969.

3 *Arthroscopic Anatomy of the Normal Knee*

For the purpose of description, the knee will be divided into four arthroscopic regions: the suprapatellar pouch, the medial compartment, the intercondylar notch, and the lateral compartment.

SUPRAPATELLAR POUCH

Properly inserted, the arthroscope when entering the knee lies beneath the patella and glides over the trochlear groove of the femur. By moving the telescope from right to left, the cavernous quadriceps bursa can be explored. The superior limits of the cavern are rounded, and the synovium is thin. The side walls of this space are frequently thrown into small vertical pleats and the synovium is thin with a prominent vascular pattern. The quadriceps bursa superiorly is contained by the quadriceps tendon (Fig. 3-1). In the majority of knees there is an incomplete transverse partition, arising from the floor of the lateral portion of the suprapatellar recess, which extends superiorly and then medially, attaching to the suprapatellar recess again inferiorly. This has been termed the *plica synovialis* (Fig. 3-2) and is an embryonic remnant of variable configuration. Occasionally this structure is seen as an imperforate fibrous mass that lies perpendicular to the long axis of the patella (Fig. 3-3) and cephalad to it.

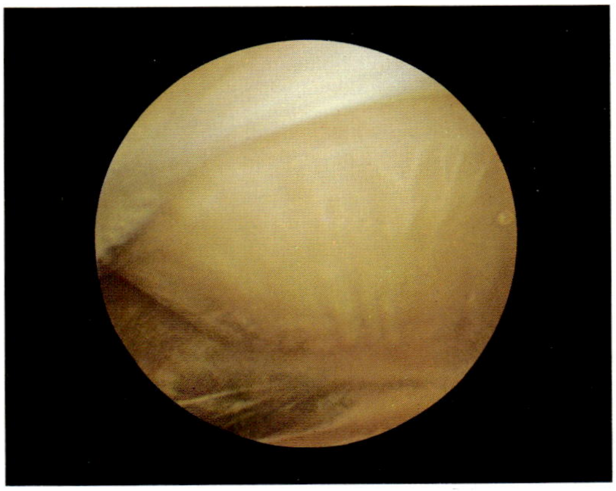

Fig. 3-1. Quadriceps tendon viewed through the 110-degree telescope. The roof of the quadriceps bursa is covered with the quadriceps tendon and a very thin layer of synovium.

The Porta. The passage between the quadriceps bursa and the knee joint proper through this fibrous arch, the plica synovialis, has been termed the *porta.* The floor of this region is the suprapatellar recess, and it is in this location that the synovium is best observed. The synovium of the suprapatellar recess is a matlike structure in the young; towards the

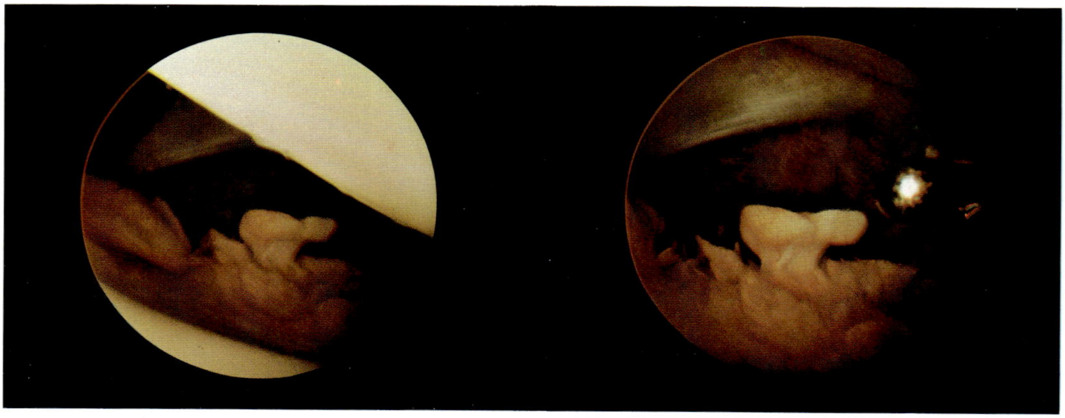

Fig. 3-2. Plica synovialis: infrapatellar approach, (right) knee. (*Left*) Lateral facet of patella above and lateral femoral condyle below. The lateral insertion of the plica synovialis is seen in the left-hand corner. (*Right*) A close-up view beneath the patella. The plica synovialis is a shiny fibrotic band surrounding the porta, which connects the quadriceps bursa and the knee joint proper.

end of adolescence, transparent villus folds appear. In the presence of intra-articular pathology, this transformation occurs much earlier. When the telescope is withdrawn slightly, the undersurface of the patella comes into view. In approximately 20 per cent of the knees I have examined, there is a fibrous structure, arising from the medial side wall of the

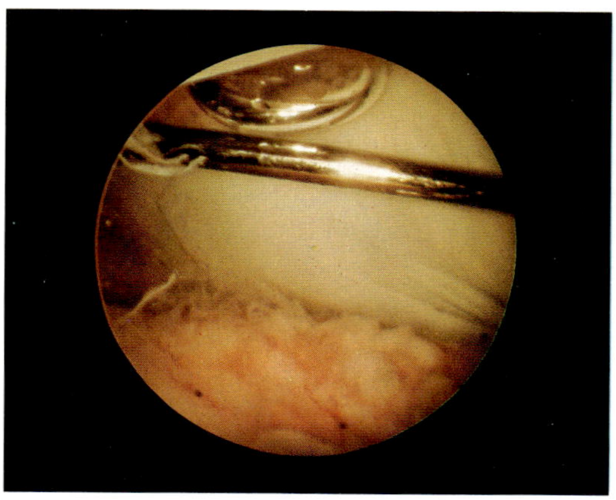

Fig. 3-3. Infrapatellar insertion. The fibrous septum is imperforate, and completely separates the quadriceps bursa from the joint.

quadriceps bursa just distal to the plica synovialis, that has been referred to as the *alar ligament, medial interarticular band,* or the *medial shelf** (Fig. 3-4). This

* Watanabe, M.: Personal communication, 1971.

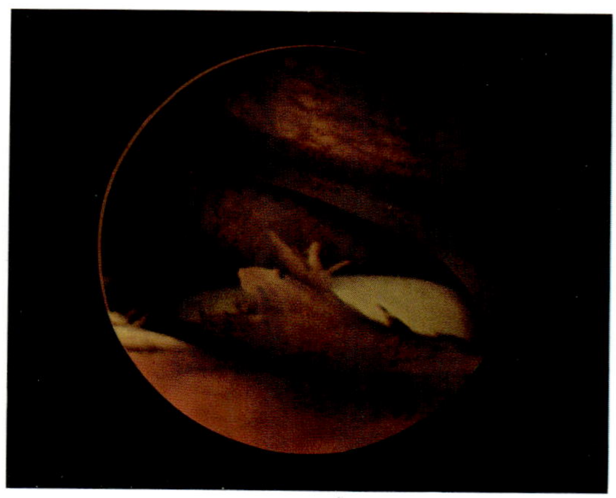

Fig. 3-4. The shelf: infrapatellar approach to the right knee. The shelf runs along the medial side wall, usually originating at the plica synovialis, and it inserts distally in the fat pad, crossing between the patella and the medial femoral condyle.

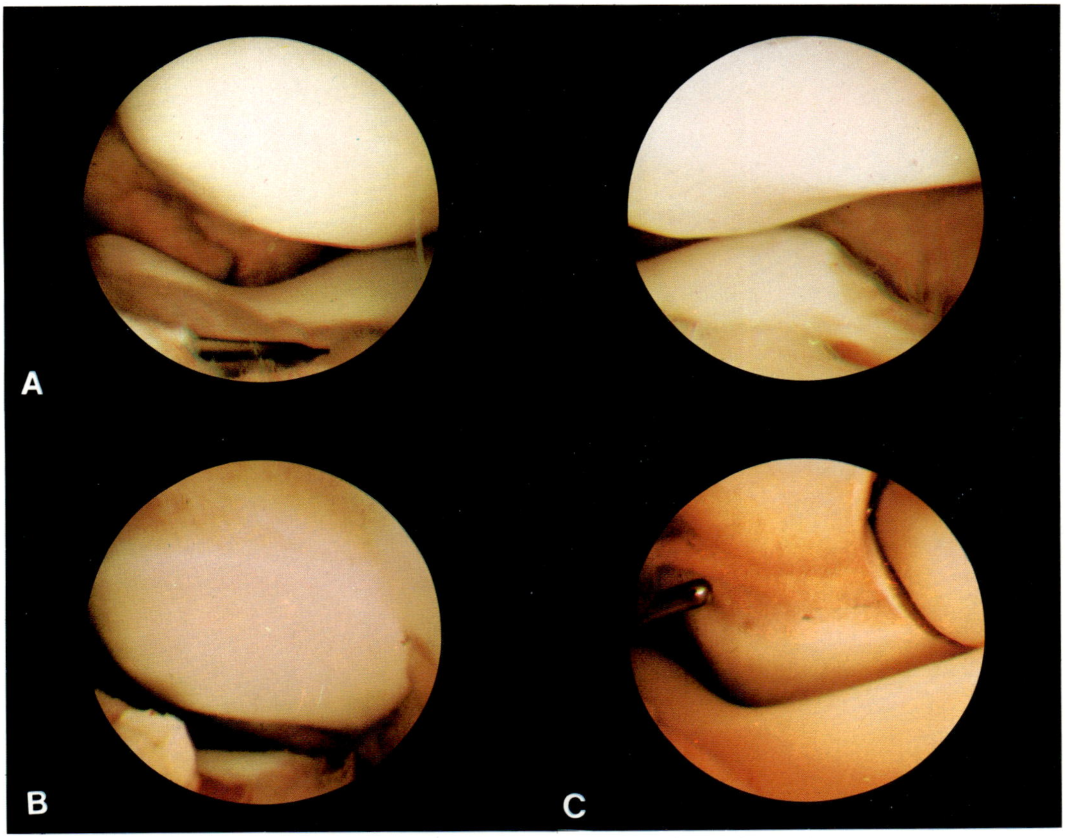

Fig. 3-5. (*A*) The patellofemoral joint of the left knee studied from a superolateral approach with a 110° telescope. The knee is in complete extension. (*Left*) The fat pad is seen between the patella and trochlear groove of the femur. The medial facet of the patella is not articulated with the medial femoral condyle. (*Right*) The patella overrides the lateral femoral condyle. (*B*) With the same telescope, using a suprapatellar approach, the knee is flexed 20 degrees. The entire superior portion of the patella is seen still partially overriding the lateral condyle. (*C*) With the same telescope, and the suprapatellar approach, the knee is flexed 30 degrees. The patella is now firmly seated in the trochlear groove of the femur. Note the superior synovial reflection above the articular surface of the patella (air bubble to the right).

fibrous band passes medially from the side wall of the quadriceps bursa, inserting into the fat pad distally. This structure, when well developed, may represent an obstacle to smooth passage of the telescope from the quadriceps bursa region over the medial femoral condyle into the medial compartment. Passage can be assured by partially withdrawing the telescope, disengaging it from the band, and then following the condyle distally into the joint line (Figs. 3-5, 3-6).

MEDIAL COMPARTMENT

Positioning of the Arthroscope. As the arthroscope follows the medial femoral

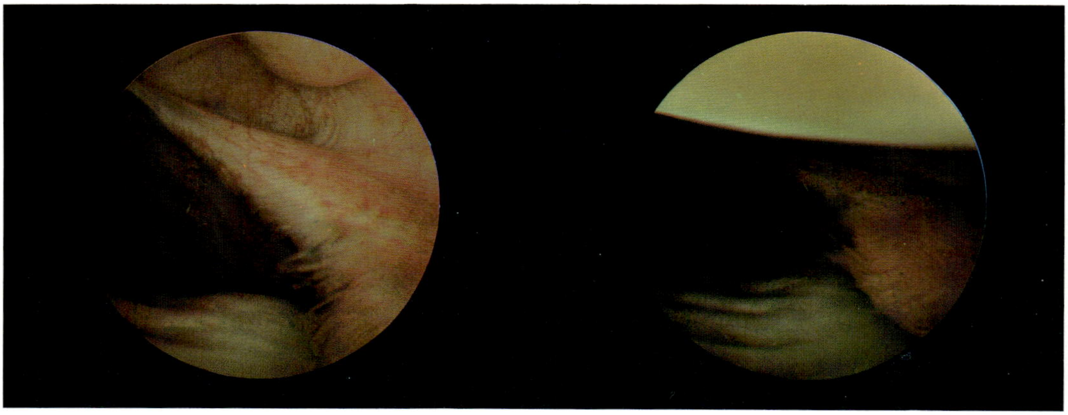

Fig. 3-6. Right knee: superior lateral approach. (*Left*) The shelf inserts into the fat pad. (*Right*) The relationship between the patella, medial femoral condyle, fat pad, and shelf.

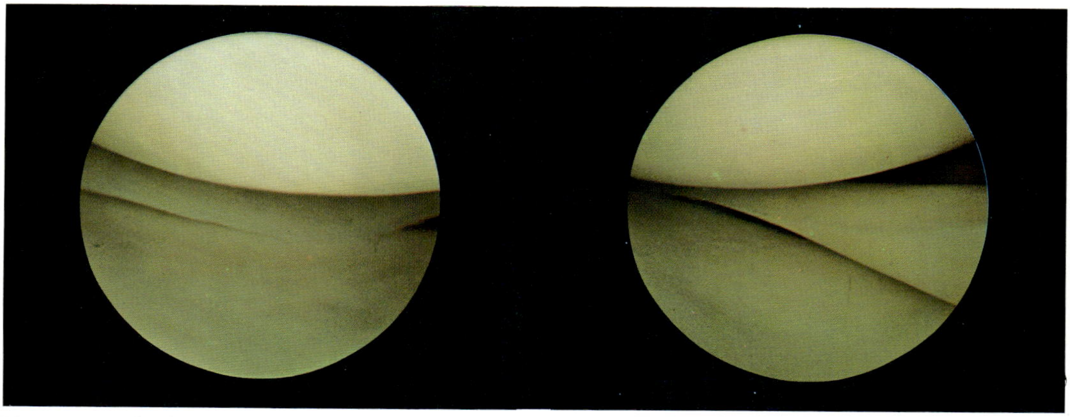

Fig. 3-7. Right knee: lateral infrapatellar approach. (*Right*) Anterior segment of the medial meniscus. (*Left*) Posterior segment of the medial meniscus.

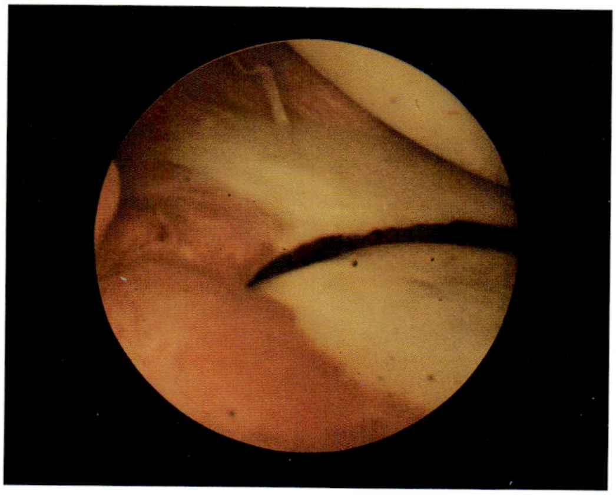

condyle posteriorly, the leg is slowly flexed over the table and the junction of the middle and posterior half of the medial meniscus is encountered. By partially withdrawing the telescope, the meniscus can be followed anteriorly (Fig. 3-7). Obstruction to vision of the superior surface of the anterior medial meniscus is

Fig. 3-8. Left knee: inferior lateral approach. The fat pad, covered with inflamed synovium, covers the superior surface of the anterior medial meniscus.

due to the overhanging fat pad (Fig. 3-8). This can be separated from the meniscus by repositioning the telescope. By increasing the amount of extension of the knee, rotating the foot externally, and applying a valgus stress, the arthroscope is brought posteriorly into the joint between the tibia and the medial femoral condyle. With gentle wedging of the arthroscope, the inner edge of the posterior medial meniscus can be viewed all the way back to its tibial insertion, in a high percentage of knees (Fig. 3-7). Internal rotation of the tibia approximates the medial tibial tubercular eminence and the medial femoral condyle, totally obscuring the posterior half of the medial meniscus. With external rotation, the inner edge of the meniscus protrudes slightly beneath the medial femoral condyle and straightens out its concave inner edge (Fig. 3-9). If valgus stress is added at this point, the meniscus assumes a serpentine configuration, but the meniscus does not protrude towards the intercondylar region (Fig. 3-10). The medial tubercular eminence obscures the view of the posterior inner edge of the medial meniscus (Fig. 3-11).

Recognition of the normal appearance and relationships of meniscus, tibia, and femur are of paramount importance because statistically the posterior horn of the medial meniscus is the most frequently involved in pathology and the anatomy conspires to keep its presence hidden. Anteriorly, the meniscus is viewed with the knee in internal and external rotation in an effort to make the medial meniscus slip off the tibial head, since in the normal knee this will not occur (Fig. 3-12). The cartilaginous surfaces of the tibia and femur are smooth, white, and glistening.

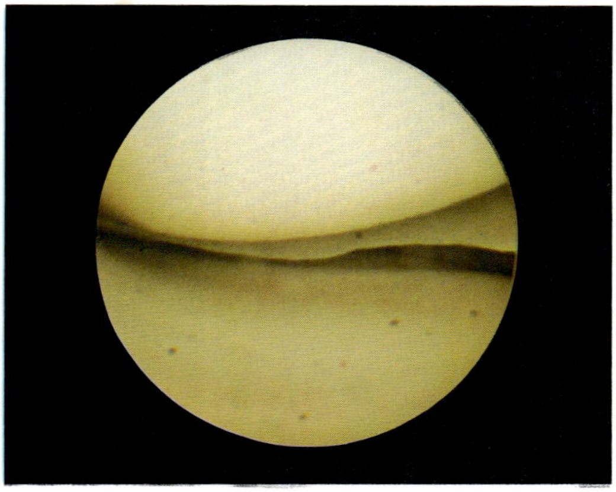

Fig. 3-9. Medial meniscus of the right knee: inferior lateral approach. With external tibial rotation, the leading edge of the medial meniscus protrudes beneath the medial femoral condyle.

INTERCONDYLAR NOTCH

The anatomy of the intercondylar notch varies from knee to knee, owing to the presence, size, and configuration of the ligamentum mucosum. As one proceeds from the medial to the lateral aspect of the joint, the synovium overlying the origin of the posterior cruciate ligament can be seen. The tendinous portion of the ligament is obscured by the anterior cruciate ligament crossing in front (Fig. 3-13). In the presence of posterior

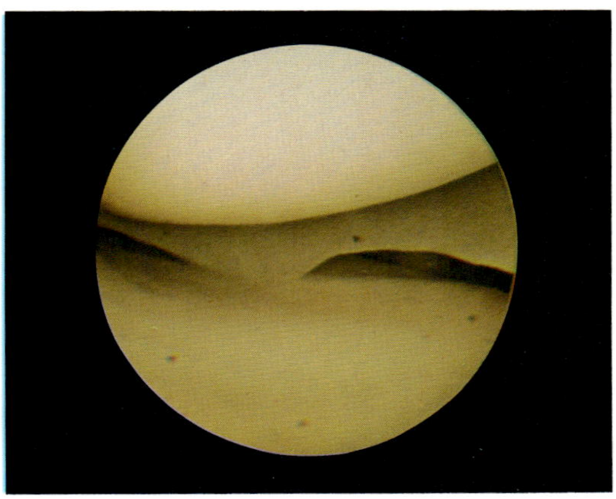

Fig. 3-10. Medial meniscus of the right knee: inferior lateral approach. A valgus strain applied to the externally rotated tibia produces a serpentine configuration of the posterior medial meniscus.

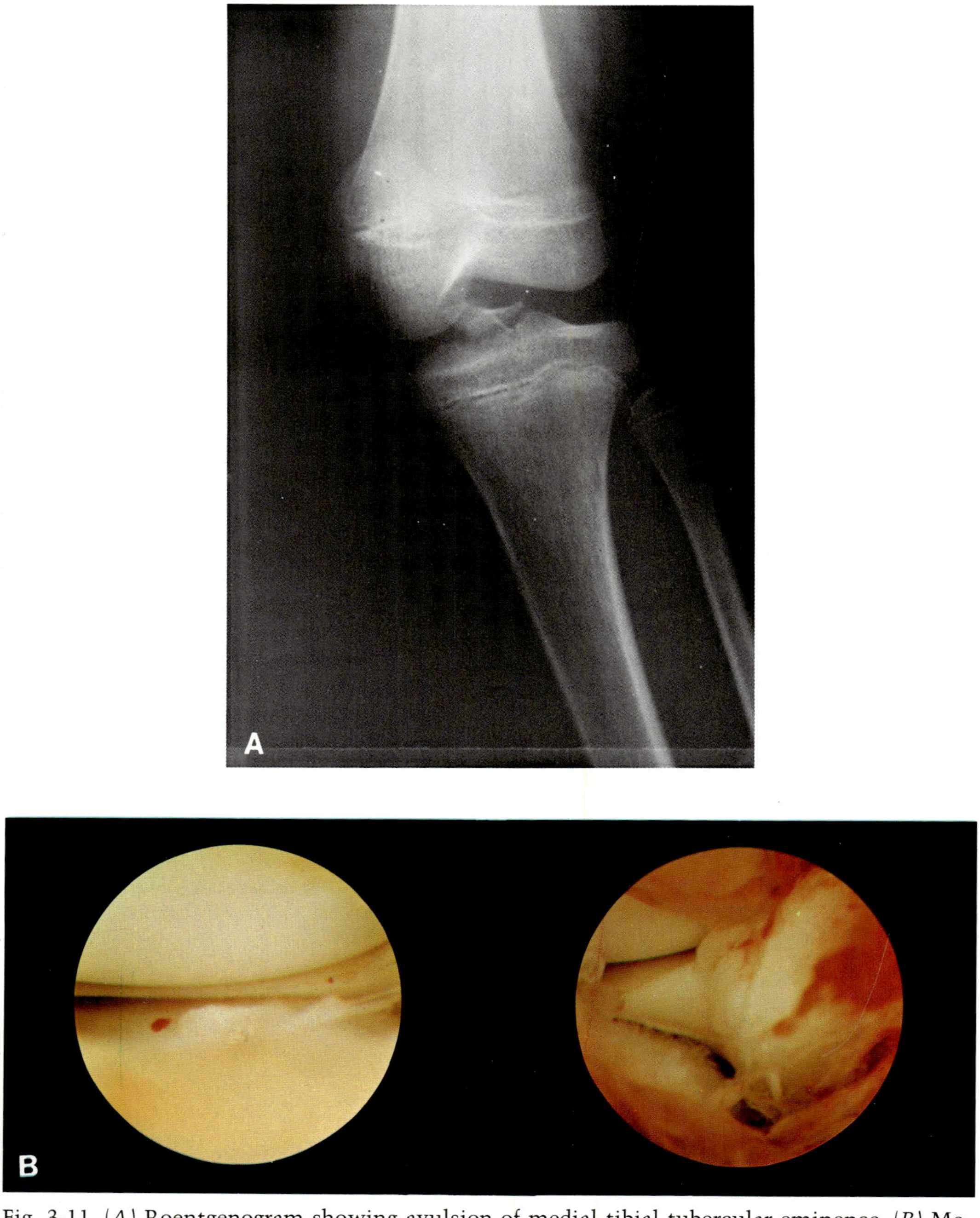

Fig. 3-11. (*A*) Roentgenogram showing avulsion of medial tibial tubercular eminence. (*B*) Medial meniscus of the left knee. (*Left*) Posterior inner edge of medial meniscus; (*Right*) posterior attachment of medial meniscus to tibia seen after pushing bony fragment anteriorly.

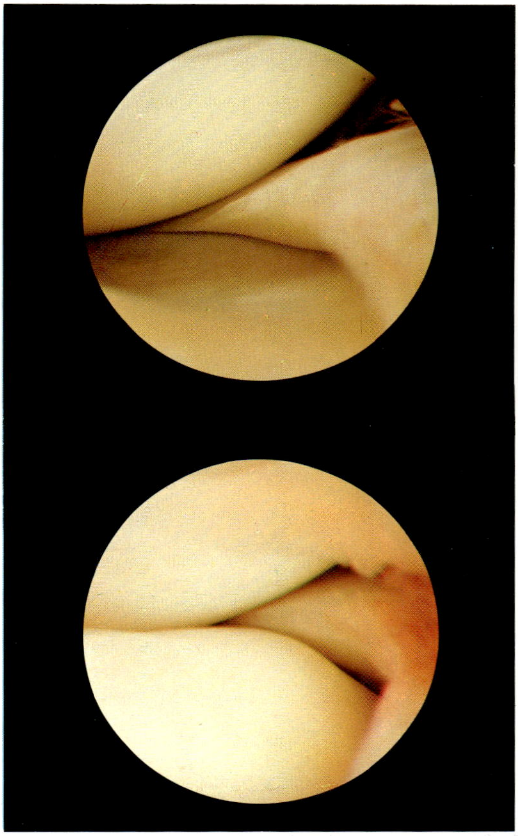

Fig. 3-12. Anterior medial meniscus of the right knee. (*Top*) Tibia in external rotation; (*Bottom*) Tibia in internal rotation. The medial meniscus slips off the tibial head.

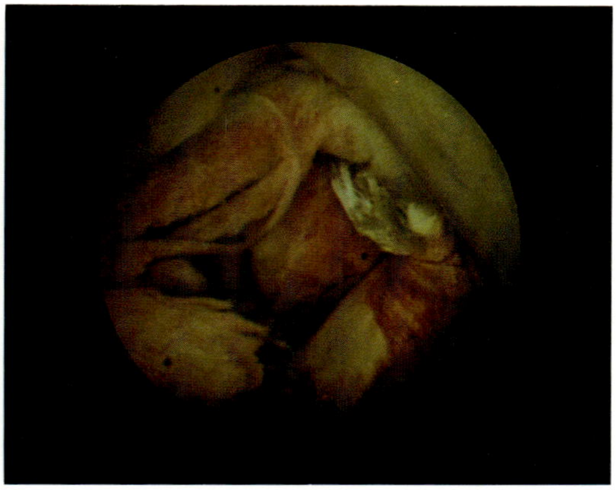

Fig. 3-13. Anatomy of the intercondylar notch of the left knee: infrapatellar approach. Medial femoral condyle is on the left. On the right is the lateral femoral condyle and the ligamentum mucosum insertion on the fat pad. In the center, the synovial cap over the origin of the posterior cruciate ligament is seen. On the lower right, the anterior cruciate ligament with a torn fasiculus of ligament is seen. Note the vascular engorgement of the synovium covering the anterior cruciate ligament.

capsular laxity however, the arthroscope may be passed from the lateral aspect across the anterior cruciate ligament and between the medial tibial plateau and the medial femoral condyle; and with rotation and using the 110-degree arthroscope, the tendinous portion of the posterior cruciate ligament can be viewed (Fig. 3-14).

The synovial cap seen covering the posterior cruciate ligament origin always appears to be well developed, even in the adolescent patient (Fig. 3-15). The instrument is moved laterally and the distal two-thirds of the anterior cruciate ligament can be visualized. Variation occurs here in synovial covering: it may be very thin in the adolescent, seeming to be absent, or (Fig. 3-16) quite thickened as age increases.

The Anterior Cruciate Ligament. There is also variation in the arthroscopic

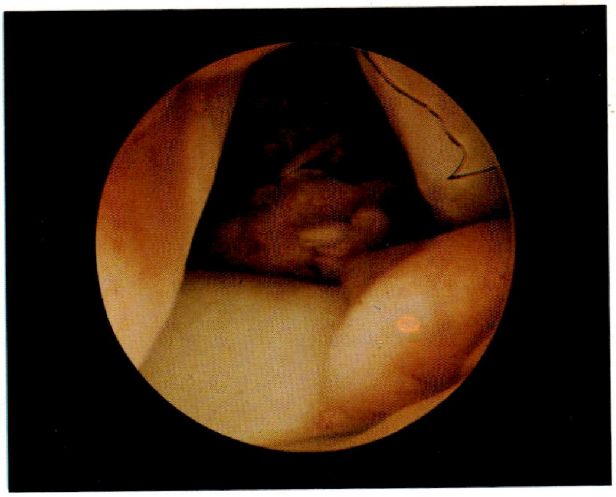

Fig. 3-14. Posterior intercondylar notch of the left knee: lateral infrapatellar approach. A triangle of posterior capsule is surrounded by the medial femoral condyle, left, posterior cruciate ligament, right, and the posterior extremity of the medial meniscus, below.

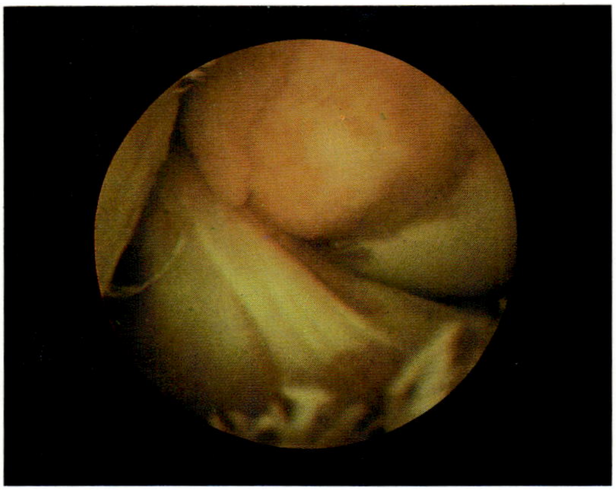

Fig. 3-15. The synovial cap is well demarcated, and covers the origin of the posterior cruciate ligament. The anterior cruciate ligament covers the ligamentous portion of the posterior cruciate ligament.

appearance of the anterior cruciate ligament itself. The bundles of fibers in this ligament may occur as vertical splits (Fig. 3-16A,B) between several segments or may appear as a tight bundle, or the spiral configuration may predominate. The integrity of the structure may be ascertained by attempting the classic anterior drawer test under direct vision. This has the advantage of detecting a tear of the anterior cruciate ligament before the drawer test becomes clinically positive. The entire proximal third of the anterior cruciate ligament may be studied by viewing from the medial infrapatellar approach.

The ligamentum mucosum runs from the intercondylar notch superior to the anterior cruciate ligament, attaching to the fat pad. A septum is sometimes formed on either side, extending distally to the fat pad, so that the insertion of the ligamentum mucosum is wider than normal.

This septum may be responsible for difficulty in passing the arthroscope into the lateral compartment, may also cause difficulty in locating a loose body in the intercondylar notch, and may possibly in-

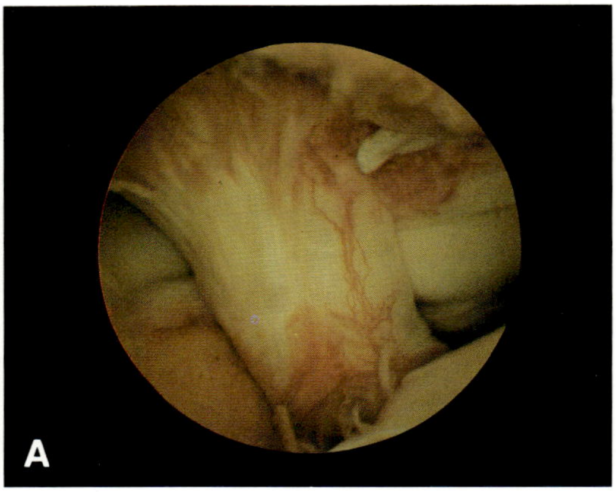

A

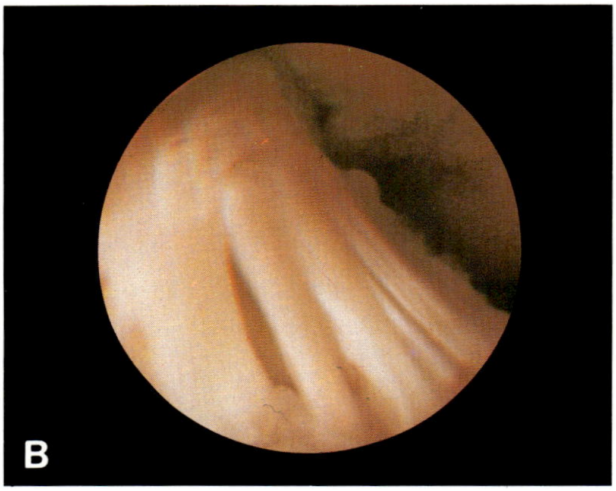

B

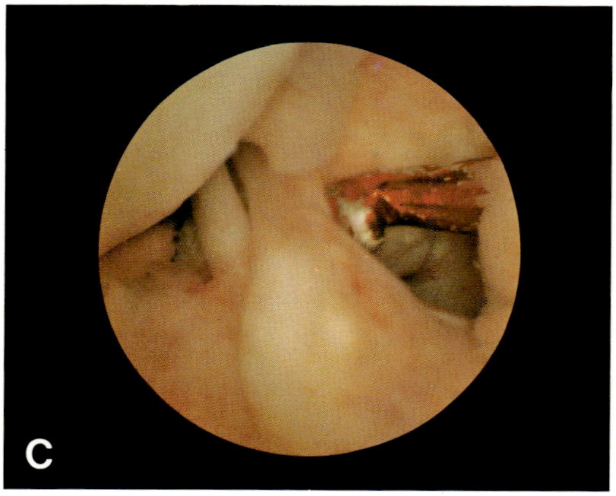

C

Fig. 3-16. (*A*) The anterior cruciate ligament seen from the lateral inferior approach with a varus stress. Note the variations in thickness of the synovial cover. (*B*) Multiple vertical splits in the anterior cruciate ligament of the right knee. (*C*) A large anomalous band of anterior cruciate ligament. Probing with a crochet hook helps evaluate its integrity.

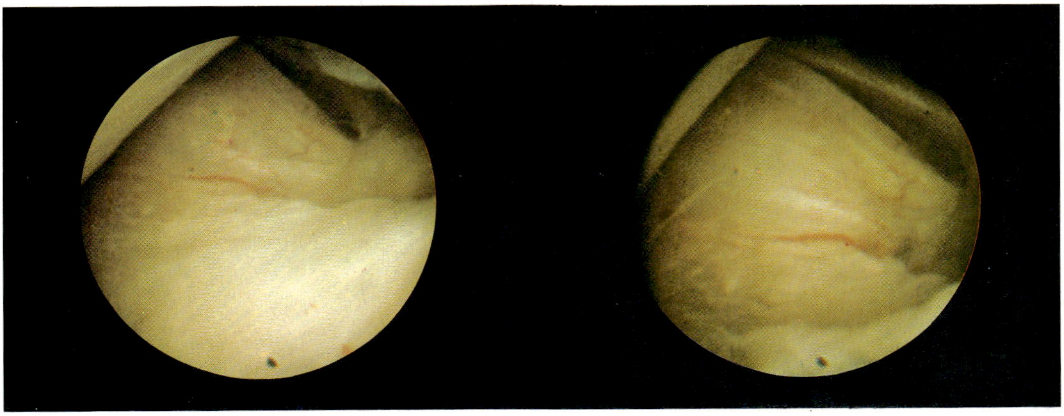

Fig. 3-17. The posterior cruciate ligament can be studied from the posterior medial approach. Posterior medial femoral condyle at upper left (left knee).

terfere with arthroscopic removal of the loose body. In one patient, visualization of a loose body known to be in the intercondylar notch was only possible after the septum was perforated to allow visualization of the medial compartment.

The fat pad is the nemesis of the arthroscopist. It seems ubiquitous and is responsible for the many technical difficulties the beginner encounters; learning arthroscopy seems to consist of learning how to deal with the fat pad. Frequently a homogenous yellow-orange color is seen; this indicates that the arthroscope has been partially withdrawn into the fat pad and at this juncture the pad is being observed from within. The fat pad lies close to the anterior horn of the medial and lateral meniscus, so in order to view these structures, the fat pad should be lifted

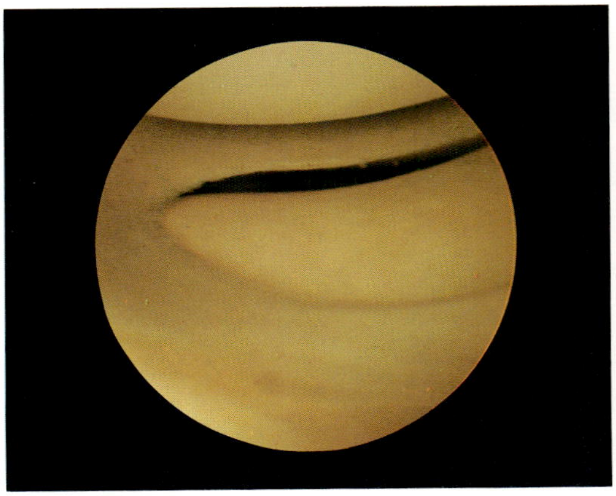

Fig. 3-18. Panoramic view of the lateral meniscus. This lateral infrapatellar approach to the right knee demonstrates the posterior, middle, and anterior segments.

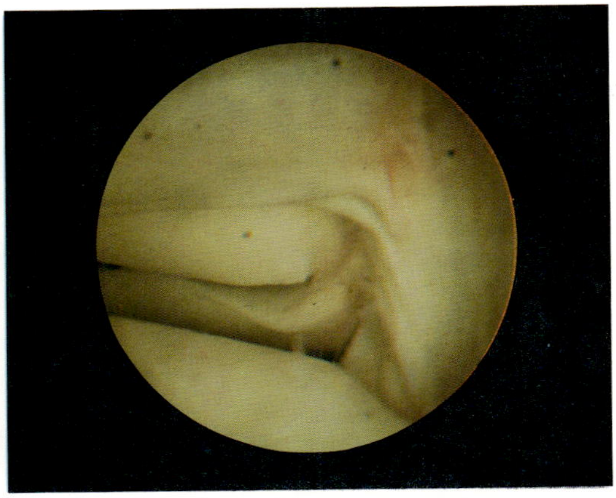

Fig. 3-19. Anterior and posterior tibial attachments of lateral meniscus of the left knee. Note the slip of meniscus gaining attachment to the anterior cruciate ligament.

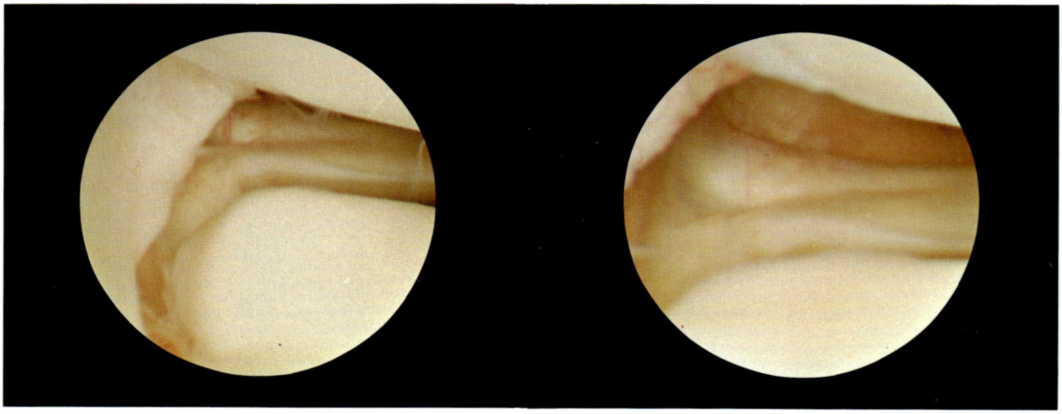

Fig. 3-20. (*Left*) Ligament of Wrisberg. The ligament of Wrisberg runs posterior and is attached to the periphery of the lateral meniscus (*right*). The ligament diverges from the meniscus, which inserts into the tibia.

from the meniscus by the telescope as it is partially withdrawn along the superior meniscal body.

LATERAL COMPARTMENT

The lateral compartment is easily studied from the lateral infrapatellar approach. The origin of the posterior horn of the lateral meniscus is followed from its posterior tibial origin anteriorly (Fig. 3-18). A normal anatomic variation is seen frequently in both the anterior and posterior tibial attachments (Fig. 3-19). The ligament of Wrisberg variation of attachment is most frequently seen arthroscopy (Fig. 3-20).

Examination of the Meniscus. The posterior third of the lateral meniscus is ideally situated for arthroscopic study, since in many instances the superior and infe-

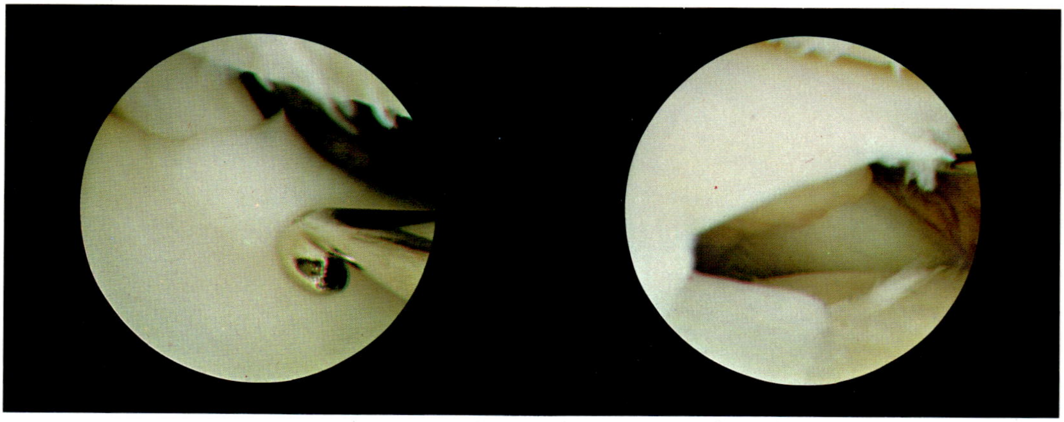

Fig. 3-21. Popliteus tendon of the right knee. The tendon is seen passing superior to the lateral meniscus (*left*) and exiting beneath the meniscus (*right*).

rior surfaces may be viewed simultaneously. However, it may be necessary to insert a separate instrument into the joint to probe the meniscus. The area beneath the lateral meniscus in the posterior third is a retreat frequently sought by the cartilaginous body. As the meniscus is studied peripherally at the posterior lateral corner of the joint, the popliteus tendon can be seen coursing obliquely and posteriorly to the lateral meniscus (Figs. 3-21, 3-22). This is usually covered by a sheath of synovium of variable thickness.

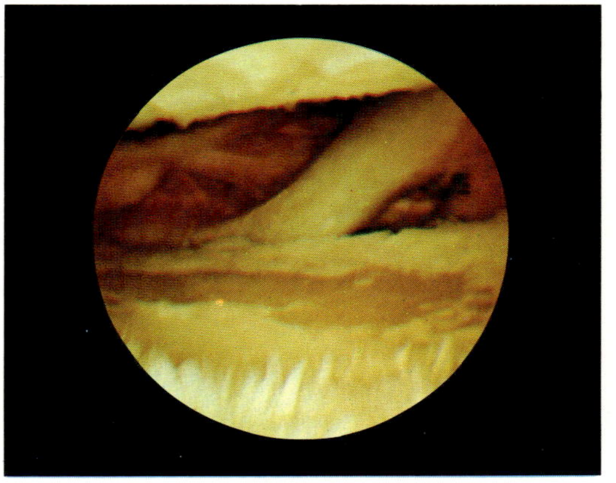

Fig. 3-22. The popliteus tendon of the left knee in the absence of the lateral mensicus, demonstrating its oblique course.

Only the superior surface of the middle and anterior third of the lateral meniscus can be viewed arthroscopically. As the instrument is moved anteriorly, the anterior inner edge of the meniscus is studied. Using the lateral approach, visualization of the anterior peripheral attachment of the lateral meniscus is inadequate, so if there is a reason to believe a tear exists, and it has not been seen, a medial insertion of the arthroscope must be performed to complete this study.

4 *The Synovium*

CHARACTER AND FUNCTION

The synovium appears to have several roles in normal and pathologic knee function, the primary one being secretion of synovial fluid for joint lubrication. With advancing age, however, the synovium is called into play in a housecleaning capacity, removing degenerative debris from the joint. The severity and chronicity of this pathologic process is mirrored by progressive alteration of the synovial lining. Not all of the synovial changes occur simultaneously; there may be severe changes adjacent to normal-appearing synovium.[1] The earliest changes occur during adolescence when the synovial mat is altered by increased villi formation, increasing the workable synovial surface area. This is usually seen towards the end of adolescence, but it may occur earlier, following an inflammation or a mechanical derangement.

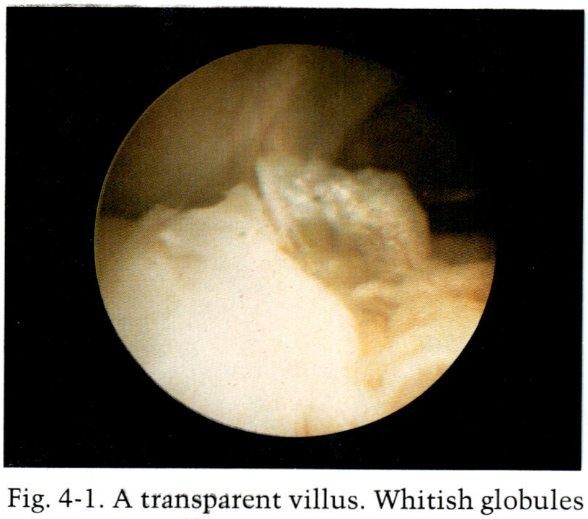

Fig. 4-1. A transparent villus. Whitish globules within the villi are imbibed saline solution. One central vessel demonstrates the normal vascularity of a transparent villus.

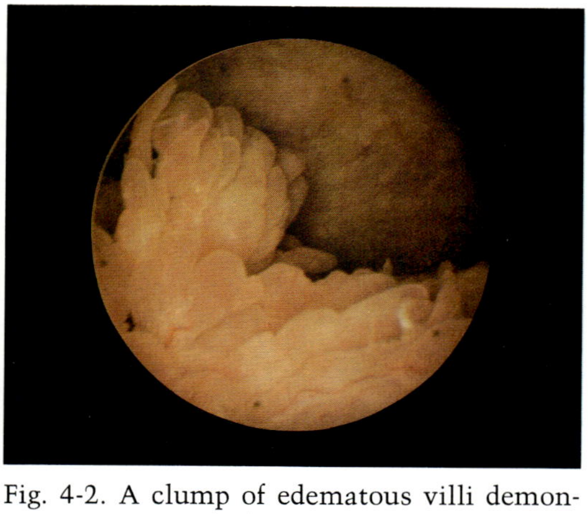

Fig. 4-2. A clump of edematous villi demonstrating a ground glass appearance and globular configuration. The vessels are still relatively sparse but become more dilated.

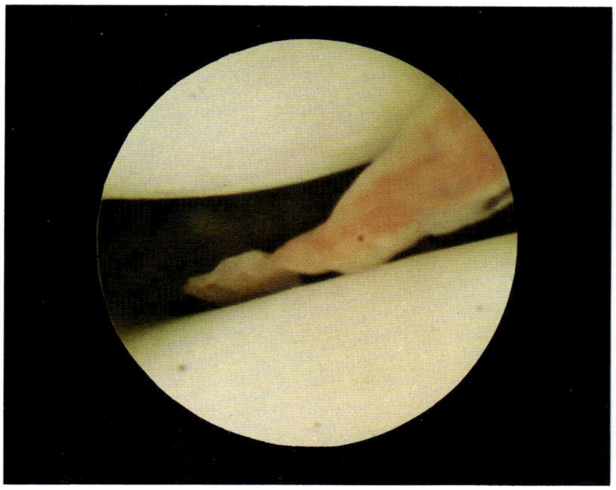

Fig. 4-3. Synovial reaction following acute injury and hemarthrosis. A synovial frond is thickened and engorged.

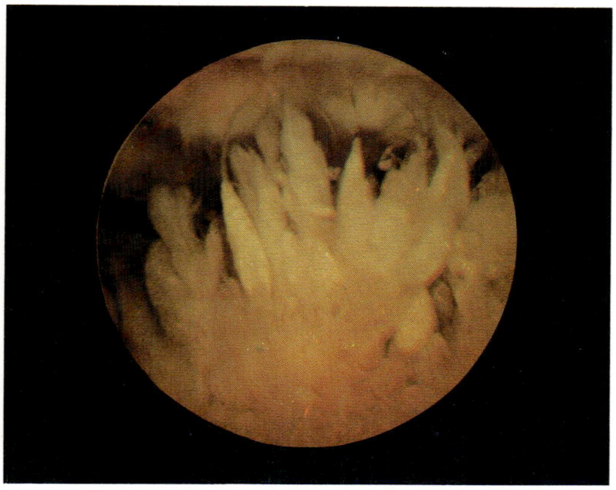

Fig. 4-4. Degenerative villi combining areas of fatty infiltration, fibrosis, and edema.

The character of the synovium may be described as matlike, transparent (Fig. 4-1), edematous (Fig. 4-2), fibrotic, opaque, vascular, degenerative, hemosiderous, or necrotic. After an acute injury or inflammatory process, it becomes swollen and has a definite globular configuration. It appears slightly pink, and the normal transparent appearance gives way to slight opacification. As the acute inflammatory process subsides, the villi revert to a hypertrophic stage, often with increased vascularity.

TRAUMATIC DISORDERS OF THE SYNOVIUM

Following an acute hemarthrosis, the synovium swells, and large fronds are created with considerable venous congestion (Fig. 4-3). As time passes, the synovium may be infiltrated with fat and increased fibrous tissue (Fig. 4-4). The fat infiltration is probably under metabolic control. The fibrous component, however, appears to be related to the severity of the cartilaginous damage and to how long the inflammatory process has been going on (Fig. 4-5). I have not had occasion to examine many rheumatoid patients (Figs. 4-6, 4-7, 4-8); however, the chronic changes of rheumatoid arthritis are not unlike the changes seen in the end stage degenerative joint, resulting in synovial replacement by fat or fibrous tissue.

Case 4-1. Cartilaginous Degeneration and Synovitis

A 25-year-old woman twisted her knee and, although she had little immediate difficulty, developed an effusion of the knee about 24 hours later that did not respond to aspiration

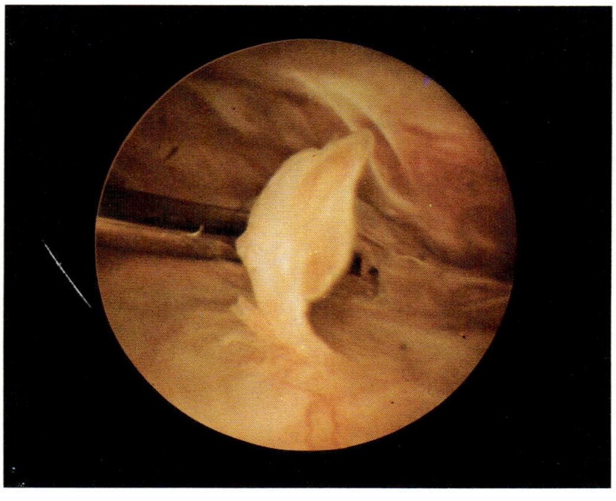

Fig. 4-5. Fibrotic villi. Note increased opacity, obscuring the vascular pattern.

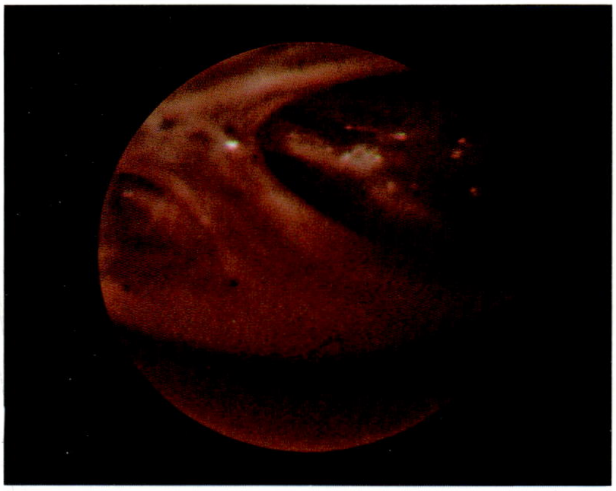

Fig. 4-6. Severe acute inflammatory response in a patient with ulcerative colitis arthritis 2 months following medial meniscectomy. The intense vascularization of the synovium surrounds islands of intense fibrotic reaction. The synovitis was controlled with antipholgistic agents.

or other anti-inflammatory agents. Arthroscopy one month following injury revealed cartilaginous degeneration in the lateral compartment, and an acute synovitis with increased vascularity and edematous villi. The patient responded slowly to arthroscopic irrigation of the joint, anti-inflammatory agents, and quadriceps redevelopment (Fig. 4-2).

The severe cartilaginous degeneration causes synovial changes as a result of sluffing of minute cartilaginous debris and the probable action of cartilaginous lysosomes. Arthroscopic evidence suggests that both the cartilaginous debris and an enzymatic component act on the synovium. At arthroscopy, many unoperated degenerative knees show areas of severe fragmentation or fibrillation and articular cartilage crater formation, but the joint is surprisingly free of cartilaginous debris. It is possible that, mechanically the debris is pulverized and then removed by the synovium. This process may occur over many years without clinical symptoms. Suddenly, the synovium becomes overburdened, either as a consequence of a sudden twisting injury or an increase in the patient's activities, and an effusion develops. Rest usually results in reabsorption of the excess synovial fluid, but the next functional overload results in exacerbation of the effusion. Eventually the capacity of the system is overloaded, owing to the fibrosis of the synovium, so the effusion remains. Arthroscopy with joint lavage frequently decreases the synovial irritation and removes considerable

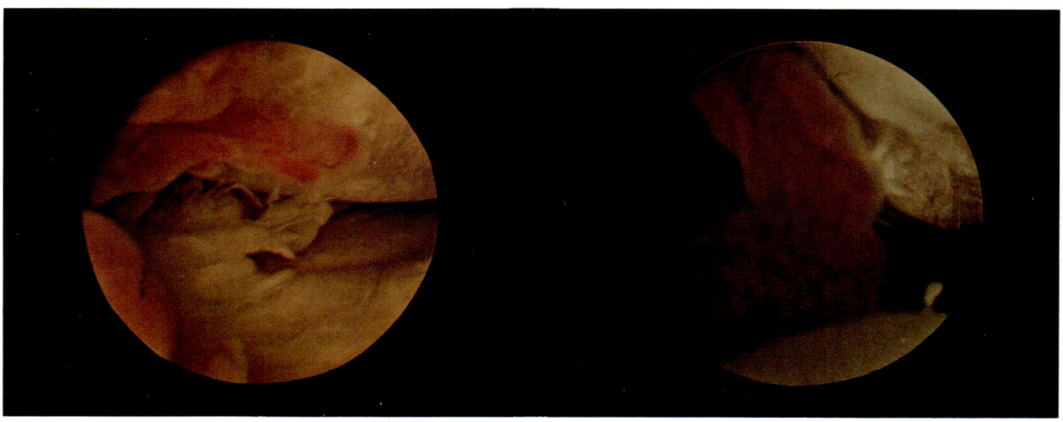

Fig. 4-7. Rheumatoid arthritis active and untreated. The patient was a 50-year-old woman with a history of left knee swelling for one year. Her range of motion was between 10 and 80 degrees of flexion with massive thickening of the synovium. Note the rheumatoid villi with intense vascular engorgement, and note degeneration of the medial femoral condyle.

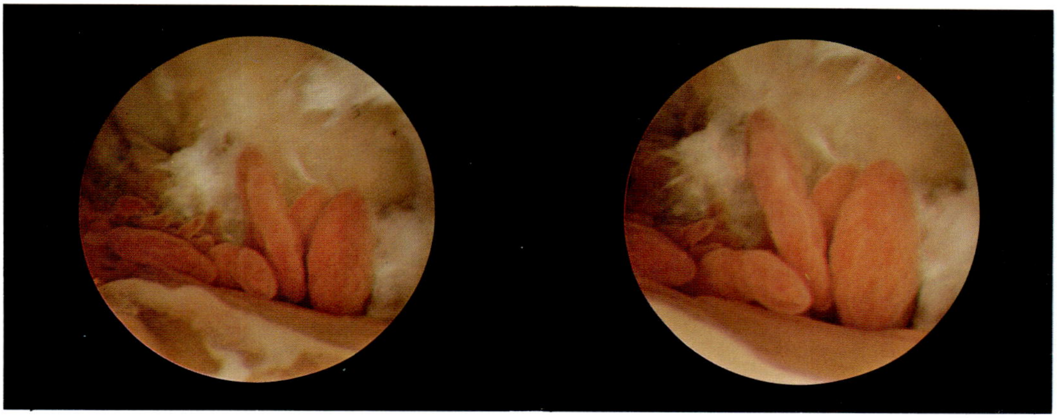

Fig. 4-8. Same patient as in Fig. 4-7, 2 months following treatment by arthroscopic partial synovectomy, intra-articular steroids, and an antipholgistic agent. The synovium now shows chronic changes with the few remaining villi rounded and club-shaped. Behind the villi is the regenerating synovium. The effusion has subsided and the range of motion is between 0 and 120 degrees of flexion.

cartilaginous debris,* and may also decrease (perhaps by dilution) an enzyme build-up. Quite frequently, pain relief and subsidence of the effusion follow arthroscopy.† The duration of this satisfactory response has been observed for as long as 3 years, but occasionally joint lavage may have to be repeated if pain and effusion recur, and on rare occasions a synovectomy is needed.

* Johnson, L.: Exhibit. Dallas, American Academy of Orthopaedic Surgeons, 1974.

† Jackson, R. W.: personal communication 1971; Watanabe, M.: personal communication, 1970.

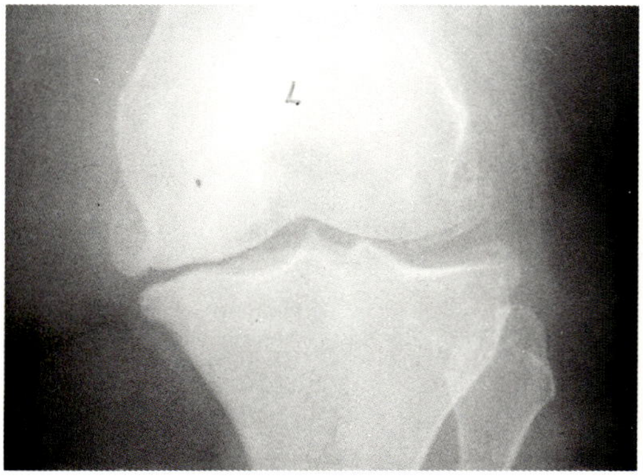

Fig. 4-9. Posterior-anterior view of the left knee in a patient with severe degenerative arthritis. Her past history suggests that this is a case of "burnt out" rheumatoid arthritis. The osteophyte rising from the medial femoral condyle can be seen in Fig. 3-11.

Case 4-2. Joint Narrowing, Subchondral Sclerosis, and Osteophyte Formation

A 50-year-old female had a history of thromboembolism and severe bilateral knee pain over the past 10 years. She was treated by a right medial meniscectomy, which resulted in

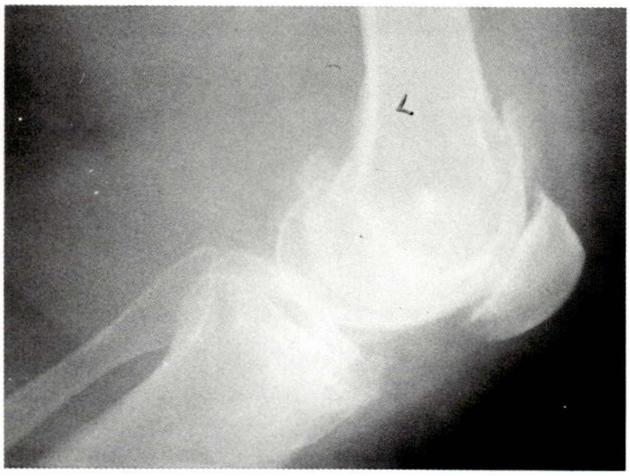

Fig. 4-10. Lateral view of the knee in Fig. 4-9.

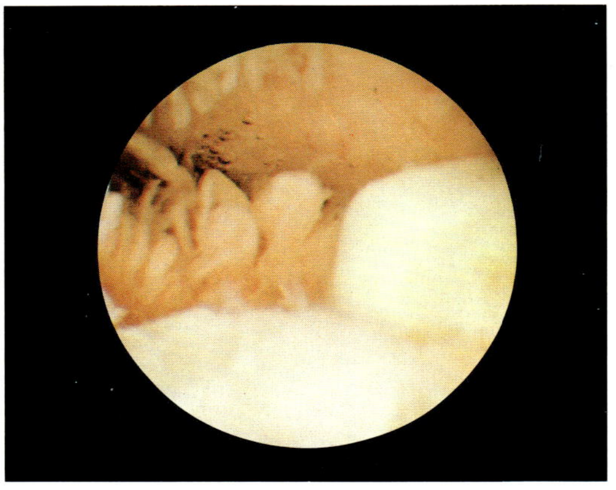

Fig. 4-11. Suprapatellar recess with fibrillation of the femur and an osteophyte on the right. The synovium presents a mixed picture with fibrotic, fatty, and edematous elements present.

pain relief for the past 3 years. Following an otherwise-inconsequential fall, both knees became painful. Roentgenograms revealed joint narrowing, subchondral sclerosis, and marked osteophyte formation. Bilateral arthroscopy resulted in moderate relief of pain, ten degrees' increase in range of motion, and it allowed an increase in activity level over the following 6 months (Figs. 4-9, 4-10, 4-11, 4-12).

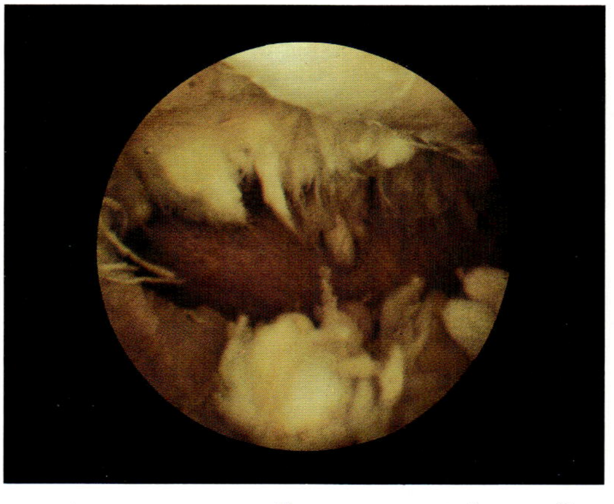

Fig. 4-12. Suprapatellar recess: infrapatellar approach. The plica synovialis shows considerable alteration with thickening, increased vascularity, and a large patch of fibrotic synovium.

CASE 4-3. JOINT EFFUSION AND DEGENERATIVE ARTHRITIS

A 64-year-old male with a 6-month history of joint effusion and limited range of motion was found to have considerable loose interarticular cartilaginous debris, including areas of cartilage in various stages of digestion by the engulfing synovium (Fig. 4-13). Rapid reabsorption of the effusion followed arthroscopic lavage.

Unfortunately not all patients with severe degenerative changes respond to joint lavage; this indicates that occasionally either chemical or surgical synovectomy is necessary.

SYNOVIAL CHONDROMATOSIS

Synovial chondromatosis is an interesting but rare synovial process.[5] In over 1500 cases in which arthroscopic examination was involved, I have seen this condition only twice.

CASE 4-4. SYNOVIAL CHONDROMATOSIS NEAR THE ANTERIOR CRUCIATE LIGAMENT

A 63-year-old male kicked a football and immediately was unable to extend his right knee completely. This condition persisted for

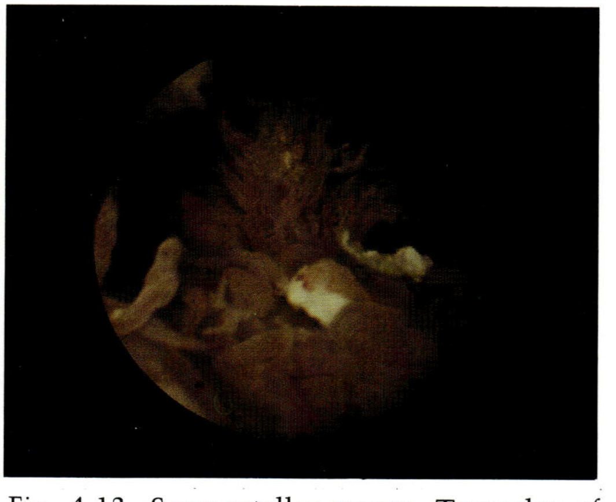

Fig. 4-13. Suprapatellar recess. Tentacles of elongated vascular villi engulf several areas of loose cartilaginous debris.

9 months before he sought medical help. Arthroscopy demonstrated that the loss of extension was due to synovial chondromatosis. This diagnosis was confirmed histologically. The only apparent area of involvement was the synovium covering the anterior cruciate ligament. Two areas of synovial outpouching arose from the medial and lateral aspects of the anterior cruciate ligament (Fig. 4-14). These resulting masses appeared as two thinly covered cocoons on a synovial pedicle attached to the anterior cruciate ligament. This condition was isolated to the synovium of the anterior cruciate ligament as seen at arthrotomy. Treatment consisted of a synovectomy of the anterior cruciate ligament and hamstring, and posterior capsular stretching exercises.

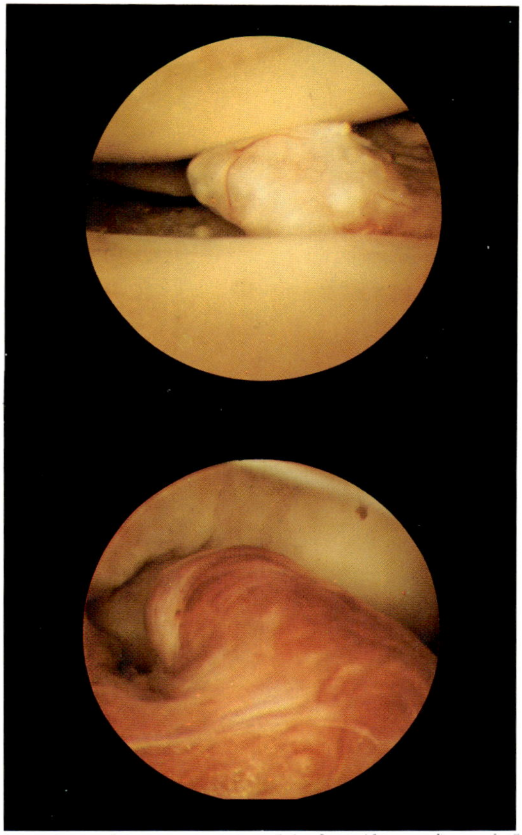

Fig. 4-14. Synovial chondromatosis. Two synovial masses project into the joint line. (*Top*) A cluster of cartilaginous nodules encased in a fibrous cocoon, project into the lateral joint line. (*Bottom*) A thickened synovial mass trapped in the medial joint line. Both rise from the synovium overlying the anterior cruciate ligament.

CRYSTAL-INDUCED SYNOVITIS

An interesting type of synovitis that has been gaining attention recently is caused by intra-articular crystals. McCarty, Hollander, and numerous others[1,3] have discussed the pathogenesis of crystal-induced synovitis and have found three types of crystals within the synovial fluid. They are: monosodium urate, calcium pyrophosphate, and certain amorphous crystals that I believe may be calcium hydroxyapatite. Definitive diagnosis of crystals depends on x-ray refraction studies, which I have not used. Arthroscopic study of joints afflicted with crystal problems shows some similarity in the sites of distribution of deposits.

In the gouty joint, crystals are deposited in the synovium and the synovial villi as well as within fibrillated and fragmented fibrocartilage or hyaline cartilage. In chondrocalcinosis, crystalline deposits are found in the synovium and within physically unaltered articular and hyaline cartilage. One significant difference between gouty arthritis deposits and calcium pyrophosphate deposits is that the former are not visible on roentgenograms. The deposits of calcium pyrophosphate crystals appear to be radiopaque and, if present in significant numbers, they may outline the cartilaginous surfaces of the femoral condyles and the tibia and meniscus. A third type of crystal, whose pathogenic properties are like those of monosodium urate and calcium pyrophosphate, is found in physically altered articular cartilage and studded within the synovium. However, its morphology and chemical composition have so far defied my analysis. These deposits are unlike those seen in calcium pyrophosphate deposits and in gout, and occur only in the elderly. They are nonradiopaque and they are only seen in severely degenerated cartilage.

I have observed 40 patients with crystalline deposition within the knee, and 2 cases of crystalline deposition in the ankle joint. The ages of these patients ranged from 18 to 72. A few were acutely affected but most were chronically diseased. A number of joints, while demonstrating crystals, had not yet exhibited an inflammatory reaction. In those joints with a history of an effusion, the onset of symptoms was heralded by either a twisting injury or a relatively minor blow on the surface of the knee. The clinical response of the injury showed no correlation to the magnitude of the cause —it was sometimes caused by a seemingly minor accident. The patients with chronic disease were usually seen on a referral basis with symptoms present continuously or intermittently for several months to several years. Usually the chronic cases of calcium pyrophosphate crystals had been previously diagnosed, and the treatment by aspiration and anti-inflammatory agents was generally ineffective. Many of the patients with chronic gout had failed to improve with the conventional remedies, colchicine, phenylbutazone (Butazolidine), and probenecid (Benemid). Those patients with work-related injuries had been out of work for many months.

The synovial fluid of all of these knees was studied under polarized light microscopy. In the acute cases, the intracellular crystals were either calcium pyrophosphate or monosodium urate, or a combination of both, and gave a positive diagnosis according to the criteria established by McCarty and Hollander. In the chronically diseased knee, and particularly in the one without roentgenographic evidence of calcification, the synovial fluid analysis was more difficult. Very rarely were intracellular crystals of calcium pyrophosphate or monosodium urate found. Occasionally, extracellular crystals were found, but they were sparse and nondiagnostic. Arthroscopy provided the means by which the diagnosis of crystal synovitis could be made and biopsy material from the involved area of crystal deposition obtained.

Of great significance was the serendipitous discovery that following arthroscopy the condition of these knees was markedly improved.[6] Many patients noted relief from the synovitis after waking up from anesthesia. At first this observation was regarded as coincidental, but later a pattern developed, allowing reasonable expectations of improvement regardless of the severity of the intra-articular pathology associated with the crystal deposition.

Case 4-5. Pain and Effusion Caused by Crystalline Deposits

A 55-year-old insurance executive gave a history of a knee injury at the age of 16 and was otherwise in good health until 3 years prior to examination. His work did not cause symptoms, but playing golf invariably brought on an episode of an effusion and pain within the knee which would take days to subside. Roentgenograms demonstrated the presence of deposits of crystalline material within the menisci and the articular cartilage. Intracellular crystals of calcium pyrophosphate were seen by polarized light microscopy. Arthroscopy revealed crystalline deposits studding the synovium and physically unaltered fibrocartilage of the medial and lateral meniscus in addition to the overlying articular cartilage. In spite of gross tearing of both menisci, marked relief of symptoms occurred, and he refused the proposed medial and lateral meniscectomy. Relief continued until his death from an unrelated cause 18 months later.

Pathogenesis

The pathogenesis of this crystal-induced synovitis has been largely described by the rheumatologists. The instigating event apparently is triggered by the chance meeting of the crystal and a polymorphonuclear leukocyte, with resultant phagocytosis of the crystal. Subsequent events are numerous and are thought to include polymorphonuclear leukocytic disintegration, releasing lysosomes and vasotrophic factors that cause increased vascular permeability of the synovium and, in turn, increase polymorphonuclear leukocytic movement across the synovial barrier. A chain reaction occurs after the initial event, rapidly increasing the joint effusion and causing severe pain.[4] In several patients, we have seen this phenomenon reaching full-blown proportions within a period of 48 hours.

The pathogenicity of crystals appears to depend on their physical rather than chemical characteristics.[2] It has been shown that:

1. Crystal size must be within the range of .5 and 20 μm to enable phagocytosis by the polymorphonuclear leukocyte to occur.
2. The crystal must be *relatively* insoluble in water or saline solution. It is well known that storage of synovium or cartilage containing crystalline deposits, in either formalin or saline solution, will cause dissolution of these crystals.

It is possible that irrigation of the joint may well decrease the crystal population both by debridement as well as by increased solubility.

Clinical Improvement After Arthroscopy

In the group of patients I have examined, the white count has tended to remain normal, but the sedimentation rate is usually elevated. Aspiration of the joint alone seems to be only minimally effective in decreasing the patient's pain. Rapid, in fact almost immediate, improvement follows arthroscopy.

Initially I considered this improvement to be due to the decrease of the crystal population within the joint. It became obvious, however, that the numerous amounts of crystalline deposits and the tiny size and relative insolubility of the crystals would be only partially and minimally affected by the irrigation of the joint. I now believe that the clinical improvement results from the removal of or dilution of the enzymes produced by leukocytic degeneration. Many theories based on laboratory experiments have been put forth to explain the increased susceptibility of the crystal to phagocytosis by the polymorphonuclear leukocytes. The probability that albumin or at least a fraction of the blood within the knee may coat the crystal and increase this susceptibility is demonstrated by the following case.

Case 4-6. Crystal-Induced Synovitis and Trauma

A 55-year-old male incurred a twisting injury while descending from a ladder. This was followed by a joint effusion, and roentgenograms demonstrated areas of calcification within the menisci and hyaline cartilage of the femoral condyles. He was treated by conservative measures for several months prior to arthroscopy, with little improvement. Only a few extracellular crystals of calcium pyrophosphate were seen by polarized light microscopy. Arthroscopy revealed numerous crystalline deposits throughout the joint as well as a degenerative tear of the medial meniscus (Fig. 4-15). Upon the patient's recovery from anesthesia, his knee pain had subsided. He was discharged from the hospital that evening, walking without artificial aids.

Forty-eight hours later he came to my office on crutches, complaining of severe knee pain—an effusion was present. Examination of the knee confirmed marked restriction of motion because of pain and the tension caused by the effusion. The joint was aspirated without significantly decreasing his pain. Microscopic study of the fluid under polarized light revealed a plethora of intracellular crystals of both monosodium urate and calcium pyrophosphate. The knee was then irrigated with 500 ml. of saline solution, which produced immediate relief of pain, and the effusion subsequently subsided.

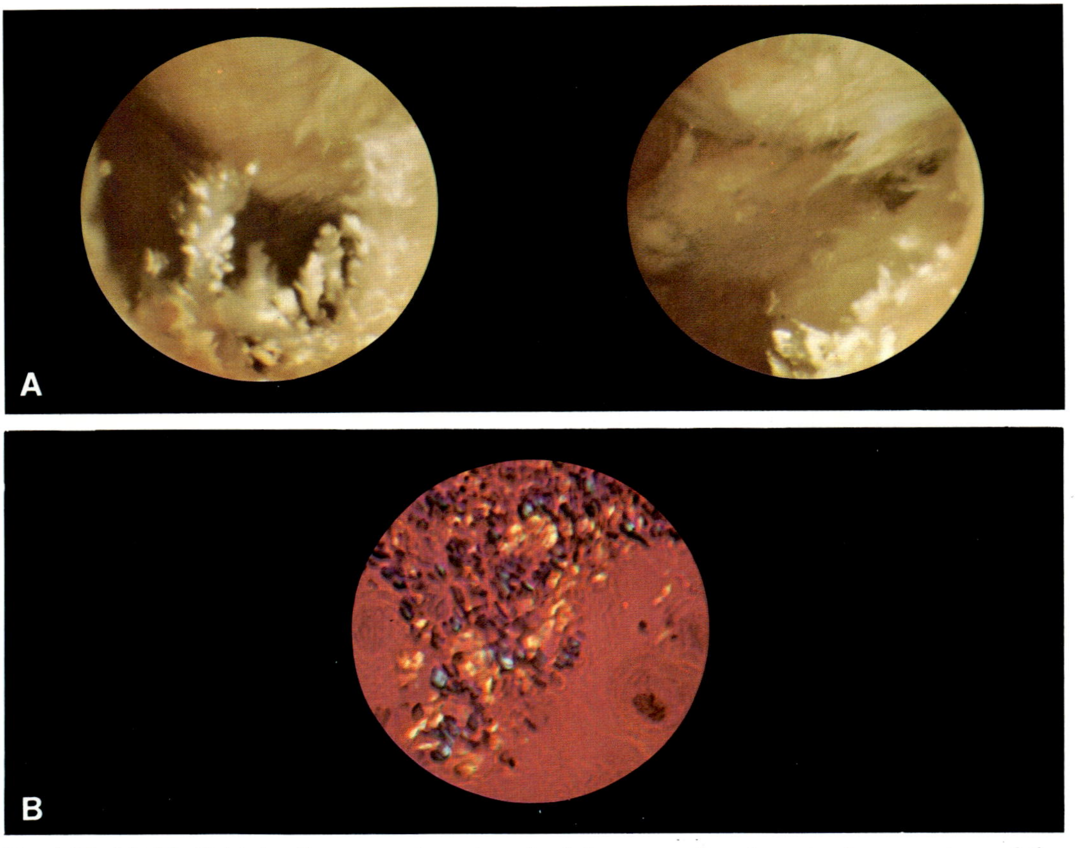

Fig. 4-15. (*A*) Medial joint line: note deposits of calcium pyrophosphate in the synovium of the intercondylar notch. Severe degeneration of the medial meniscus and the medial femoral condyle is present. (*B*) Biopsy specimen of medial meniscus under polarized light and a unit retardation crystal. These crystals are calcium pyrophosphate, and are characterized by their rhomboid configuration. Note that as the position of the crystal changes, the color changes. When light passes through the polarizer, crystal, and a unit retardation plate, the relationship of the axis of the crystal studied to the unit retardation crystal either speeds or retards the light wave, thus producing either yellow or blue light. Rotation of the specimen studied by 90 degrees will cause the color to change.

This patient's course demonstrates the many characteristics of crystal-induced synovitis:

1. The chronic crystal-induced synovitis improved rapidly with treatment by joint irrigation.

2. Bleeding into the joint is one of the initiating mechanisms of acute crystal-induced synovitis.

3. The lag phase between the initiation of the phagocytic process and the effusion started at the time of arthroscopy or shortly thereafter and resulted in a full-blown acute attack within 24 hours caused by the intra-articular bleeding at arthroscopy.

4. A marked alteration of the synovial fluid characteristics occurred with the

presence of large numbers of intracellular crystals of monosodium urate and calcium pyrophosphate.

5. Immediate relief followed irrigation of the joint.

The next case illustrates the necessity for arthroscopic examination in a patient who has continuing postoperative knee complaints.

Case 4-7. Recurrent Episodes of Crystal-Induced Synovitis

In 1968, a 45-year-old male patient complained of medial jointline pain, tenderness, and giving way. Clinical examination revealed a torn left medial meniscus, which was verified by a positive arthrogram. At the time of arthrotomy and medial meniscectomy, severe chondromalacia of the patella was noted. Five days following surgery he developed podagra of the right great toe. The serum uric acid was elevated, and the patient was treated with colchicine and probenecid, which improved or relieved his acute gouty diathesis.

One year later, because of retropatellar pain that restricted his activities, a patellectomy was performed. Three months following patellectomy, the patient presented with acute severe knee pain with marked distention of the joint. The white blood count was 10,500; sedimentation rate 43 mm. per hour, and the synovial fluid white count 50,000. Gram stain revealed no organisms, and the culture produced no growth. The serum and synovial fluid uric acid was elevated. Crystal analysis of the joint fluid was not done. His effusion responded to aspiration of the joint as well as oral colchicine, but he still had severe knee pain. Rehabilitation of the quadriceps was inhibited by the continuing pain; a brace was applied that extended from the pelvis to foot, and the patient became dependent upon it for ambulation. This sorry situation continued for approximately one year, at which time another acute flare-up occurred.

By this time, experience had been gained in treating crystal problems. In the office, the joint was irrigated with 200 ml. of saline solution, which gave immediate relief, but only for about 3 days. Several months later, arthroscopy was performed, revealing degeneration within the lateral compartment and areas of crystalline deposition in both the synovium and the lateral meniscus (Figs. 4-16, 4-17). The pain subsided after arthroscopy, and the patient was able to re-educate his quadriceps and soon discarded the brace he had worn for over a year.

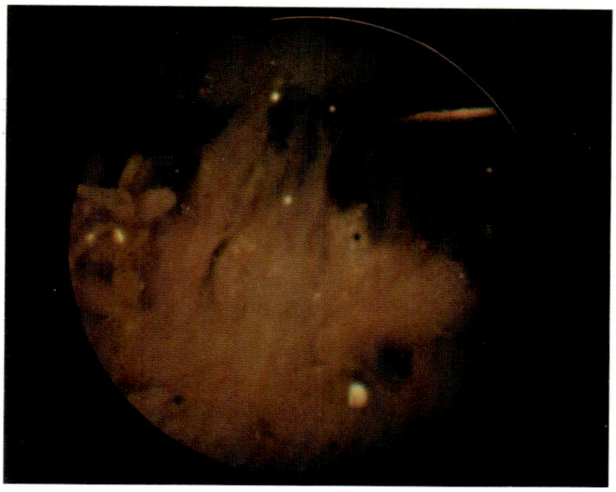

Fig. 4-16. Suprapatellar recess: note the tiny deposits of uric acid crystals in the synovium.

Case 4-8. Subacute Crystal-Induced Synovitis

The patient, a 40-year-old high school principal, had been playing tennis regularly every Sunday for 4 months. On the evening after each game his knee would begin to swell. Pain and swelling would last for the next 4 to 5

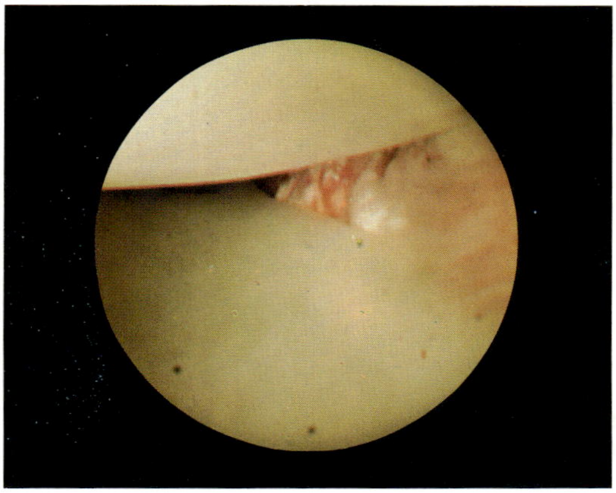

Fig. 4-17. Larger deposits of urate crystals in the synovium cover the popliteus tendon.

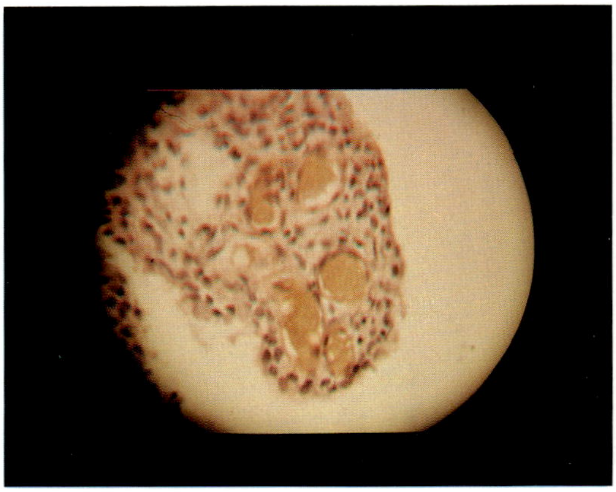

Fig. 4-18. Synovial villus with dilated veins: h and e.

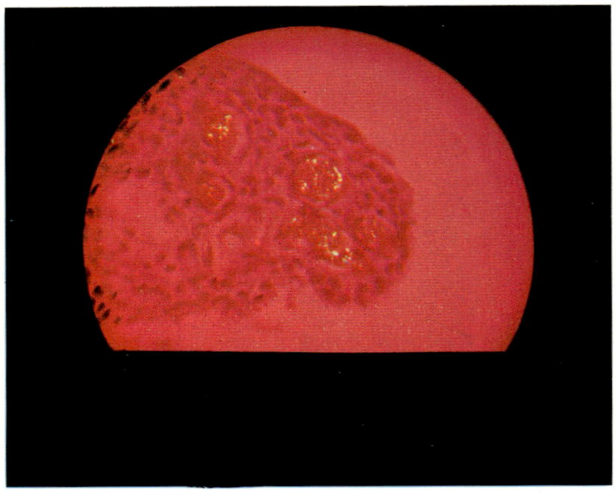

Fig. 4-20. The same villus as in Fig. 4-19, with polarized light and a unit retardation crystal.

days, showing improvement towards the end of the week. Playing tennis the following Sunday would bring on the symptoms again. Arthroscopy performed 4 months after the original episode revealed only a few crystalline deposits within the synovium. Extracellular calcium pyrophosphate crystals were identified within the synovial fluid. Synovial biopsy revealed areas of crystalline deposition within the veins of the synovium (Figs. 4-18—4-20). The patient's response to arthroscopy was gratifying, and he was able to return to playing tennis. Indeed, at last report, he was playing almost daily during the summer, up to 5 hours a day without difficulty.

Case 4-9. Atypical Chronic Crystal-Induced Synovitis

A 72-year-old female had a history of bilateral knee pain for 20 years. The pain in the left knee was more severe than that in the right. On examination, there was diffuse swelling of both knees with only a minimal amount of synovial fluid present. Aspiration of the synovial fluid revealed a crystal whose morphology

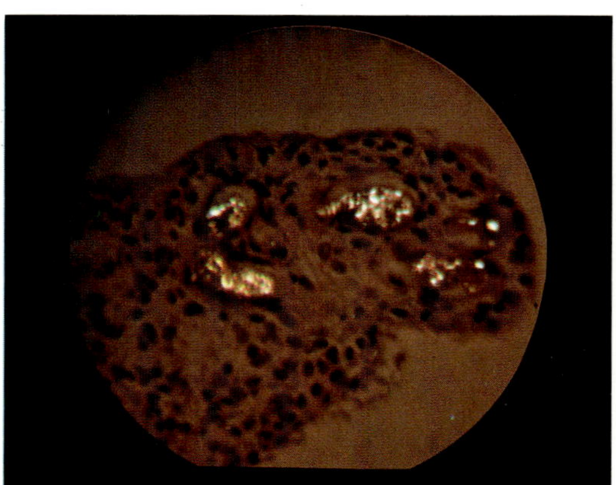

Fig. 4-19. The same villus as in Fig. 4-18, with the addition of polarized light.

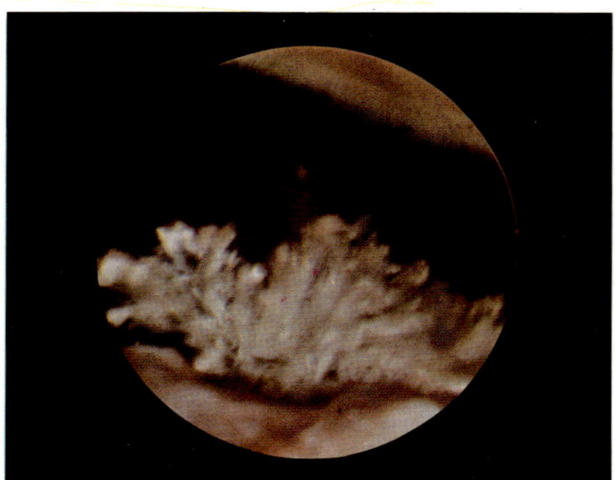

Fig. 4-21. The synovium is completely studded with crystalline deposits thought to be hydroxyapatite. Note the eburnation of the patella.

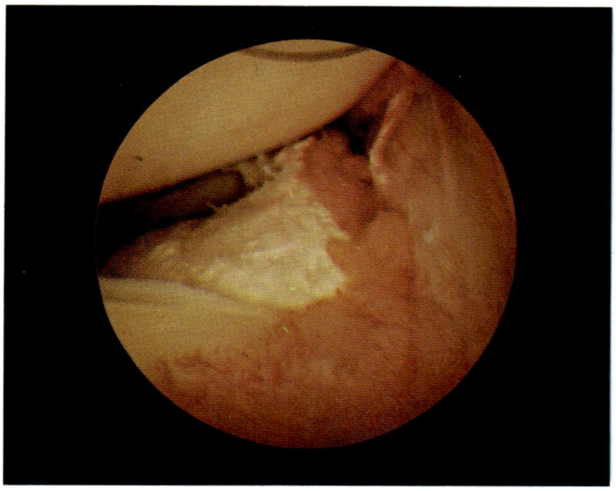

Fig. 4-22. Lateral joint line demonstrating chalky deposits of calcium pyrophosphate in the synovium, lateral tibial cartilage, and posterior lateral meniscus.

could not be determined. Roentgenograms revealed moderately severe genu varum with generalized joint degeneration. Arthroscopy revealed marked evidence of crystalline infiltration of the synovium (Fig. 4-21) as well as the hyaline cartilage of the patella, femoral condyles, and tibia. The menisci were torn, and in areas of fragmented articular cartilage and fibrocartilage large crystalline deposits were present. The serum uric acid level was normal, but the serum and synovial fluid calcium level was elevated. This woman responded to irrigation of her joint, and has had no further pain within her knee. In spite of the severe degenerative changes, she has not required repeat arthroscopy for over a 3-year period. She was seen on one occasion, 2 years following arthroscopy, complaining of pain in the contralateral knee and in the ankle, which responded to anti-inflammatory agents.

Case 4-10. Intra-Articular Surgery in the Presence of Crystal-Induced Disease

A 32-year-old fireman was participating in a physical fitness program and twisted his knee while arising from a squatting position. He was off work for several months with a subsequent effusion of the knee that did not yield to conservative measures. Roentgenograms revealed extensive crystalline deposition of the femoral condyle, tibia, and menisci (Fig. 4-22). An arthrogram was obtained, which was felt to be equivocally positive, demonstrating a tear of the medial meniscus. Arthroscopy was then performed, establishing the diagnosis of a displaced bucket-handle tear of the medial meniscus. He was treated by arthrotomy and excision of the inner rim of the meniscus. His postoperative course was uneventful, with the exception of a continuous effusion of the knee that necessitated weekly aspiration for a 2-month period. Polarized-light microscopy revealed rare intracellular crystals but abundant extracellular crystals of calcium pyrophosphate.

Two months after the operation, the joint was again aspirated and irrigated with 2,000 ml. of saline solution. The effusion cleared dramatically, and the patient was able to return to work shortly thereafter. Again, surgical trauma was thought to be responsible for the continuing effusion. The cycle was interrupted by joint lavage.

Case 4-11. Decrease of Crystal Population by Irrigation of a Joint

A young man of 18 was injured while playing basketball. For several months he complained of pain over the lateral aspect of his knee, and an effusion was present. An arthrogram failed to reveal a tear of the lateral meniscus, but this diagnosis was made clinically. Arthroscopy revealed a tear of the lateral meniscus as well as degeneration of the lateral femoral condyle. Of greater interest, however, was a relatively opaque yellow crystalline deposit within the synovium overlying the anterior cruciate ligament, and scattered deposits within the villi of the suprapateller recess. These deposits were photographed. The effusion decreased quickly, and the patient redeveloped his quadriceps and returned to competitive basketball. Because of repeated giving way of the knee, however, arthroscopy was performed again a year later. At this time no evidence of crystalline deposition could be seen within the joint. He was treated by surgical excision of the meniscus, and had no further episodes of effusion. Unfortunately the synovium was not biopsied. The serum urate level was found to be elevated after surgery.

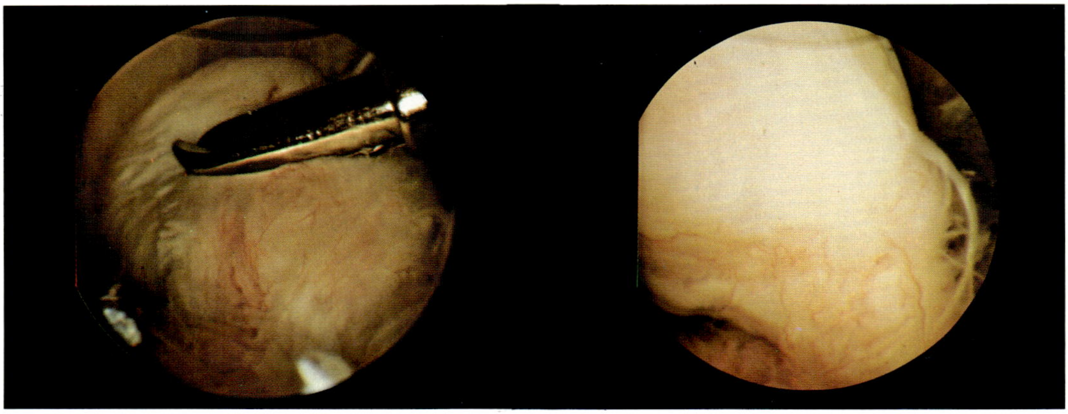

Fig. 4-23. (*Right*) Nodular mass rising from the floor of the quadriceps bursa. (*Left*) Top of the mass, with 5 mm. meniscal scissor to demonstrate relative size.

PIGMENTED VILLONODULAR SYNOVITIS

I have not encountered any cases of generalized pigmented villonodular synovitis arthroscopically, but I have seen this condition in localized form in 4 patients. In one patient, a small brownish mass arising from the fat pad at arthrotomy was noted and excised. Localized pigmented villonodular synovitis may simulate a loose body.

Case 4-12. Localized Pigmented Villonodular Synovitis

A 45-year-old male complained of a locking sensation along the medial patellar border during flexion and extension. Roentgenograms failed to reveal an osteochondral loose body. Arthroscopy demonstrated a pedunculated soft tissue mass arising from the floor of the suprapatellar pouch that interfered with patellar motion (Fig. 4-23). The lesion was excised with biopsy scissors, relieving the locking symptoms. Histological examination demonstrated numerous giant cells and hemosiderin-stained matrix (Fig. 4-24).

An unusual location for localized pigmented villonodular synovitis is at the joint line. In one patient the "buckling," rather than being caused by a meniscal tear, was due to a small nodular mass arising from the lateral capsule and protruding

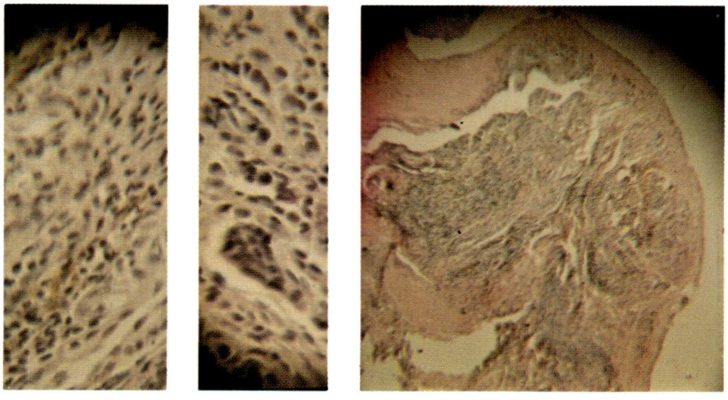

Fig. 4-24. Histologic section demonstrating nodular mass. The mass is surrounded by abundant stroma, multinucleated giant cells, and hemosiderin.

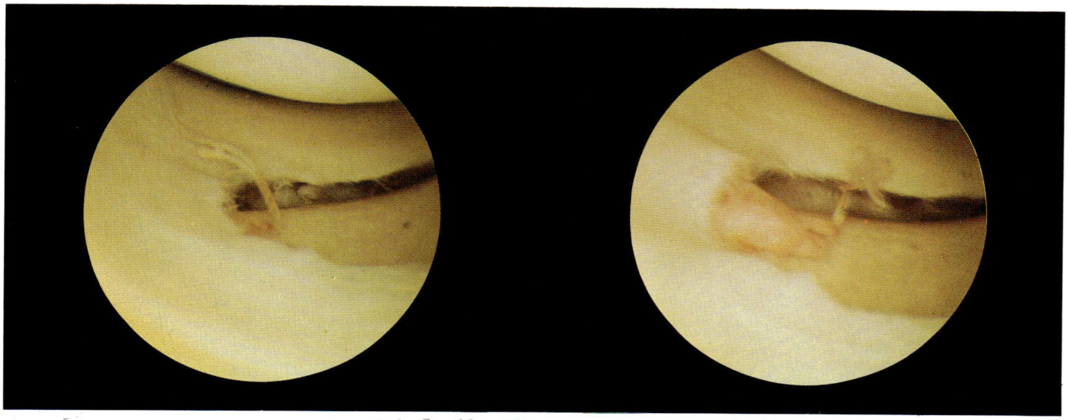

Fig. 4-25. Mass beneath lateral meniscus in various positions of tibial rotation. The "antennae" seem to be a feature of localized pigmented villonodular synovitis, as we have seen it on one other occasion.

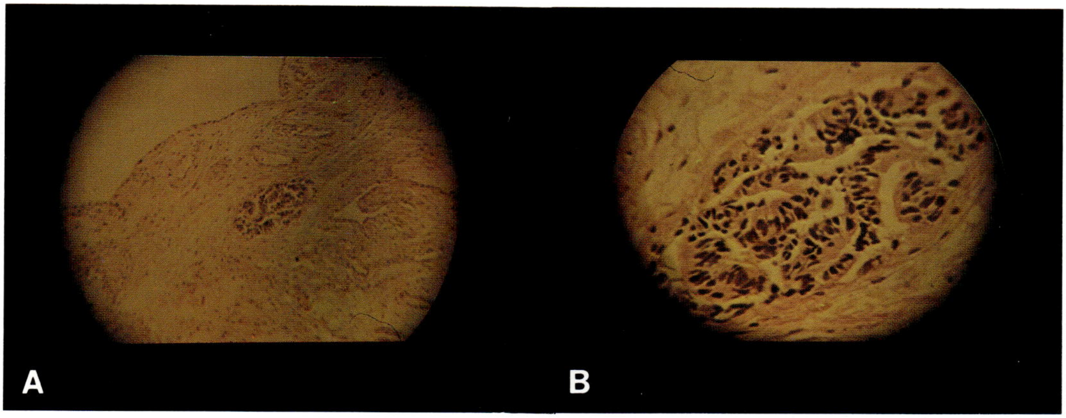

Fig. 4-26. (*A*) A nest of tumor cells beneath the synovial lining. (*B*) Magnification of this nest allows the diagnosis of its colonic origin.

centrally beneath the lateral meniscus (Fig. 4-25). Histologic examination of the arthroscopically excised specimen was interpreted as pigmented villonodular synovitis.

METASTASES INVOLVING SYNOVIUM

Obscure causes of synovitis have been discovered by arthroscopy and synovial biopsy. A 59-year-old woman, with a history of adenocarcinoma of the colon 5 years prior, developed an insidious right-knee pain associated with a 10-degree flexion contracture and a marked synovitis. The significant work-up was a tomogram of the femur, which demonstrated a cystic lesion of the femoral condyle. Arthroscopy provided the diagnosis by allowing direct biopsy of the altered synovium. The carcinoma had invaded the femoral cortex (Fig. 4-26).

REFERENCES

1. McCarty, D. J. Jr. and Gatter, R. A.: Pseudogout syndrome (articular chondromatosis). Bull. Rheum. Dis., *14:* 331, 1964.
2. McCarty, D. J. Jr. and Hogan, J. M.: Inflammatory reaction after intrasynovial infection of microcrystalline and adrenocorticosteroid esters. Arthritis Rheum., *7:* 359, 1964.
3. McCarty, D. J. Jr. and Hollander, J. L.: Identification of urate crystals in gouty synovial fluid. Ann. Int. Med., *54:* 452, 1961.
4. Mann, T. S.: Acute calcific synovitis of the knee. J. Bone Joint Surg., *48B:* 56, 1966.
5. Murphy, F. P., Dahlin, D. C., and Sullivan, C. R.: Articular synovial chondromatosis. J. Bone Joint Surg., *44A:* 77, 1962.
6. O'Connor, R. L.: The arthroscope in the management of crystal induced synovitis of the knee. J. Bone Joint Surg., *55A:* 1443, 1973.
7. Takeda, S.: On the relationship between arthroscopic findings and histological changes of the synovial membrane. J. Jap. Orthop. Assoc., *34:* 373, 1960.

5 *Meniscal Tears*

The diagnosis of meniscal tears by arthrography has been difficult, but with careful technique and application, arthrography can complement arthroscopy in many cases. The technique for obtaining high-quality double contrast arthrograms is well established; unfortunately, the expertise demonstrated by some arthrographers in obtaining consistently high-quality arthrograms has not been universally duplicated. Since the posterior third of the medial meniscus is partially sheltered by the over-hanging medial femoral condyle, discovery of peripheral marginal tears, inferior splits, or tears within the body of the meniscus—when suspected by arthroscopic observation of deviant meniscal motion—may be confirmed by arthrography. However, arthrography is less reliable for detecting tears of the posterior third of the lateral meniscus. (This, and the fact that tears in this area are often clinically silent, certainly *more* silent than tears in the medial meniscus, may be responsible for the statistical prevalence of medial tears over lateral ones.) The combination of both these modalities in appropriate cases should increase the degree of diagnostic certitude.[1] When performing arthroscopy for meniscal tears, the questions one should ask are:

1. Is the tear significant in that it causes mechanical obstruction to motion?
2. Is it a degenerative tear not requiring surgical excision?
3. Is it a tear that can be removed under arthroscopic visualization through a small ancillary half-inch stab wound?

APPEARANCE OF THE MEDIAL MENISCUS

The Normal Meniscus

The medial meniscus viewed from the lateral infrapatellar approach demonstrates the superior surface of the medial meniscus, covered anteriorly by the fat pad. As the arthroscope passes posteriorly between the medial femoral condyle and medial meniscus, a valgus stress is applied to the leg and external rotation of the foot allows passage of the arthroscope between the medial tibial tubercular eminence and the medial femoral condyle. The leg is gradually extended and the inner edge of the meniscus appears beneath the medial femoral condyle. Since the peripheral portion of the posterior third of the medial meniscus is sometimes hidden from view by the overhanging medial femoral condyle, the

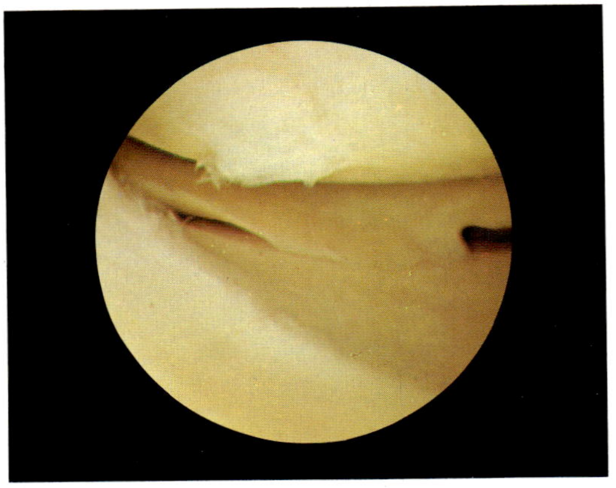

Fig. 5-1. Reversal of the concave inner meniscal border. If an arthrogram has not been obtained, this area should be investigated with a small-diameter arthroscope passed superior or inferior to the meniscus.

amount of meniscus that protrudes is variable; but normally, in spite of the amount of valgus and external rotation of the tibia, the inner edge retains a suggestion of a concave or straight border. However, the total surface area of the meniscus edge varies, the greatest amount being seen in the adolescent with hyperextensible knees.

Deviant Meniscal Patterns

When the inner-edge assumes a convex configuration, pathology within the meniscus or deep capsular ligament is usually present. There are several deviant meniscal patterns that I have found associated with the tears of the posterior third of the medial meniscus:

Protrusion of the meniscus beneath the medial femoral condyle, causing a reversal of its concave border to a convex one,[6] is by far the most common pattern observed.* The actual tear may not be seen, as it may lie deep within the substance of the meniscus or may be an actual separation of the meniscus from the deep capsular ligament, a tear of the superior or inferior meniscal surface, or a tear of the deep capsular ligament above or below the joint line. Only rarely have I noted this arthroscopic finding associated with the clinical symptoms of locking of the knee. Usually, the patient's complaints consist of giving way and tenderness to palpation of the posterior medial corner. This pattern is frequently seen in lax hyperextensible knees follow-

* Jackson, R. W.: Personal communication, 1973.

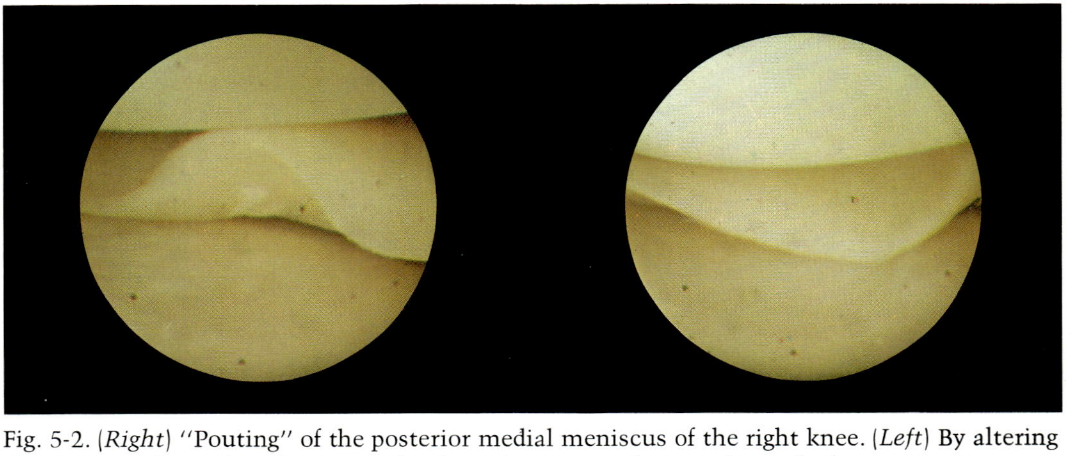

Fig. 5-2. (*Right*) "Pouting" of the posterior medial meniscus of the right knee. (*Left*) By altering the amount of rotation, flexion, and valgus the tear can be seen beneath the meniscus.

ing a valgus injury associated with mild capsular laxity and a negative arthrogram or associated with a parameniscal tear and an arthrogram showing contrast material between the capsule and the body of the meniscus. One also sees this pattern in the degeneration of the posterior third of the meniscus, when still confined to the interior of the meniscus, not having broken through to the surface. At arthrotomy, the defect in the parameniscal tissue can be palpated with a nerve hook, and with minimal dissection of the posterior medial corner the meniscus shifts beneath the medial femoral condyle and into the intercondylar notch. To increase the certitude of diagnosis in this region, the arthrogram is important (Figs. 5-1, and 5-2).

Ninety-degree rotation of the inner edge of the meniscus is another common abnormality (Fig. 5-3). This arthroscopic finding is associated clinically with complaints of locking of the knee and is caused by a small longitudinal tear confined to the posterior third of the meniscus. The tear occasionally may be identified by the combined maneuver of external rotation of the leg and a valgus stress applied to the knee. If a tear is not seen, external rotation will displace the inner edge of the meniscus, rolling it beneath the medial femoral condyle and wrapping it around its lateral surface. Again the actual tear may not be seen—just the abnormal behavior of the meniscus.

Acute angulation of the inner edge of the medial meniscus is still another common pattern (Fig. 5-4). A tear of the posterior third of the periphery of the medial meniscus is seen when external tibial rotation and valgus stress is applied, causing the acute angulation. Clinically, this is associated with locking of the knee, and when this lesion is found, the tear will be demonstrated in the specimen. On occasion, when the arthroscope can be maneuvered behind the medial femoral condyle, the capsular portion of the tear may be seen. This tear, as previously mentioned, is rarely demonstrated

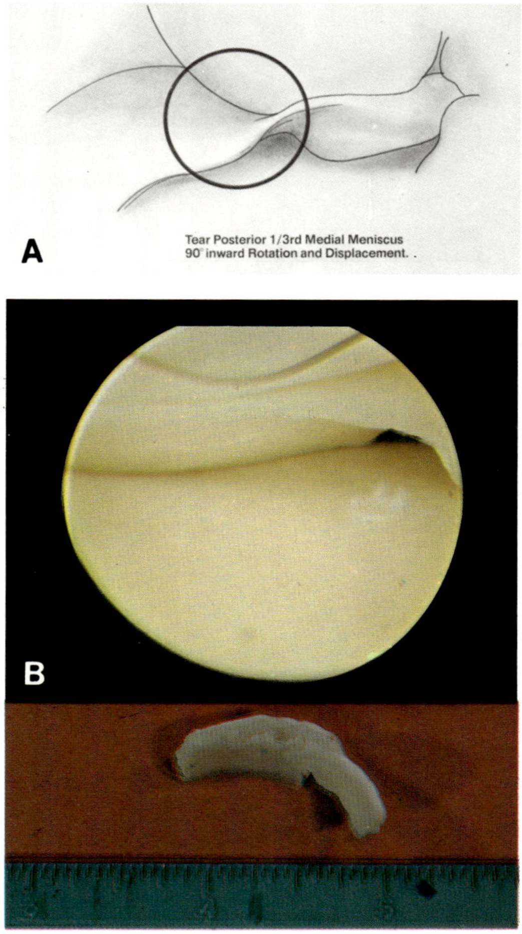

Fig. 5-3. (*A*) Diagrammatic demonstration of the meniscal dynamics in a left knee. (*B*) The same situation seen arthroscopically. (*Top*) Posterior medial meniscus of the right knee. An indirectly pathognomonic sign of a peripheral tear of the posterior medial meniscus is obtained by externally rotating the tibia and applying a moderate valgus stress. The inner edge rotates 90 degrees, hugging the medial femoral condyle. The inner meniscal fragment is actually separated towards the intercondylar notch by the rotation of the medial femoral condyle. (*Bottom*) Excised meniscus demonstrating tear through peripheral segment of the meniscus.

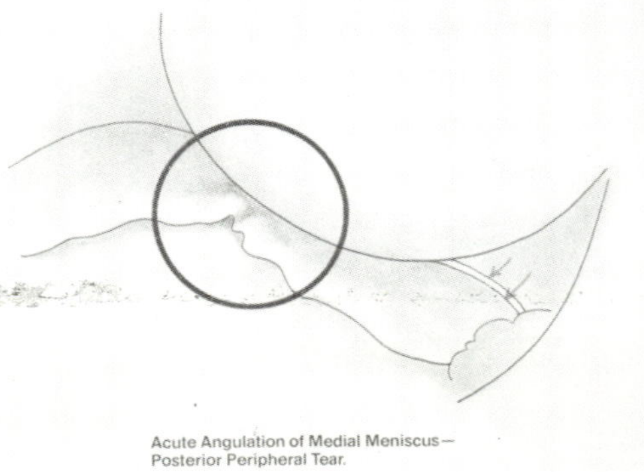

Fig. 5-4. Medial meniscus of the left knee. Another indirect sign indicative of a tear of the periphery of the medial meniscus is demonstrated schematically: acute angulation of the inner edge of the medial meniscus. A small-diameter arthroscope passed beneath the medial femoral condyle demonstrates this tear.

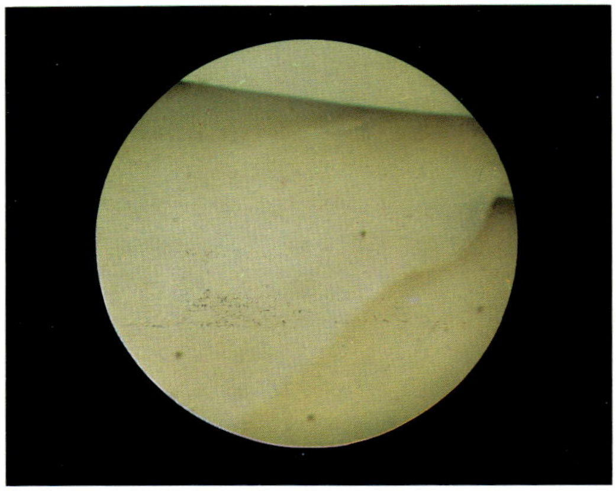

Fig. 5-5. Medial meniscus of the left knee. A faint line is perceived just beneath the medial femoral condyle. The medial femoral condyle covers the remaining extent of the tear.

by the arthroscope, but the abnormal behavior of the meniscus is almost pathognomonic of the tear. Recently, some investigators have observed[3]* the superior surface of the meniscus posterior to the medial collateral ligament with the use of a small-diameter arthroscope. This technique certainly has importance in locating, with the highest possible degree of certitude, tears of this region. The inferior surface of the meniscus is made visible by insertion of a smaller arthroscope between the tibia and the meniscus. Unfortunately, with the use of the smaller arthroscope, orientation may be confusing and the magnification factors may cause distortion and, in turn, improper and incorrect interpretation.

The vertical split in the direction of the long axis of the body of the meniscus is another common meniscal rupture seen in the posterior third of the medial meniscus. At times it does extend far enough anteriorly so that the edge of the tear can be seen beneath the medial femoral condyle (Fig. 5-5). Significantly, this lesion is so situated that abnormal behavior may not occur with associated valgus stress and external rotation. This tear is associated with locking episodes. If the rupture is situated midway between the peripheral margin and the inner edge of the posterior third of the meniscus, the tear is easily seen beneath the normally obstructive medial femoral condyle.

Bucket Handle Tear. The most common tear in the adolescent and the young adult is the displaced bucket handle tear, which results from an anterior extension of the previously mentioned tears (Fig. 5-6). When the meniscal tear is displaced, there is little difficulty in diagnosis. However, when the meniscus is returned to its proper location (i.e., reduced beneath the medial femoral condyle) the actual rupture may not be seen. One may see only a ragged line in the superior surface of the meniscus.

A fracture of the inner rim may result from the prolonged dislocation of the inner rim of the bucket handle tear (Fig. 5-7). When this occurs posteriorly, the junction between the posterior and middle two-thirds of the posterior frag-

* Watanabe, M.: Personal communication, 1972.

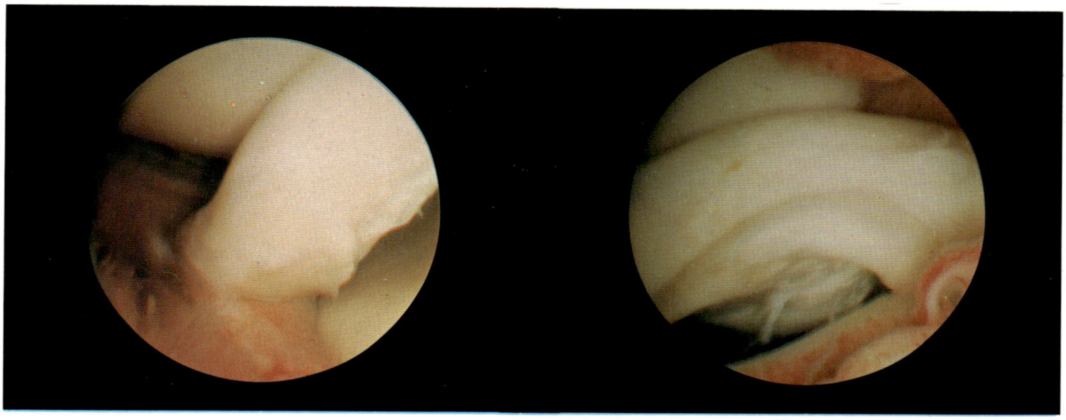

Fig. 5-6. Medial meniscus of the left knee: lateral infrapatellar approach. Displaced bucket handle tear of medial meniscus. (*Left*) The anterior attachment of the displaced inner rim. (*Right*) The main body of the displaced fragment disappearing between the medial femoral condyle and the medial tibial spine.

ment remains dislocated and becomes rounded, appearing as a globular mass. The anterior fragment may rotate 90 degrees, and the anterior attachment can extend into the suprapatellar region and lie along the medial femoral condyle in the medial gutter. This situation definitely interferes with tibial rotation, because of the displaced posterior third of the meniscus. Tenderness to palpation is noted over the anterior fragment along its course superiorly. Clinically, this tear could not be ascertained with any degree of certitude preoperatively, and the arthrogram has been nondiagnostic in several of these cases. This type of tear has been removed under arthroscopic control.

Case 5-1. Displaced Anterior Fragment of the Medial Meniscus

A 21-year-old male who for several years complained of giving way of his knee, medial joint line tenderness, and discomfort had an arthrogram one year prior to arthroscopy, which was positive for both medial and lateral meniscal tears. At arthroscopy no tear was seen in the lateral meniscus, but in the medial compartment a large displaced anterior fragment of the medial meniscus rotated 90 degrees to the long axis of the meniscus; the posterior remnant remained displaced between the medial tibial tubercular eminence and the medial femoral condyle. Under direct arthroscopic visualization, these fragments were severed with scissors and removed from the joint (Fig. 5-8A,B). The postoperative course was uncomplicated, and the patient has returned to full activities.

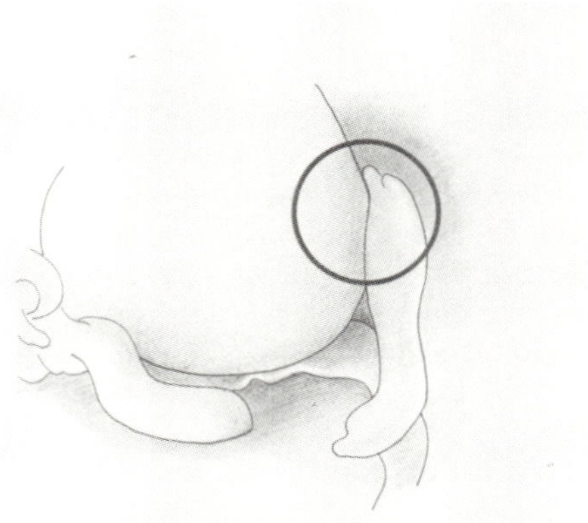

Fig. 5-7. Right knee: drawing demonstrating a rupture of the displaced inner rim of the bucket handle tear of the medial meniscus. The anterior fragment rotates 90 degrees to its long axis, and lies in the medial gutter.

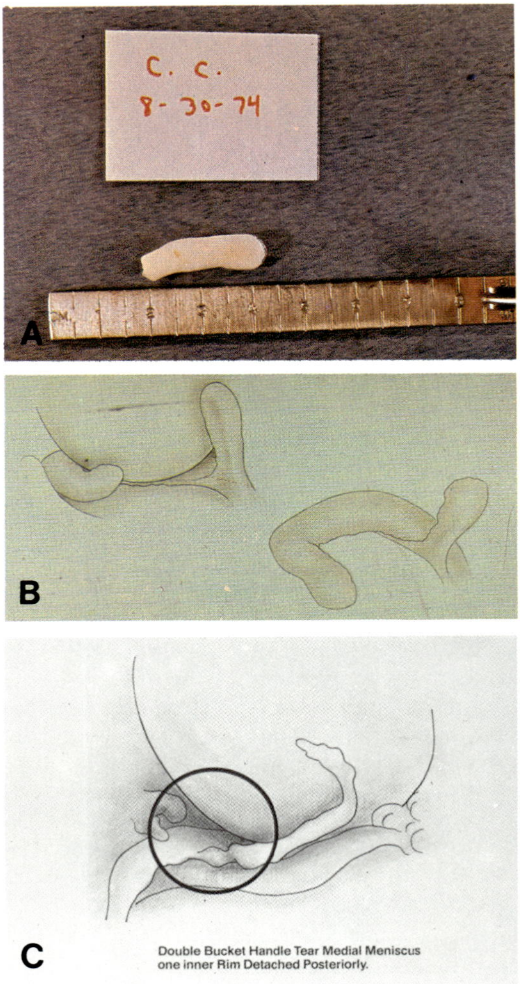

Fig. 5-8. (*A*) Anterior fragment of torn displaced bucket handle tear of medial meniscus. Specimen measures 2.4 cm. Note the rounding of the free tip. (*B*) Arthroscopic impression of the specimen prior to surgical excision. (*C*) Arthroscopic impression of 2 displaced fragments, one of which is detached from its posterior attachment.

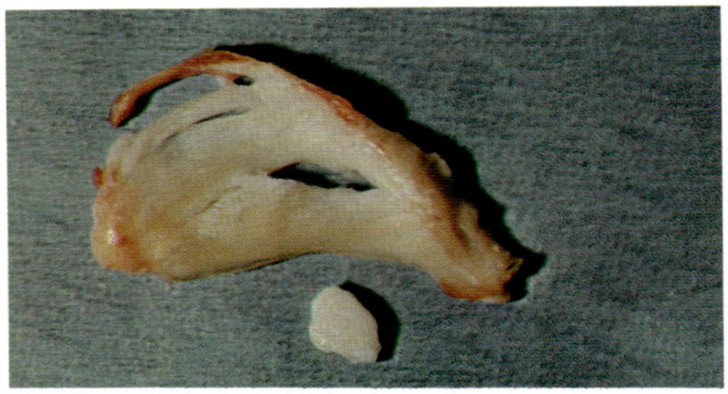

Fig. 5-9. Specimen of right medial meniscus. The patient's history included multiple episodes of giving way and locking. As the peripheral rim was not stable, the entire meniscus was excised.

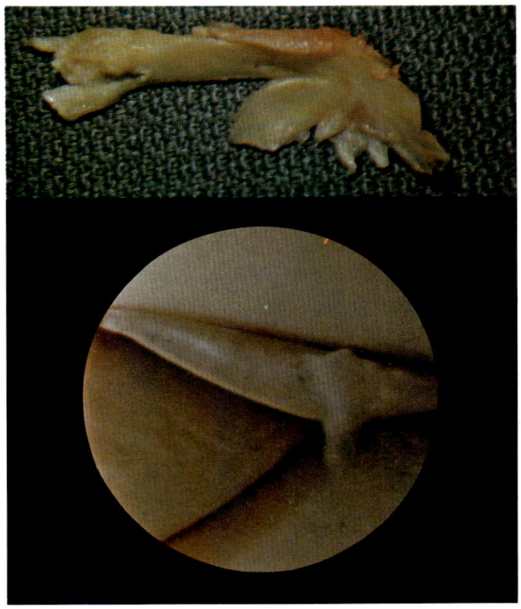

Fig. 5-10. Medial meniscus of the left knee. (*Bottom*) A large flap of medial meniscus is horizontally torn from the posterior third of the medial meniscus and rotated anteriorly to lie superior to the meniscus. (*Top*) Specimen demonstrating the superior surface of the medial meniscus.

Another variety of tear that has been observed is a double displaced bucket handle tear with one of the displaced inner rims separated posteriorly (Fig. 5-8C). This has been treated by excision of both inner rims. The classical objection to surgical excision of the displaced bucket handle tear is that this may result in incomplete removal of the torn meniscus,[5] and that further locking may also result. The clinical history and the arthroscopic appearance of the tear together should provide enough information when

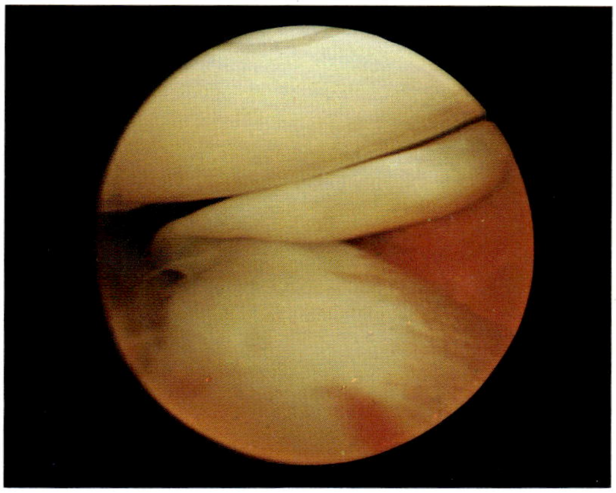

Fig. 5-11. Medial meniscus of the right knee: medial infrapatellar approach. A horizontal cleavage tear is rotated to lie between the medial femoral condyle and the main body of the medial meniscus.

more than an inner rim excision is necessary.

Case 5-2. Multiple Longitudinal Tears of the Medial Meniscus

A 32-year-old male gave a history of 8 years of giving way and locking of his right knee. He had undergone a meniscectomy of his left knee 10 years previously. The patient sought medical help because the locking was becoming more frequent. An arthrogram confirmed the presence of a tear of the posterior medial meniscus, but the periphery appeared to be abnormal as well, since there was some question whether another fragment was present. Excision of the entire meniscus was carried out (Fig. 5-9).

If, after removal of the displaced inner meniscal rim arthroscopically or at arthrotomy, a doubt exists whether another tear remains posteriorly, the arthroscope should be reinserted into the joint for further examination. On one occasion when this procedure was carried out, reexamination revealed a flap of meniscus remaining posteriorly, which was then easily removed under arthroscopic control with a rongeur.

Horizontal Cleavage Tears. The arthroscope is very reliable in demonstrating horizontal cleavage tears, especially when the tear has reached the surface of the meniscus and has rotated as a flap. This tear is not associated with clinical locking, as would be anticipated when one visualizes the large size of the displaced fragment. Symptoms associated with a horizontal cleavage tear, as described by Smillie,[5] include severe medial joint line pain and a complaint that the patient is unable to obtain comfort in bed at night and frequently needs to place a small pillow between his knees. Episodes of buckling of the knee are common in this type of tear. Smillie's observation of a palpable mass seen at the joint line has occurred infrequently in my experience.

Case 5-3. Displaced Meniscal Fragment After Twisting Injury

A 38-year-old male suffered a twisting injury of his knee at work and complained of medial joint line pain and tenderness beneath the medial collateral ligament superior to the joint line. An effusion was present and was aspirated. Because of persistent tenderness beneath the medial collateral ligament, the area was injected with lidocaine, which gave relief. The patient had no further difficulties for 18 months, but then presented with medial joint line pain. This time he did not respond to lidocaine injections of the region, and an arthrogram of poor technical quality failed to reveal the presence of a meniscal tear. Arthroscopy was performed, which showed a large displaced fragment of the medial meniscus rotated anteriorly (Fig. 5-10).

The meniscal flap may arise from either the superior (Fig. 5-11) or inferior (Fig. 5-12) surface. Arising from the inferior surface, it may be displaced between the meniscus and medial tibial plateau. The prominent symptom with this type of tear is medial joint line pain. Such displaced flap tears have been removed under arthroscopic control with scissors.

Hypermobile Anterior Medial Meniscus. This debatable clinical entity does

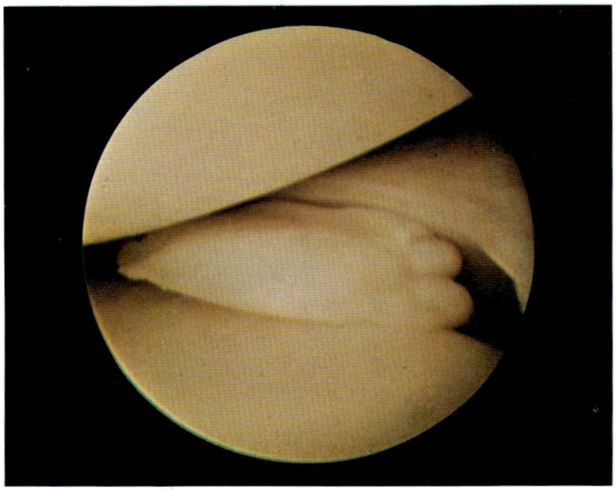

Fig. 5-12. Medial meniscus of the right knee: lateral infrapatellar approach. A horizontal cleavage tear of the medial meniscus is displaced anteriorly to lie between the medial meniscus and the medial tibial plateau. Note the rounding of the torn surface (Figs. 5-10, 11, and 12).

exist and can be observed arthroscopically. It may well represent a partial detachment of the anterior insertion of the medial meniscus, as claimed by Helfet.[2] The anterior portion of the medial meniscus may seem to be displaced peripherally off the medial tibial plateau with internal rotation of the tibia. It is repositioned with external rotation. Normally, such hypermobility of the meniscus does not occur. Occasionally, this is associated with some scuffing of the underlying articular cartilage of the tibia.

Case 5-4. Meniscal Subluxation and Cartilaginous Degeneration

A 29-year-old male gave a history of 18 years of difficulty with his knee. The symptoms were produced by such activities as mountain climbing and tennis. He had been examined by many consultants and had several arthrograms that failed to reveal any evidence of meniscal pathology. There was persistent tenderness to palpation over the medial joint line anterior to the medial collateral ligament. Arthroscopy revealed subluxuation of the meniscus off the head of the tibia in internal rotation (Fig. 5-13). There was also a mild degree of cartilaginous degeneration of the overlying medial femoral condyle and the tibial plateau, with fraying of a portion of the meniscus.

It is well recognized that meniscal tears produce degeneration of the overlying articular cartilage of both the tibia and femur. The apparent sequence is first the loss of ground substance, then subsequent

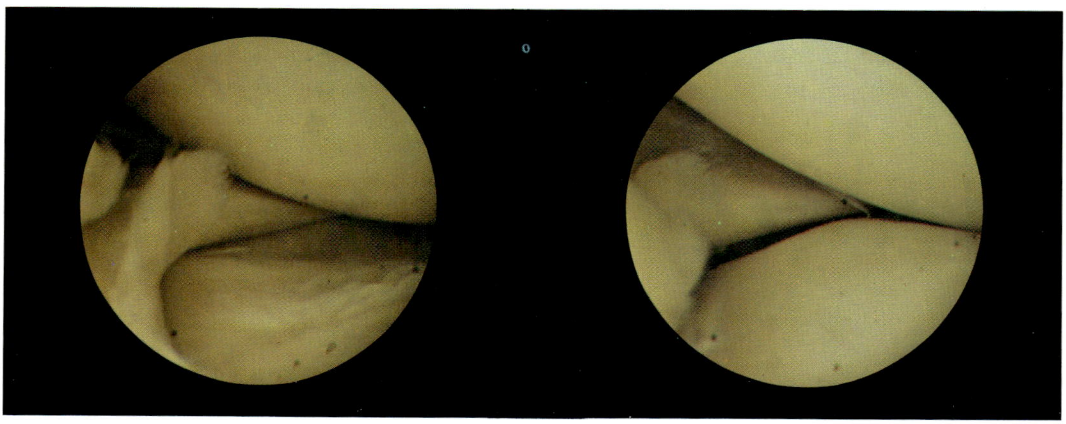

Fig. 5-13. Medial meniscus of the left knee. (*Left*) Anterior medial meniscus with tibia in neutral rotation. (*Right*) Anterior medial meniscus with tibia in internal rotation, subluxing off the medial tibial plateau.

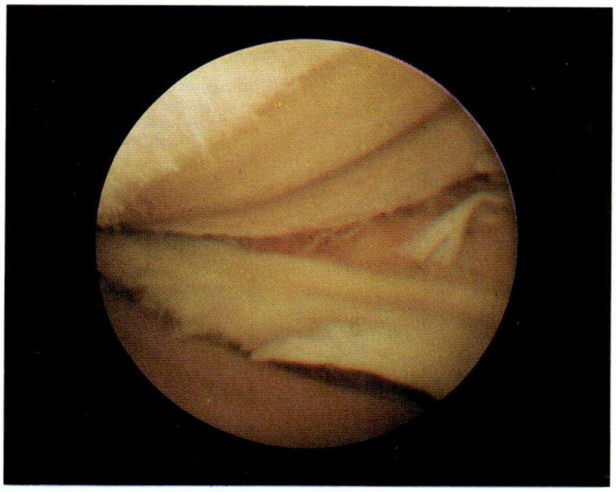

Fig. 5-14. Right knee: degenerative tear of medial meniscus with severe articular cartilage changes. Note the "sled runner" defect in the medial femoral condyle with complete eburnation of the medial femoral condyle and the medial tibial plateau.

fibrillation and fragmentation, and eventually eburnation. In many degenerative knees, the defect corresponds amazingly well with the site of the meniscal tear and may include a cartilaginous lesion in both the femoral condyle and tibial plateau in the vicinity of the tear. The meniscus in the degenerative knee may cause indentation on the medial femoral condyle that looks much like that caused by a sled runner (Fig. 5-14).

APPEARANCE OF THE LATERAL MENISCUS

Problems in the Observation of Lateral Meniscal Tears

Arthroscopy has been found to be of much greater value in the lateral compartment than the medial because of the anatomic configuration of the compartment, particularly the laxity of the lateral ligaments. The lateral femoral condyle does not provide the meniscal cover that the medial condyle does. The posterior third of the meniscus (i.e., the portion between the popliteus tendon at the posterior lateral corner and the posterior tibial attachment) can be viewed almost entirely on the superior and inferior surfaces (see Fig. 2-19). The middle third of the meniscus can only be viewed on the superior surface, and the anterior third is obscured by the overhanging fat pad and may require an ancillary medial infrapa-

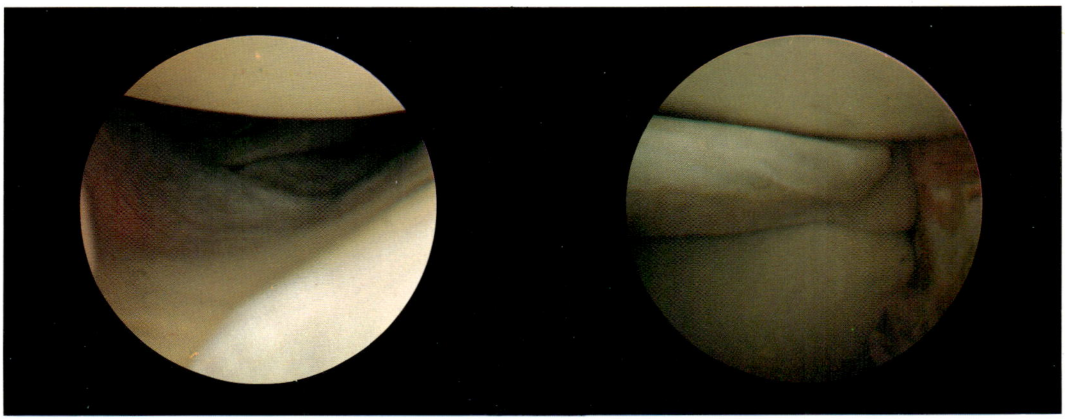

Fig. 5-15. Lateral infrapatellar approach to the right knee: displaced bucket handle tear of lateral meniscus. (*Left*) Lateral attachment of displaced fragment. The rounded peripheral rim over the popliteus tendon can be seen in the background. (*Right*) Displaced fragment and posterior attachment.

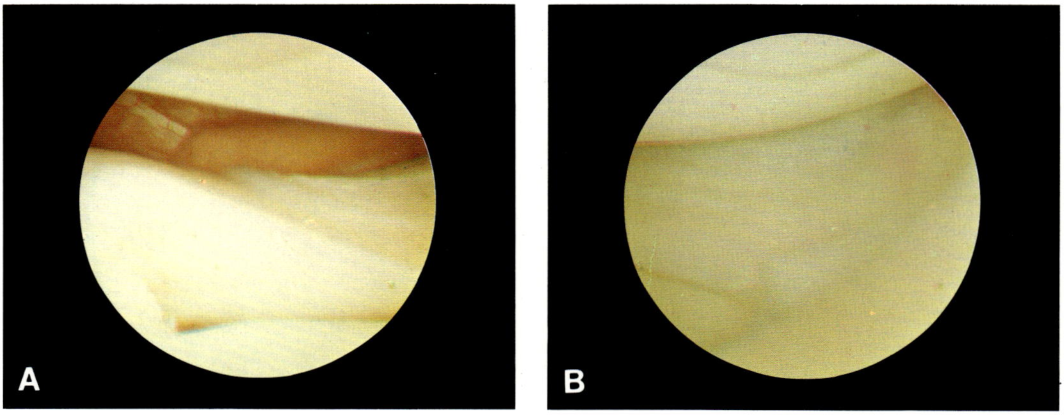

Fig. 5-16. Left knee, lateral infrapatellar approach. Tear confined to posterior third of lateral meniscus, extending from the posterior tibial attachment (*A*) to the popliteus tendon (*B*).

tellar approach to reveal its peripheral portion. Displaced bucket handle tears of the lateral meniscus are not infrequently seen, and most often the area of tear extends no further anteriorly than the vicinity of the popliteus tendon (Fig. 5-15). When displaced, these tears are very tight and may not release spontaneously, even during arthroscopy.

The undisplaced tears noted on the superior surface of the posterior third of the lateral meniscus are easily visualized, but may appear only as a straight line, the depth of which is not always apparent. An additional instrument may be introduced into the joint to probe the depth of the tear.

Case 5-5. Arthroscopic Confirmation of a Lateral Meniscal Tear

A 16-year-old female complained of locking of her knee after sitting Indian fashion. An arthrogram did not confirm the suspected lateral meniscal tear. Prior to arthroscopy, she was able to lock and unlock her knee in the presence of the author. At arthroscopy a tear was seen, limited to the posterior third of the lateral meniscus (Fig. 5-16).

Often, however, with internal rotation of the tibia and a varus stress, the inner segment of the tear of the posterior third of the lateral meniscus protrudes slightly into the center of the joint. Occasionally vertical tears of the meniscus, starting in the vicinity of the periphery, but not extending into its superior surface, may be detected inferiorly.

Case 5-6. Partial Observation of a Lateral Meniscal Tear

A 32-year-old female complained of locking of her knee intermittently for 16 years. At

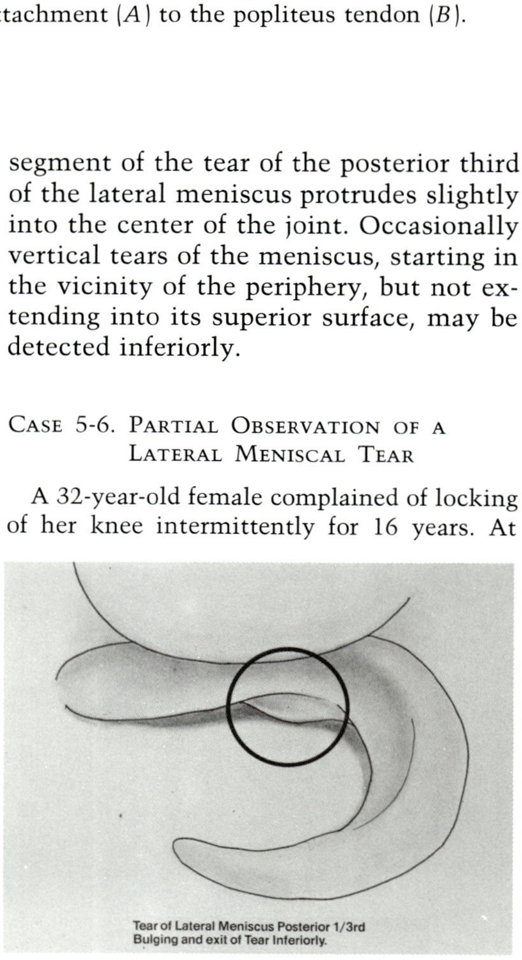

Fig. 5-17. Left knee: lateral infrapatellar approach. Tear of the lateral meniscus with bulging of the posterior third. The tear exits inferiorly.

arthroscopy a tear was noted inferiorly in the posterior third of the meniscus. The superior edge of the rupture was not seen, but varus stress and internal rotation caused protrusion of the posterior superior portion of the meniscus into the joint (Fig. 5-17).

Tears of the Middle Segment of the Lateral Meniscus

Unlike the medial side of the joint, the middle segment of the lateral meniscus is frequently the site of a meniscal tear that may occur as a simple transverse tear. This may extend posteriorly, resulting in a defect in the middle third of the meniscus. Examination of such a specimen erroneously suggests that the tear is in the anterior third. At arthroscopy it can easily be seen that this tear is in the middle third. The meniscus is normally under tension, and after it is severed from the peripheral attachment it contracts considerably so that the specimen then suggests that the tear is confined to the anterior third. I believe that this tear occurs as an innocuous-appearing transverse split; when the specimen is examined, it appears that it is an iatrogenic tear. This tear may cause lateral joint line pain and may be associated with persistent effusion.

Case 5-7. Transverse Tear of the Middle Third of the Lateral Meniscus

A 32-year-old draftsman incurred a twisting injury of his right knee. This was followed by an effusion that persisted for 9 months. A complete rheumatology work-up failed to yield a diagnosis. However, the orthopaedic examination revealed marked quadriceps atrophy and a moderate effusion, with mild lateral joint line tenderness. The arthrogram failed to reveal a tear. Arthroscopy demonstrated a transverse tear of the middle third of the lateral meniscus (Fig. 5-18). The rest of the joint appeared normal. Recovery was rapid following lateral meniscectomy.

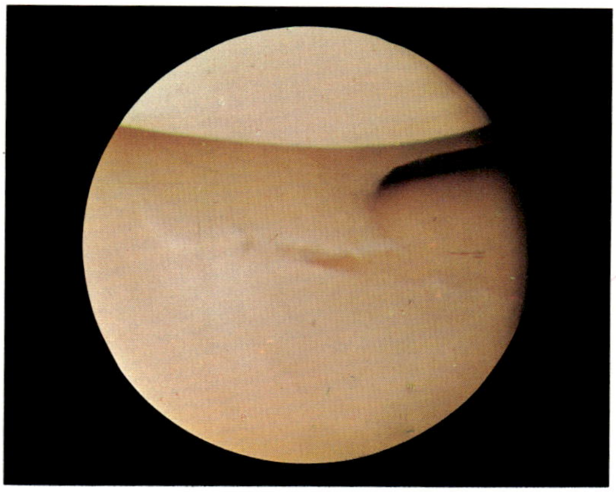

Fig. 5-18. Right knee: lateral infrapatellar approach. A simple transverse tear of the lateral meniscus is seen through the middle segment.

With the passage of time, and repeated episodes of meniscal trapping, this type of tear extends farther peripherally and splits anteriorly and posteriorly. In one instance, the tear extended transversely through the peripheral rim, dividing the meniscus in half (see below).

Case 5-8. Extension of Meniscal Tear Through the Peripheral Rim

A 17-year-old male twisted a knee playing baseball, and for 4 months complained of intermittent lateral joint line pain. Examination revealed lateral joint line tenderness. Two months later, while playing football, he was hit from the side as he was kicking for an extra point. Examination disclosed a mild hemarthrosis, and again lateral and medial joint line tenderness. The meniscal tests were negative. An arthrogram suggested medial meniscus involvement. Arthroscopy demonstrated a normal medial meniscus, a partial tear of the anterior cruciate ligament, and a complete separation of the anterior and posterior half of the lateral meniscus, with synovium separating the meniscal halves (Fig. 5-19). Arthrotomy confirmed this arthroscopic observation. No meniscal substance was present between the anterior and posterior halves of the meniscus.

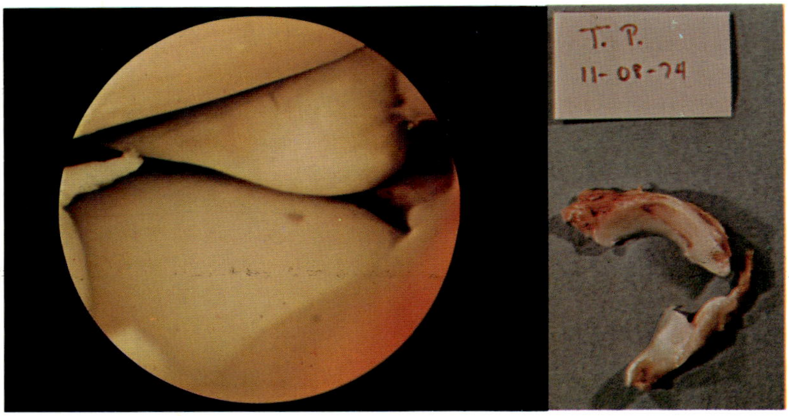

Fig. 5-19. Lateral meniscus of the left knee: complete separation of anterior and posterior lateral segments. The rounded posterior segment shows no evidence of the synovial ingrowth said to occur when the tear through the meniscus segment reaches the synovium. Rotation of the tibia has inhibited this process. The specimen demonstrates the defect.

A rupture of the anterior attachment of the lateral meniscus is not often seen but appears to be more common laterally than medially.

Case 5-9. Rupture of the Anterior Attachment of the Lateral Meniscus

A 43-year-old female complaining of lateral joint line pain was seen in consultation. This pain interfered with her routine activities. Extensive work-up, including an arthrogram, myleogram, and a phlebogram, failed to disclose any cause. Arthroscopy revealed a peripheral marginal tear of the lateral meniscus extending from the anterior cruciate ligament anteriorly to the middle third of the meniscus (Fig. 5-20). Arthrotomy resulted in clinical improvement.

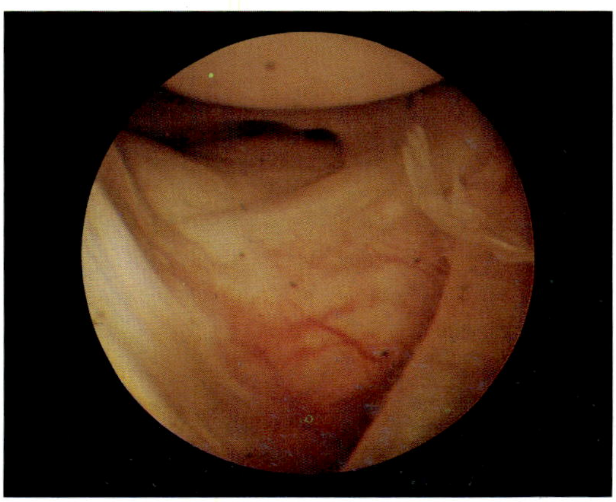

Fig. 5-20. Lateral meniscus of the left knee: medial infrapatellar approach. The split between the peripheral marginal fibers extended halfway around the meniscus.

Occasionally, incomplete tears of both the anterior lateral meniscus and the anterior medial meniscus attachments are seen following a tibial plateau fracture. These appear as ragged tears with retraction of the anterior attachments.

Meniscal Tears Associated With Tears of the Anterior Cruciate Ligament

An unusual tear of the posterior third of the lateral meniscus has been seen in 12 of my patients. I have found this to be invariably associated with a complete tear of the anterior cruciate ligament from its femoral origin, or after several episodes of a stretch injury of the anterior cruciate ligament that did not rupture the overlying synovial sheath. (Arthrotomy performed 3 months after injury in one of these patients revealed complete fibrosis of the anterior cruciate ligament with marked laxity.) Initially, the benign appearance of this tear did not suggest any indication for surgery. As time passed and clinical symptoms became more pronounced, it became obvious that this assessment was erroneous. Some of these patients were able to lock their knee at will. All complained of giving way and instability when running or turning to the side. These were deceleration injuries with the knee partially flexed, the foot externally rotated, and an abduction stress applied. All of these patients initially complained of medial joint line pain and tenderness to palpation localized over the medial joint line. Little or no laxity was noted to valgus stress, and minimal external rotary laxity was noted during Slocum's maneuver in several patients. Motion picture films taken during arthroscopy showed the tear of the lateral meniscus separated in external rotation of the tibia and approximated in internal rotation, lending credence to the inference that external rotation of the tibia was involved in the production of this lesion. Initially these patients were treated conservatively; later, when they were arthroscoped again, they were found to have incurred some secondary changes that included:

1. Rounding off of the central fragment, or the posterior tibial insertion of the lateral meniscus.
2. Chondral fractures, as a result of translocation of the tibia on the femur.
3. One patient had osteocartilaginous loose bodies that had become trapped in the popliteus recess, causing locking of the knee.
4. The posterior lateral meniscus became trapped between the tibia and femur, incurring secondary tears in its posterior third.
5. A strain of the medial capsule, which may erroneously direct the examiner's attention initially to the medial joint line. Not included in this series of 12, but seen recently, have been several patients who in addition to the above also had a bucket handle tear of the medial meniscus.

Some patients could feel the joint line tenderness transferred from the medial aspect to the posterior lateral joint line. Arthrotomy yielded a normal-appearing lateral meniscus if the operation was undertaken early after injury. However, when the knee was positioned with a varus stress, 20 degrees of flexion, and 20 degrees of internal tibial rotation so that the lateral tibial plateau and lateral femoral condyle could be separated, the tear could be seen. After the large meniscal fragments had been removed, the central nubbin could be seen; a rongeur was then introduced into the joint to remove it.

Seven of these patients were treated surgically with excision of the lateral meniscus and three with minimal rotary instability had additional pes anserinus transplantation. The short-term course has been gratifying.

Case 5-10. Torn Anterior Cruciate Ligament and Lateral Meniscus, and Osteochondral Fracture

An 18-year-old basketball player was seen after a mild twisting injury associated with an effusion. His medial joint line pain resolved after a negative arthrogram. Six months later, he was seen after an external rotation deceleration injury, and he again complained of medial joint line pain and was unable to extend his knee the terminal 20 degrees. A hemarthrosis was present. Arthroscopy revealed a chronic tear of the posterior lateral meniscus and a reabsorbing torn anterior cruciate ligament. The immediate cause of discomfort was a recent osteochondral fracture, displaced from a craterous defect of the medial femoral condyle. He was treated by intra-articular excision of the fragmented cartilage from the medial femoral condyle and by removal of the loose bodies under arthroscopic control. He responded well to quadriceps exercises and a derotation brace, and has returned to competitive basketball using this appliance.

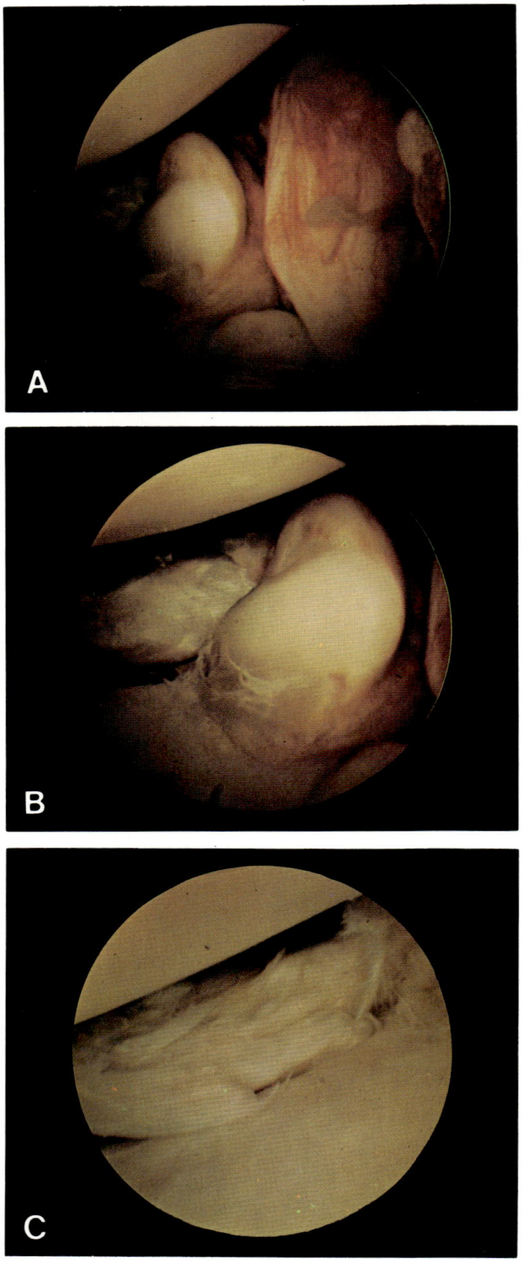

Fig. 5-21. Lateral meniscus of the right knee: lateral infrapatellar approach. (*A*) Stretched anterior cruciate ligament with thickened synovium adjacent to a nubbin of the lateral meniscus, lying perpendicular to the long axis of the meniscus. (*B*) Junction of tear of posterior tibial attachment of the lateral meniscus. (*C*) Posterior segment of the lateral meniscus with multiple secondary tears.

CASE 5-11. STRAINED MEDIAL CAPSULE, TORN ANTERIOR CRUCIATE LIGAMENT, AND TORN LATERAL MENISCUS

A 27-year-old paramedic incurred a twisting injury followed by a hemarthrosis. Initially, tenderness was localized to the medial aspect of the knee. A cast was applied for a month. Examination one year following injury revealed medial joint line tenderness, and the Drawer test was minimally positive in internal and external rotation. Arthroscopy revealed a rounded mass posterior and central to the lateral meniscus, which rotated with the tibia. Secondary tearing was obvious in the posterior lateral meniscal body. The anterior cruciate ligament was covered by synovium and was considerably lax (Fig. 5-21). At arthroscopy, the tibia could be brought forward from beneath the lateral femoral condyle. The patient was treated with quadriceps exercises and a derotation brace, and surgery has not been necessary to date.

I feel that the disabling factor here is external rotary instability and anterior tibial displacement under high-demand situations. Normally these patients can do well in a situation not requiring strenuous activity or sudden stops.

This unusual combination of pathologic findings may cause considerable clinical confusion. Reliance on clinical examination and the arthrogram will probably result in misdiagnosis. Initially, there is strong clinical evidence of a tear of the medial capsule or medial meniscus but minimal laxity to valgus stress. Arthrography should be performed, but total reliance on this technique to the exclusion of others results in sacrifice of the medial meniscus, unless this tear is seen on a high-quality arthrogram in multiple projections. Arthroscopy easily detects the cruciate ligament abnormality and the lateral meniscal tear, but may overlook a peripheral marginal separation of the posterior medial meniscus. Rotary stress involves the medial compartment, the cruciate ligaments, and the lateral compartment, and on the basis of this small

Fig. 5-22. Left knee. (*A*) Incomplete discoid lateral meniscus: a small area of lateral tibial plateau can be seen. (*B*) Discoid medial meniscus with small posterior tear (*left*). (*Right*) Specimen of medial meniscus.

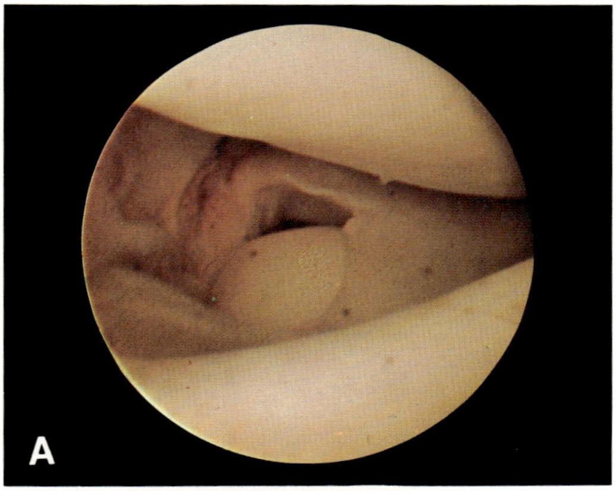

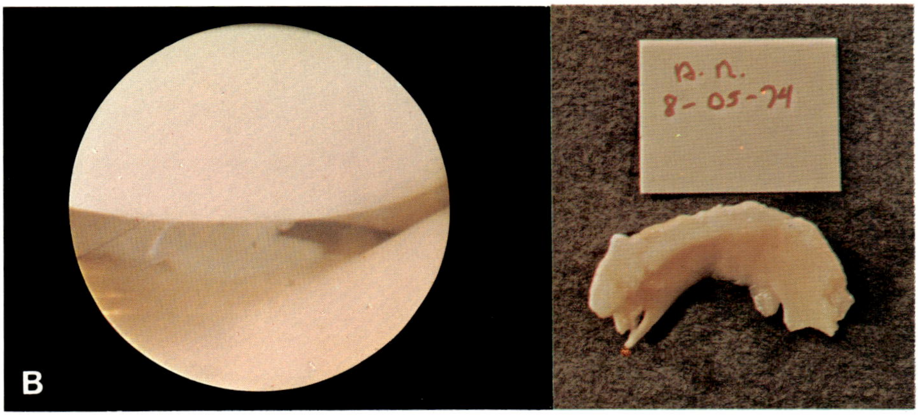

series it appears that the medial ligament complex escapes *major* injury initially. But if correction of the instability is delayed and further deceleration injuries occur, the medial meniscus may subsequently be torn.

Discoid Meniscus

Several examples of discoid lateral menisci have been seen, which probably should be classified as incomplete rather than complete discoid lateral meniscus, since a small area of tibia is visible.

Case 5-12. Incomplete Discoid Lateral Meniscus and Torn Medial Meniscus

A 32-year-old male was involved in an industrial injury. This was a twisting injury associated with medial joint line tenderness and pain, which kept him from returning to work. The arthrogram revealed a discoid lateral meniscus. Arthroscopy revealed an incomplete discoid lateral meniscus (Fig. 5-22A) and a transverse tear of the posterior medial meniscus (Fig. 5-22B). The medial meniscus protruded much further beneath the medial femoral condyle than would be normally anticipated.

Case 5-13. Torn Discoid Lateral Meniscus

A 39-year-old male complained of right lateral joint line pain and tenderness. An arthrogram was interpreted as normal. Arthroscopy revealed a torn discoid lateral meniscus (Fig. 5-23). He was treated by surgical excision and returned to work shortly thereafter.

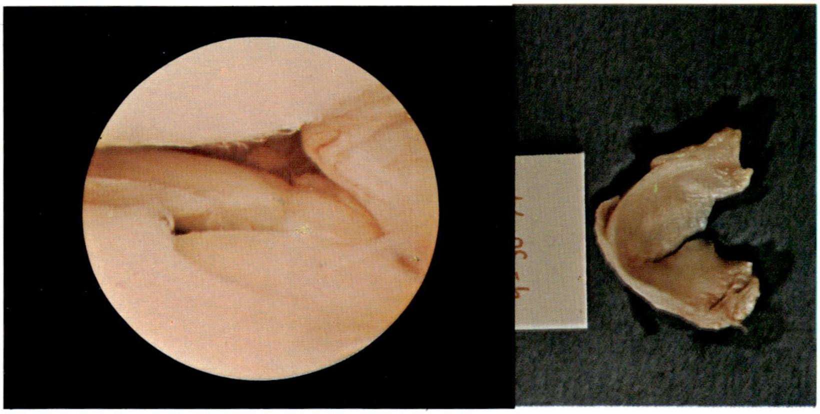

Fig. 5-23. Right knee: torn incomplete discoid lateral meniscus (*left*) and specimen (*right*).

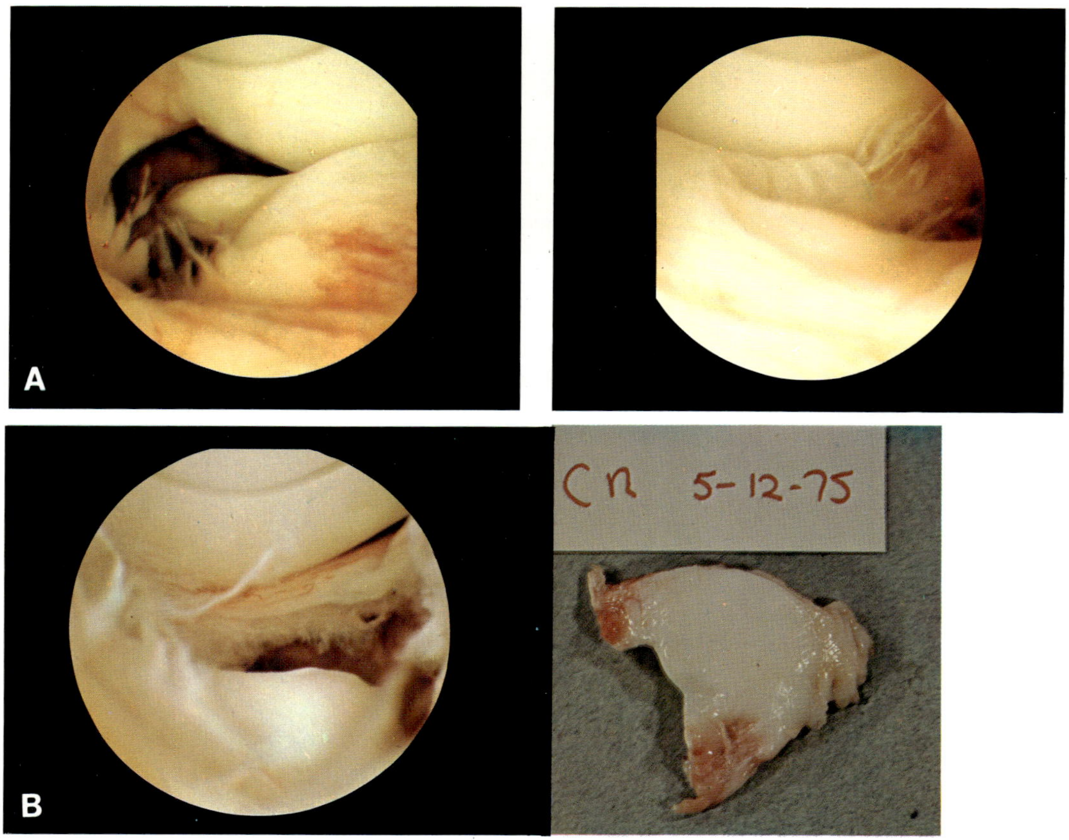

Fig. 5-24. (*A*) Left knee: complete discoid lateral meniscus completely covering the central lateral tibial plateau (*left*), with a posterolateral marginal tear (*right*). (*B*) Posterolateral corner demonstrating the peripheral rim of the tear. The lattermost lateral tibial plateau is uncovered. Specimen: complete discoid lateral meniscus.

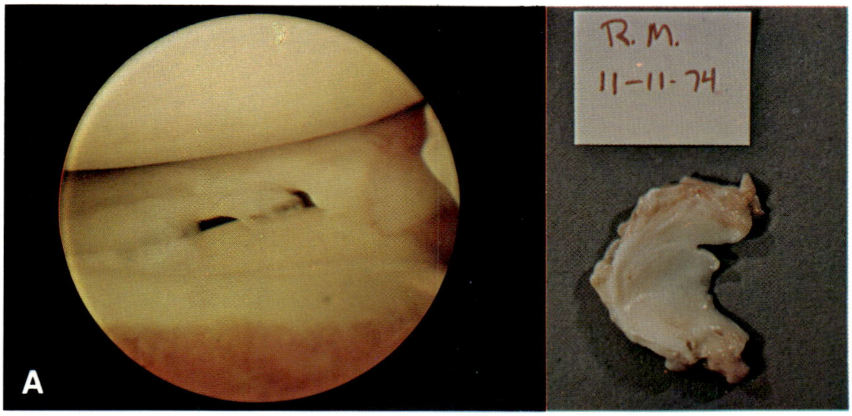

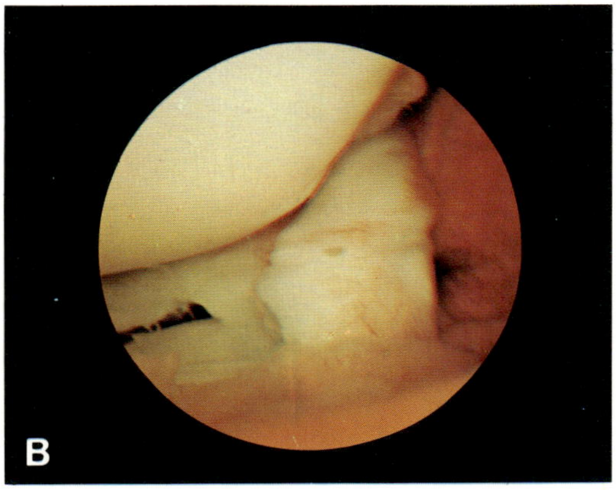

Fig. 5-25. (*A*) Specimen: tear of inner edge incompletely extends to the periphery of the disk. (*Left*) Incomplete discoid meniscus with a tear at the posterior inner edge. On the far right is a fibrotic band that runs from the anterior horn of the lateral meniscus to the lateral femoral condyle. (*B*) Close-up view of the anomolous band.

Rarely, a discoid lateral meniscus tears at its peripheral attachments and is displaced, as illustrated by the following:

CASE 5-14. DISCOID MENISCUS TORN FROM THE POSTERIOR LATERAL PERIPHERAL ATTACHMENT

A 10-year-old male, learning karate, kicked his opponent and experienced a sharp pain over the anterior lateral aspect of his left knee. Observation of flexion and extension revealed that the knee would lock at 30 degrees of flexion and unlock as the patient attempted to extend the knee. Arthroscopy revealed a complete discoid lateral meniscus torn from the posterior lateral peripheral attachment. At arthrotomy, the entire meniscus could be dislocated anterior to the lateral femoral condyle (Fig. 5-24).

CASE 5-15. DISCOID MENISCUS WITH AN ANOMOLOUS BAND

A 17-year-old male complained of lateral joint line discomfort. There was a buckling sensation and tenderness over the middle and lateral joint line. An arthrogram was negative. Arthroscopy demonstrated a torn discoid lateral meniscus. The patient was treated by surgical excision. Of interest was an anomalous band extending from the anterior attachment of the lateral meniscus to the lateral femoral condyle (Fig. 5-25).

CASE 5-16. DISLOCATED TEAR OF DISCOID LATERAL MENISCUS

A 49-year-old female fell from a loading dock, injuring her right knee. She was able to continue working for several days. Five months later, examination revealed loss of the

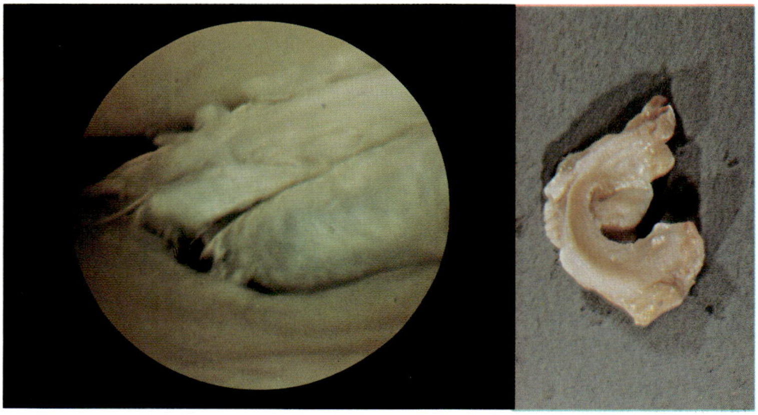

Fig. 5-26. Right knee: torn incomplete discoid lateral meniscus. The appearance at arthroscopy suggested a displaced bucket handle tear. These tears in discoid menisci, because of their increased volume of fibrocartilage, fill up the joint line, making detailed observation of the tear difficult.

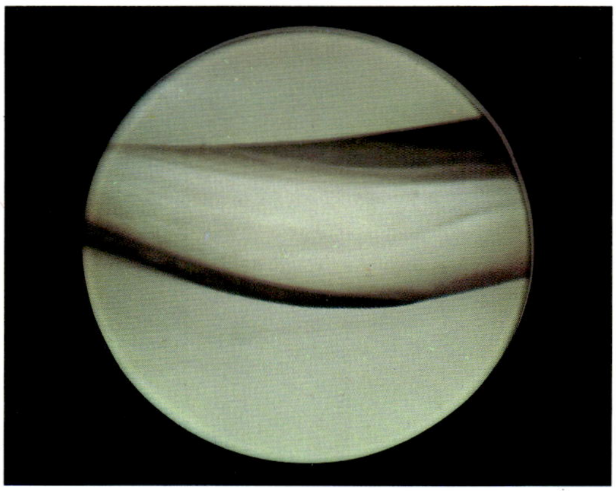

Fig. 5-27. Lateral meniscus of the right knee. A 28-year-old man, one year after arthrotomy and removal of a flap tear of the lateral meniscus, complained of recurrent locking episodes. A repeat arthrogram was negative, and the patient was referred for arthroscopy. A tear of the posterior horn of the retained lateral meniscus could be made to dislocate at arthroscopy. He was treated by subtotal lateral meniscectomy.

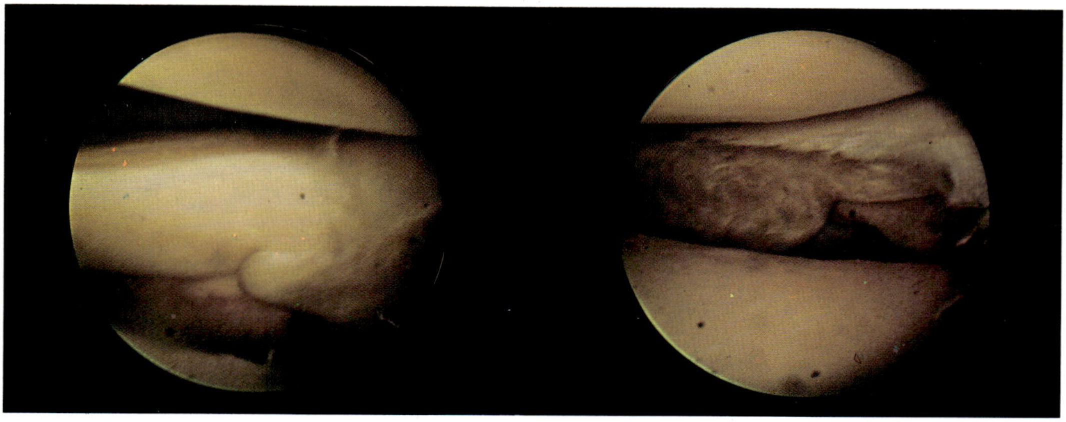

Fig. 5-28. Lateral meniscus of the left knee, demonstrating cystic degeneration in the posterior third, elevating the free meniscal edge. The meniscus was not visibly torn.

Fig. 5-29. Cystic degeneration may be concealed. Following arthroscopic excision of a bucket handle tear of the medial meniscus and a flap tear of the lateral meniscus, final joint line assessment revealed a mass of gelatinous material not previously present. The significance of this occurrence is not known.

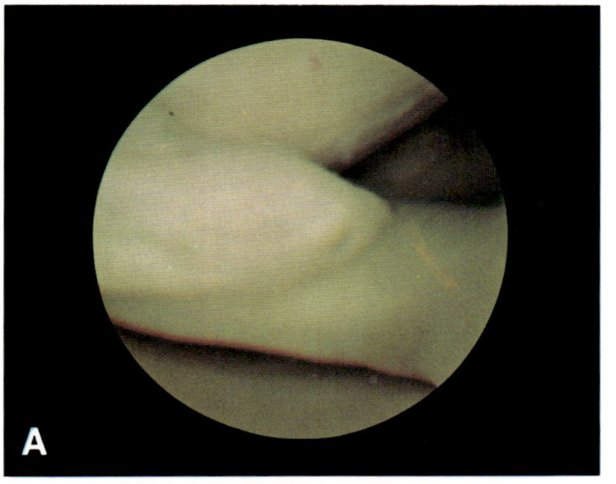

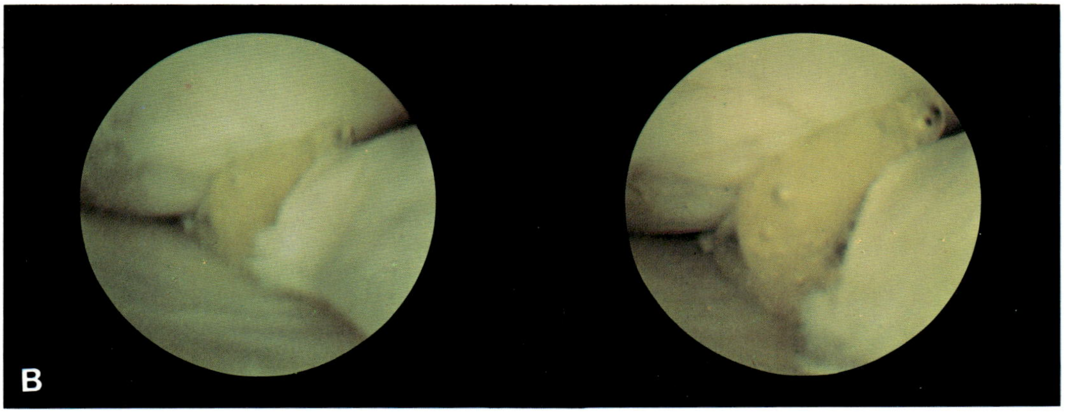

terminal 20 degrees of extension and 15 degrees of flexion. A mild effusion and lateral joint line tenderness were noted as well. The arthrogram confirmed a tear of the lateral meniscus. Arthroscopy revealed a heaped-up torn mass dislocation between the lateral femoral condyle and lateral tibial plateau. The patient was treated by lateral meniscectomy (Fig. 5-26).

Case 5-17. Tear of Retained Posterior Horn of the Lateral Meniscus

If partial meniscectomy performed by arthrotomy fails to relieve symptoms, arthroscopy is indicated, as illustrated by the following. A 28-year-old male complained of recurrent locking episodes, one year after arthrotomy and removal of a flap tear of the lateral meniscus. Arthrography failed to yield a diagnosis, but at arthroscopy the tear of the posterior third of the lateral meniscus remnant was quite apparent (Fig. 5-27).

Case 5-18. Cystic Degeneration of the Lateral Meniscus

Popliteal pain was the complaint of this young adult male. Several arthrograms were obtained with various interpretations. At arthroscopy no tear of the lateral meniscus was seen, but a large cystic mass was found to be elevating the posterior third of the lateral meniscus. The mass was found to contain gelatinous material at arthrotomy (Fig. 5-28).

Case 5-19. Cystic Degeneration of the Medial Meniscus

Following arthroscopic excision of a displaced bucket handle tear of the medial meniscus, final joint line inspection unexpectedly revealed a mass of gelatinous material indicating cystic degeneration within the peripheral rim (Fig. 5-29). In spite of this, the patient has had no further symptoms.

REFERENCES

1. De Haven, K. E., and Collins, H. R.: Diagnosis of internal derangements of the knee. J. Bone Joint Surg., *57A:* 802, 1975.
2. Helfet, A. J.: Disorders of the Knee. Philadelphia, J. B. Lippincott, 1974.
3. Johnson, L.: Unpublished paper. American Acad. of Orthopedic Surgeons Meeting. New Orleans, 1976.
4. Nicholas, J. A., Freiberger, R. H., and Killbran, P. J.: Double contrast arthrography of the knee—its value in the management of two hundred and twenty-five knee derangements. J. Bone Joint Surg., *52A:* 203, 1970.
5. Smillie, I. S.: Injuries of the Knee Joint. Baltimore, Williams & Wilkins, 1971.
6. Watanabe, M., Takeda, S., and Ikeuchi, H.: Atlas of Arthroscopy. ed. 2. Tokyo, Igaku Shoin, 1969.

6 *Osteochondritis Dissecans*

ARTHROSCOPIC ASSESSMENT AND TREATMENT

My arthroscopic experience with osteochondritis dissecans is limited, representing only 15 knees. Arthroscopy aids the physician in noting the amount of loosening of the osteochondral fragment, in determining the status of the overlying articular cartilage, and in assessing the degree of healing. Occasionally, the osteochondritic loose body may be removed from the joint, and, when necessary, an undisplaced necrotic and fragmented osteocartilaginous loose body can be removed during arthroscopy. The use of the arthroscope in osteochondritis dissecans will be illustrated by several cases.

CASE 6-1. OSTEOCHRONDRITIS DISSECANS WITH INTACT CARTILAGINOUS COVER

A 16-year-old male presented a history of pain in both knees following athletic endeavors. He gave no history of giving way or locking

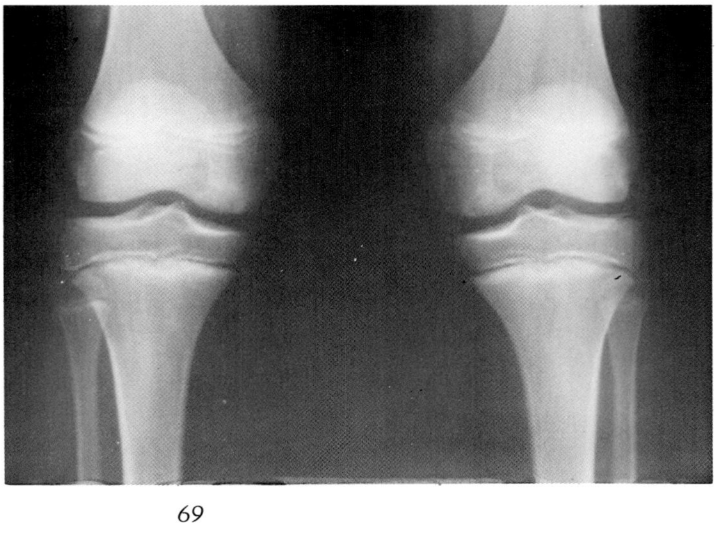

Fig. 6-1. Bilateral osteochondritis dissecans. The fragments were firmly held by intact hyaline cartilage at arthroscopy. The medial femoral condyle of the left knee was drilled at arthrotomy.

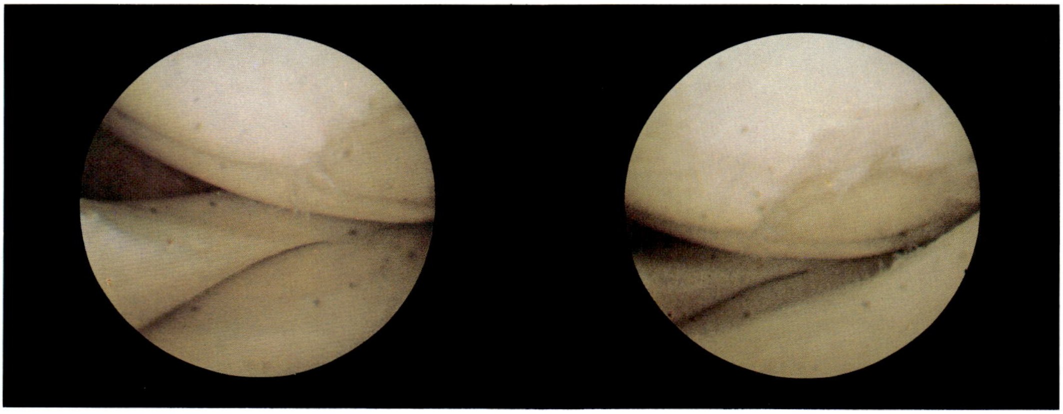

Fig. 6-2. Medial femoral condyle of the left knee. Osteochondritis dissecans in situ with color change of the covering articular cartilage (*right*). (*Left*) A linear depression extends anterior to the circumscribed defect. The fragment was hinged, allowing it to rotate. It was loosened with a small periosteal elevator, cut in half with a ronguer, and removed.

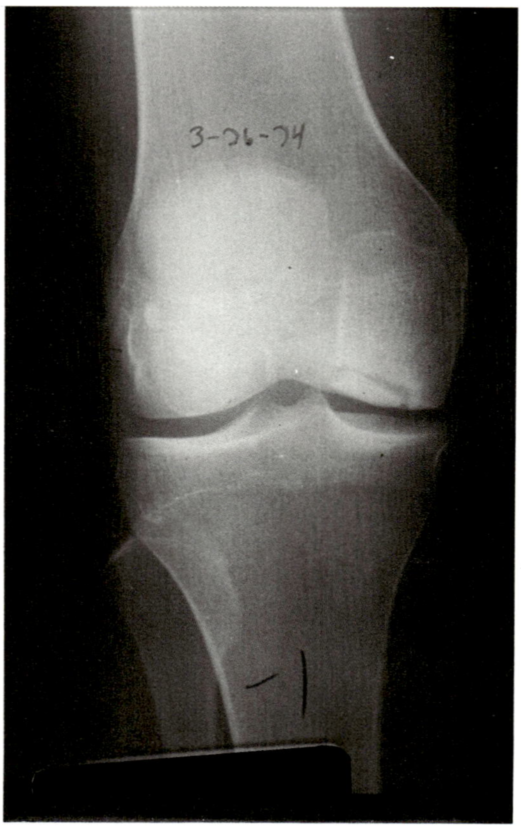

but did complain of an ache deep within the knee. Roentenograms showed the typical lesions of bilateral osteochondritis dissecans of the medial femoral condyles. Bilateral arthroscopy was performed. The left knee revealed normal articular cartilage overlying the defect, which was tightly held in place. In palpation with an obturator there was no abnormal mobility of the loose fragment. The roentgenographic appearance (Fig. 6-1) of the medial femoral condyle and the arthroscopic confirmation of the intact cartilaginous cover indicated that this patient was a good candidate for drilling the crater alone, with no necessity for the use of Smillie nails. The defect healed without incident.

Case 6-2. Extraction of Osteochondritic Fragment During Arthroscopy

A 24-year-old male with a history of previous knee surgery for osteochondritis dissecans,

Fig. 6-3. This roentgenogram demonstrates a large osteochondritic fragment in situ, occupying a large surface area. (Posterior-anterior view of the right knee.)

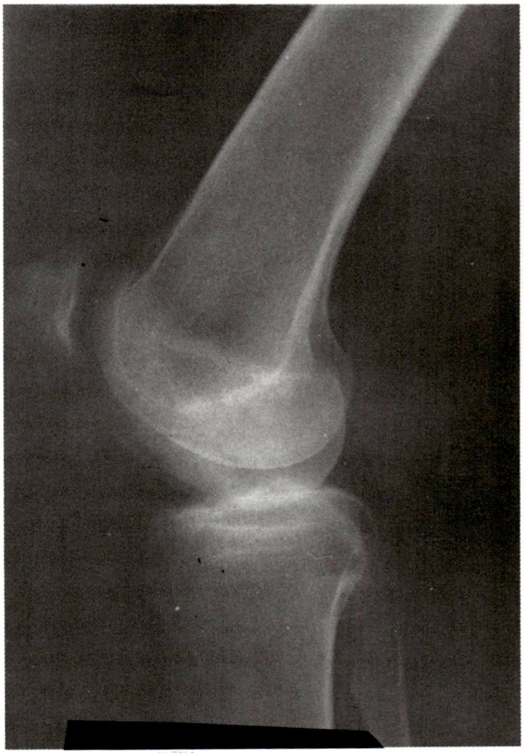

Fig. 6-4. Lateral view of the knee in Fig. 6-3.

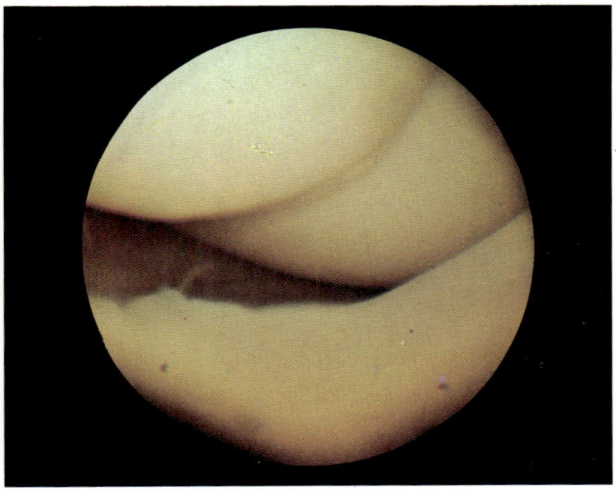

Fig. 6-5. The appearance of the healed crater of the left medial femoral condyle several years following removal of a large osteochondritic fragment. No treatment was given to the crater at that time.

incurred a twisting injury and felt something dislocate within his knee. This was followed by hemarthrosis and intermittent locking episodes. The locking episodes persisted following arthrocentesis. Examination revealed a surgical scar on the medial aspect of the knee, and roentgenograms showed a fragmented defect on the medial femoral condyle with sclerosis of the base. The loose body appeared to be in proper position.

Arthroscopy revealed a slightly brownish-yellow discoloration of the cartilage of the osteochondritic fragment (Fig. 6-2), which was found to be hinged on one surface, thus allowing limited mobility. He was treated by the double-puncture technique, and a small Key periosteal elevator was placed medially in the joint line, and under direct vision the osteochondritic fragment was removed from the bed in the medial femoral condyle, cut in half with a rongeur, and extracted from the joint. The patient was back at heavy work within 3 weeks.

Case 6-3. Arthroscopic Extraction of Osteochondritic Fragments in Both Knees

A 17-year-old girl was first seen in 1971, having been treated conservatively for osteochondritis dissecans of both medial femoral condyles. The osteochondritic fragments were large with sclerotic craters. She had little difficulty until the fragment in the *left* knee dislodged and was found lying in the intercondylar region. The loose body was easily grasped through a single-puncture technique and extracted from the joint. The patient was discharged from the hospital the evening of surgery and, aside from several follow-up office visits, was not seen again until 1974.

At that time, the patient stated that she had intermittent locking and instability of her *right* knee, associated with an aching pain towards the end of the day. Examination revealed a full range of motion with good ligamentous stability. Roentgenograms demonstrated osteochondritis dissecans of the medial femoral condyle with marked sclerosis of the base of the crater and necrosis of the central fragment (Figs. 6-3, 6-4). Arthroscopy of both knees was performed. The previous defect in the left medial femoral condyle, treated only by excision of the osteocartilaginous fragment, showed only a groovelike defect unassociated with fibrillation or fragmentation (Fig. 6-5).

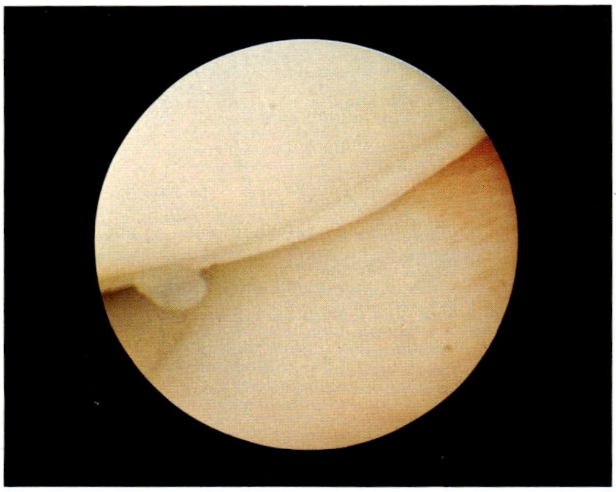

Fig. 6-6. Arthroscopic view of the right medial femoral condyle. Note the faint shadow running obliquely beneath the tuft of articular cartilage. This is the appearance of osteochondritis dissecans in situ, and can be easily missed with the arthroscope if the examining light is too bright.

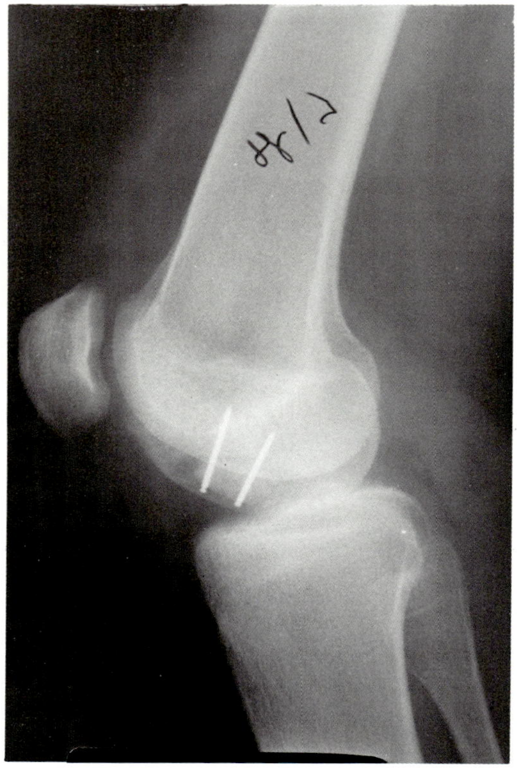

Fig. 6-7. Lateral view of the right knee. The osteochondritic fragment is held firmly by two Smillie nails.

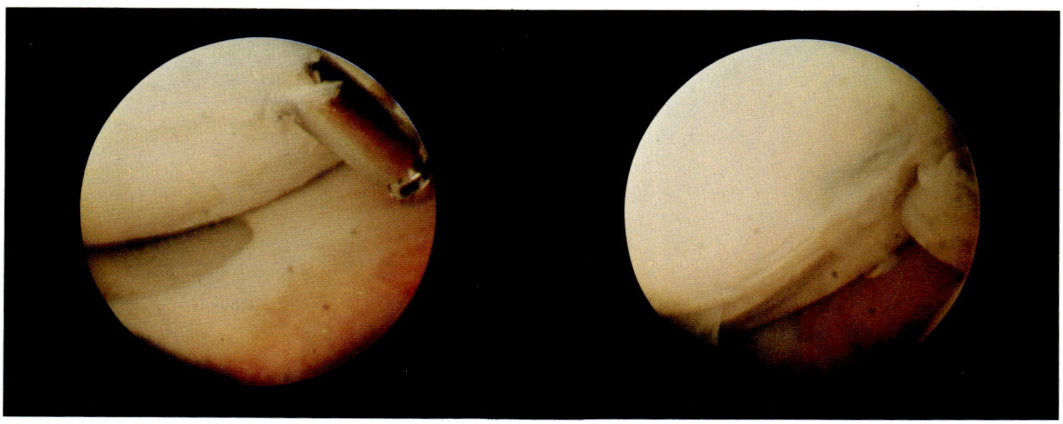

Fig. 6-8. (*Left*) Right knee. The defect is now healed, as revealed by palpation. The Smillie nail is being partially removed under arthroscopic control. (*Right*) Right knee. Medial femoral condyle prior to removal of Smillie nails. The small bluish area is the nail, partially seen beneath the articular cartilage.

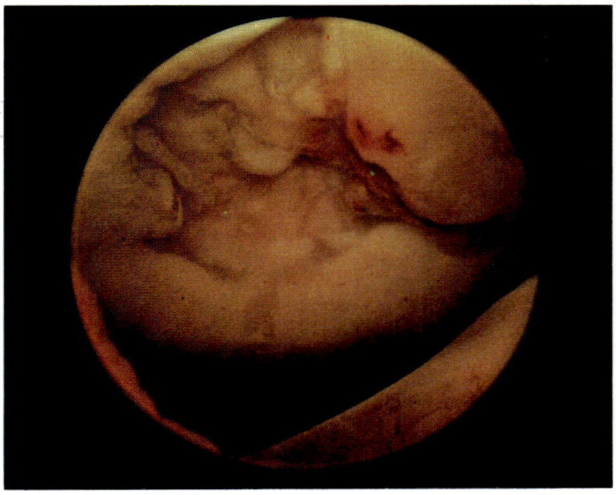

Fig. 6-9. New defect in the left medial femoral condyle; compare with Fig. 6-5.

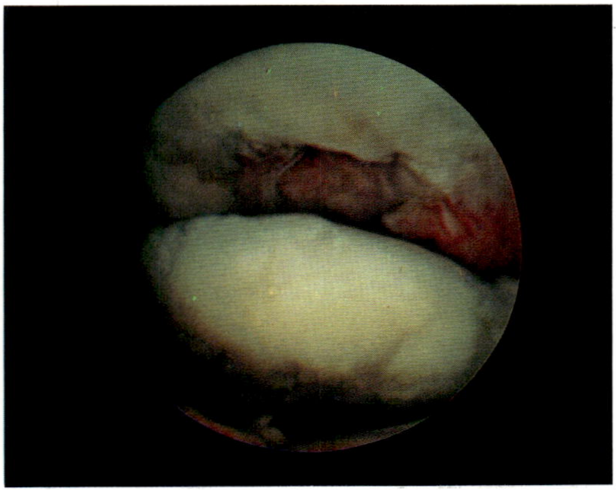

Fig. 6-10. An 18-year-old soccer player incurred a twisting injury, followed by a hemarthrosis. Roentgenograms were negative. Arthroscopy revealed osteochondritis dissecans of the medial femoral condyle. The loose fragment was removed arthroscopically.

Arthroscopic examination of the right knee, however, revealed an osteochondritic fragment with a normal-appearing articular cartilage having no evidence of discoloration. The osteocartilaginous body was found to be reduced within the medial femoral condyle, but the area of fracture through the articular cartilage could easily be appreciated arthroscopically (Fig. 6-6). Palpation of this fragment with an obturator through a medial incision revealed that it was loose. Arthrotomy was performed and the osteochondritic fragment was found to be attached by a posterior hinge, which was left in place. The fragment was raised as a leaf in a book, and the crater was drilled. The fragment was then replaced and held with two Smillie nails (Fig. 6-7). The patient wore a

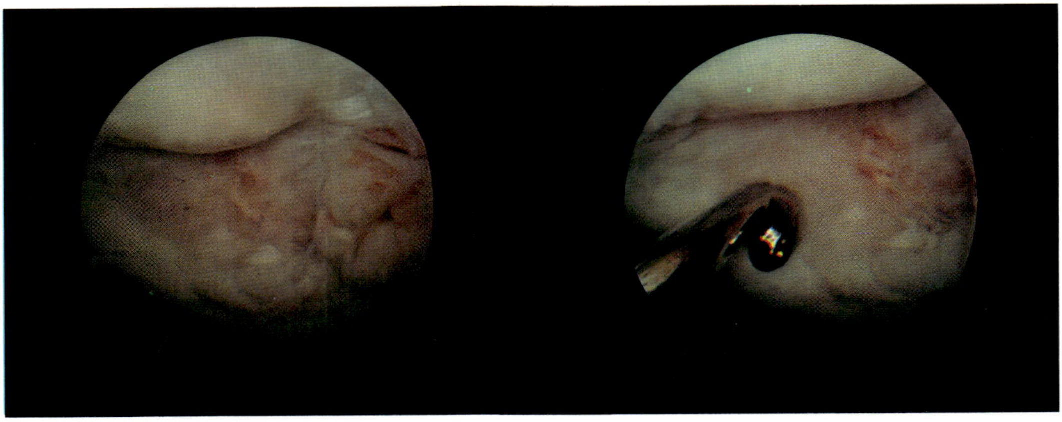

Fig. 6-11. The patient returned to the soccer field one week following arthroscopy, and afterwards complained of a new loose body in the quadriceps bursa. Repeat arthroscopy 3 weeks later allowed the removal of a second fragment, and the crater of the medial femoral condyle was found to be filling in. (*Right*) A crochet hook was used to palpate the defect and adjacent articular cartilage, to be certain that no loose fragment was still present.

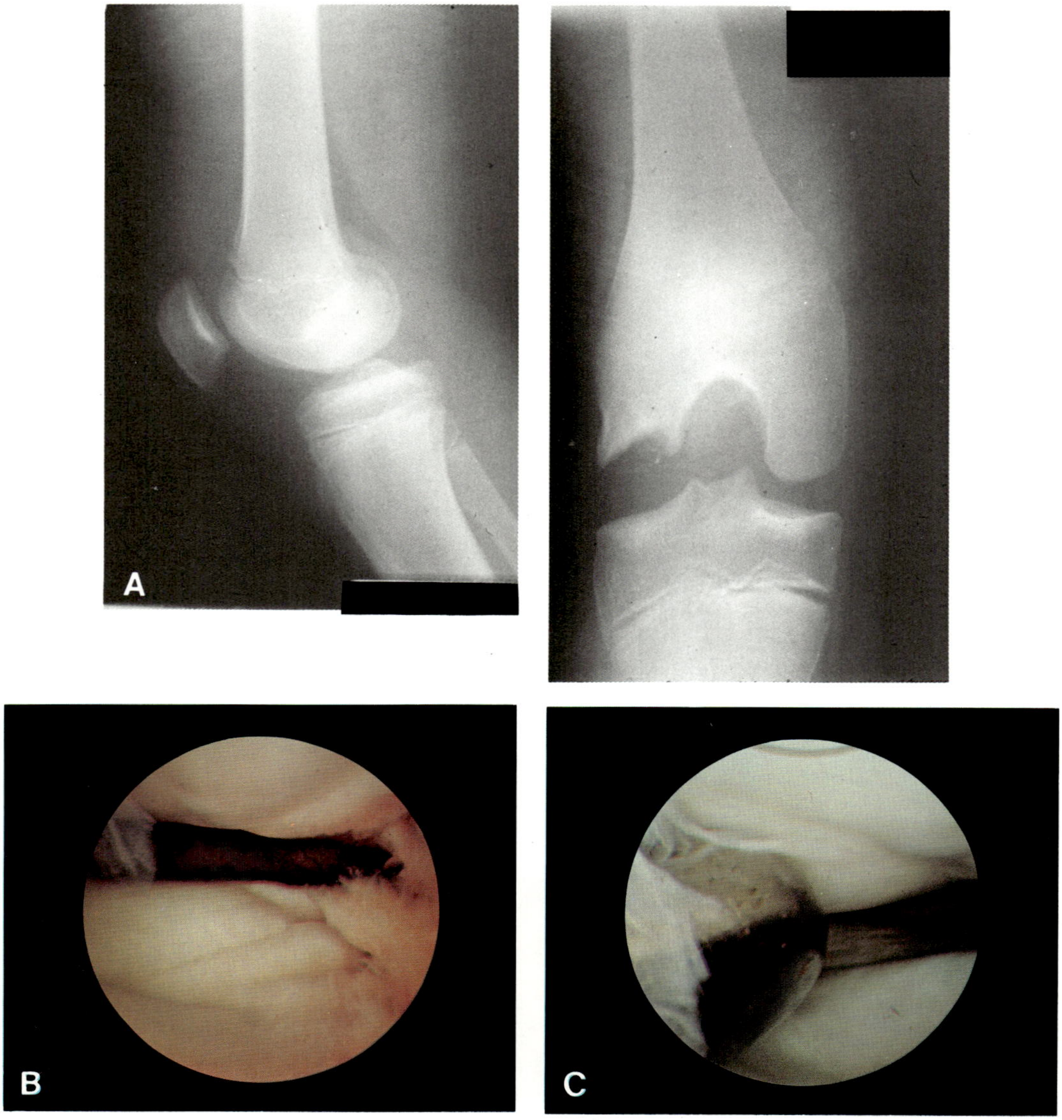

Fig. 6-12. (*A*) Roentgenogram of the right knee demonstrating a large unossified portion of the lateral femoral condyle. This was thought to be a vascular phenomena that would correct with growth. The patient complained of snapping in his knee, and pain over the lateral joint line. (*B*) Lateral joint line. Note defect of the femoral articular cartilage overlying a large discoid lateral meniscus. (*C*) Lateral joint line: medial infrapatellar approach. Methalene blue has been introduced to outline the defect. A blunt obturator has been introduced from the inferior lateral approach to palpate the defective area. The articular fragment was solidly held and the lesion was treated by drilling under arthroscopic control.

cast for three months, then underwent several weeks of nonweight and mobilizing exercises. Then arthroscopy was again performed. The Smillie nails were removed through a small stab wound, and an obturator was inserted to palpate the replaced fragment (Fig. 6-8, *right*). The typical "ping pong ball" feel was no longer present, and the osteocartilaginous fragment appeared to be solidly united, although this was not the impression one would get from viewing the roentgenograms.

Four months later, the patient complained of a sensation of a loose body in her left knee, which could be easily palpated and was extremely mobile. She denied having any recent injury. Roentgenograms were obtained which showed the loose body in the suprapatellar pouch (Fig. 6-8, *left*). This was removed with a double-puncture technique under arthroscopic visualization. A defect was now noted in the base of the medial femoral condyle, which was not seen at arthroscopy several months previously (Fig. 6-9).

This case describes the obvious advantages that arthroscopy may offer in the treatment of this condition. Multiple orthopaedic procedures were done that would ordinarily require formal arthrotomy, and the joint was opened only on one occasion.

In the future it will be possible to develop techniques of treatment that range from drilling the base to insertion of Smillie nails under direct vision. Arthroscopy used in conjunction with standard roentgenographic techniques increases the ease of care (Figs. 6-10, 6-11), improves the quality of care, and decreases the morbidity of osteochondritis dissecans (Fig. 6-12).

7 *Loose Bodies*

DIAGNOSIS

The diagnosis of osteocartilaginous loose bodies, larger than 8 mm., in the knee is usually proven by standard roentgenograms,[2,3] and the classic treatment is arthrotomy. The diagnosis of cartilaginous loose bodies, however, is often impossible with the available modalities. An arthrogram often adds little information of a positive nature. Arthroscopy may facilitate the removal of an osteocartilaginous loose body and provide as well the initial diagnosis of a cartilaginous loose body and allow its removal.[1] The mobility of these fragments may make attempts at removal frustrating, since the cartilaginous fragment is the more buoyant of the two. The flow of the irrigating fluid causes a whirling effect, so it is wise when attempting to remove the cartilaginous loose body to cut the irrigating fluid down or off to avoid time wasted in pursuit. Obstacles, such as synovial fronds or villi, though small in size, frequently hide the loose body from view and so complicate the problem.

The greatest obstacle is the ligamentum mucosum, with its synovial ramifications and connections to the fat pad. Secondly, a well-developed plica synovialis may offer sanctuary to the loose body. The loose body may well migrate through the porta into the quadriceps bursa and become hidden behind the pillar of the plica synovialis, particularly the lateral origin of the plica. The loose body often moves into an area not usually viewed, either the medial or lateral gutter, or retreats anteriorly beneath the fat pad. The area always to be searched, if difficulties are encountered locating the loose body, is that beneath the lateral meniscus between the lateral meniscus and tibia posteriorly. Loose bodies have also been found beneath the anterior medial meniscus. Frustration is increased, during the search and seizure, by synovial fronds obscuring the tip of the arthroscope. Although the cartilaginous loose body is generally much more mobile than the heavier osteocartilaginous fragment, both may move rapidly. On numerous occasions these cartilaginous loose bodies clinically mimic the behavior of a locking meniscal tear; however, the differentiation can be established by arthroscopy. When clinical suspicion is high, a thorough search is indicated and requires several insertions of the arthro-

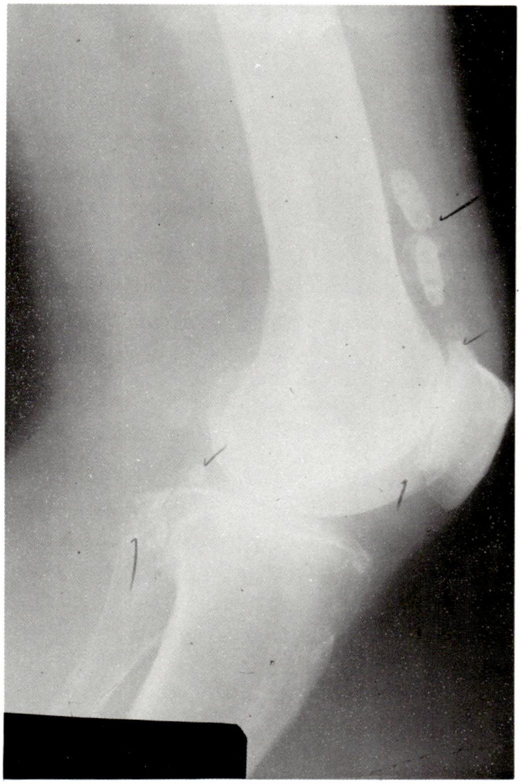

Fig. 7-1. Lateral roentgenogram: several osteocartilaginous loose bodies may be seen in the quadriceps bursa and a large fragment in the intracondylar notch.

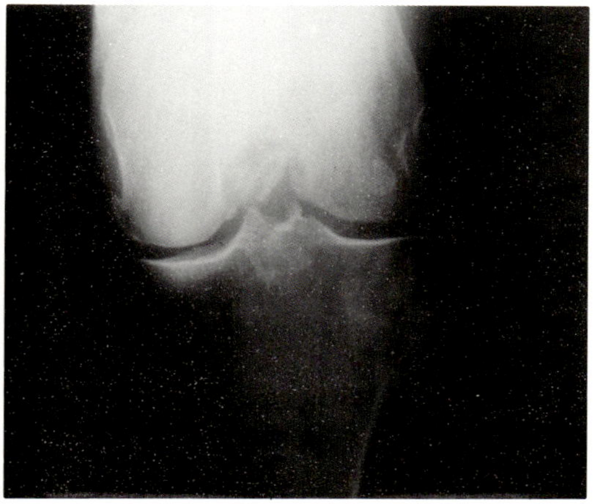

Fig. 7-2. Posterior-anterior view: a large osteocartilaginous body occupies the medial portion of the intracondylar notch.

scope to view both the medial and lateral gutters (see list on p. 78).

The multiplicity of loose bodies also poses a problem, and any joint with more than 3 osteocartilaginous bodies seen on the roentgenogram may require repeated attempts at removal (Figs. 7-1–7-4). Since a secondary puncture is often made in these instances, escape of saline solution over a period of time will cause swell-

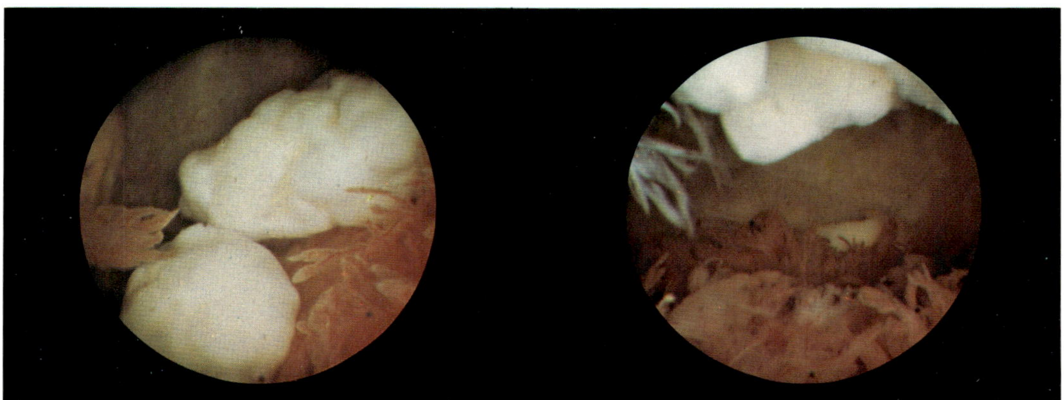

Fig. 7-3. Osteochondritic fragments in the quadriceps bursa. (*Left*) The retropatellar surface was the origin of these loose bodies. At the proximal end of the quadriceps bursa, a loose body is seen partially covered by synovium. (*Right*) 2 osteocartilaginous loose bodies in the quadriceps bursa.

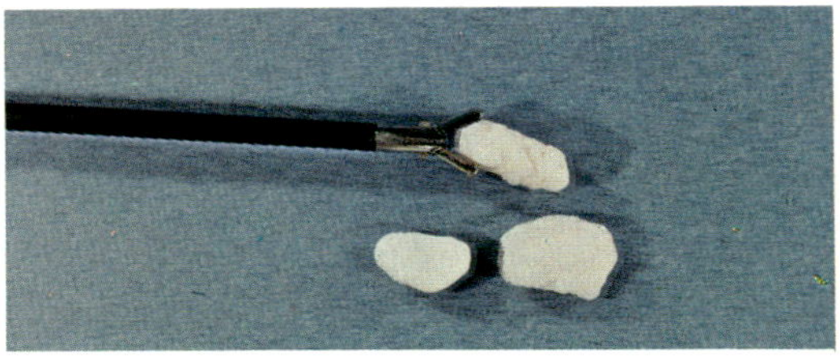

Fig. 7-4. The specimen: 3 osteocartilaginous loose bodies, one held by a 5 mm. extracting forceps with teeth. This forceps is essential for removal from the joint; if the blades of the forceps are too sharp, they will bite through the loose body; the teeth give a secure purchase.

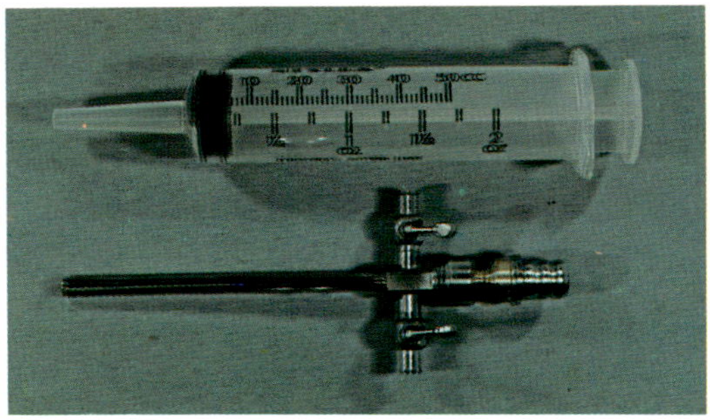

Fig. 7-5. Toomey syringe with adapter to fit the water sleeve. A great deal of negative pressure can be generated with this syringe.

Findings in Arthroscopy of 746 Knees

48 knees (6.4%) had loose bodies
26 knees (3.4%) contained cartilaginous loose bodies
22 knees (3.0%) contained osteocartilaginous loose bodies

ing of the subcutaneous tissue, which will dissect up and down the fascial planes and eventually obliterate the suprapatellar recess and thus make recovery and removal much more difficult.

TECHNIQUES FOR REMOVAL

Single-Puncture Technique

The single-puncture technique is particularly applicable for removal of a large osteocartilaginous loose body that is trapped in the intercondylar region between the tibial condyle, medial femoral condyle, or cruciate ligament or a large loose body in the suprapatellar recess that can be forced against the proximal extent of the quadriceps bursa, or (occasionally) a loose body in the recesses of the medial and lateral gutter. This technique has the advantage of not necessitating a second stab wound, but it is not always successful. When the loose body has been trapped, the water flow is stopped and the telescope is slowly removed from the water sheath while the examiner continues to peer down the tube to ascertain whether the loose body has moved. The arthroscope should be approximately 1 cm. from the loose body. While rigidly holding the water sleeve in one hand, the examiner takes hold of the special forceps designed for retrieval, places it down the water sleeve, and grasps the loose body. The entire water sleeve and forceps are then withdrawn to the skin level. The use of this particular forceps insures that when the osseous portion of the loose body is grasped the loose body will not be cut and that adequate purchase is afforded. The loose body is twisted from side to side to allow its smallest diameter to tent the skin. The skin incision as well as the soft tissue beneath it is then gradually enlarged and the loose body removed.

Irrigation Technique

This technique is only applicable for removal of cartilaginous loose bodies, especially those lying in the joint line. The irrigation flow is turned off, and the water sheath and telescope are partially withdrawn approximately 5 mm. from the loose body. The telescope is gently removed, and the thumb is placed over the end of the water sheath. The assistant then attaches a syringe to the irrigating needle and distends the joint with between 50 and 100 ml. of saline solution, depending on joint capacity. The thumb is then removed from the water sleeve, and a rapid burst of saline solution from the tube occasionally will float the loose body out of the joint. This technique has worked only rarely with osteocartilaginous loose bodies because of their size and density. An improvement of this technique is afforded by the use of a Toomey syringe (Figs. 7-5, 7-6), familiar to the urologist, and is the most common method we use to remove these fragments. The joint is distended with saline via the Toomey syringe connected to the water sleeve by the Toomey adapter, and the outflow and inflow valves are occluded. Negative pressure on the barrel of the syringe often removes more cartilaginous fragments than were suspected to be present within the joint.

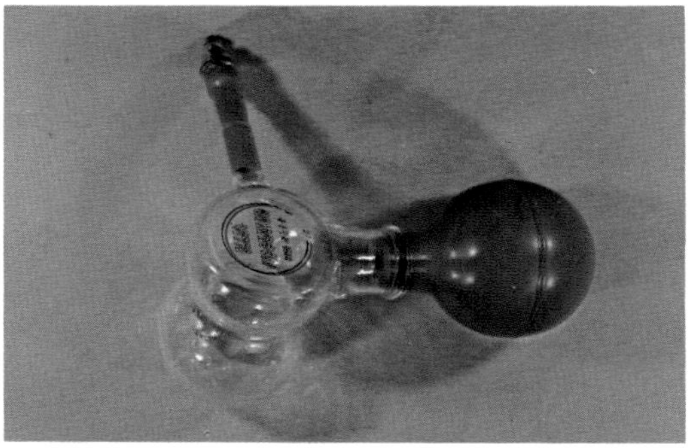

Fig. 7-6. An Ellick syringe may be used in place of the Toomey; the cartilaginous particles fall into the bottom of the syringe. Less saline is lost from the joint using this device, but greater negative pressure is produced by the Toomey.

Double-Puncture Technique

This technique works very well, particularly in the case of the very immobile osteocartilaginous loose body. This is probably the most successful technique of retrieving medium-sized foreign bodies from within the joint. After the loose body is located in the suprapatellar pouch, a second incision is made either superiorly, medially, or laterally to the patella. If the loose body is found within the intercondylar notch, the medial or lateral joint line or the medial or lateral gutter, the second incision should be on the side of the joint line opposite to the side of insertion of the telescope. The loose body is then grasped and brought to the surface, and the incision enlarged if necessary for its removal.

When multiple osteocartilaginous loose bodies are present, they usually tend to gravitate to the same region in the quadriceps bursa. Unfortunately, the attempt to remove one of these often scatters the loose bodies throughout the knee, complicating complete removal. Inviting as it may appear in some cases, the tendency to place the incision through the quadriceps tendon for removal decreases the mobility of the forceps, and hence decreases the rate of recovery. Therefore, perforation of the quadriceps tendon should be avoided.

Obstruction by Soft Tissue Structures

As previously mentioned, the soft tissue structures occasionally obstruct the line of sight and make removal difficult. Several remedies may help overcome these problems. In the intercondylar notch, the prime offenders are the ligamentum mucosum and the fat pad. The Watanabe No. 21 arthroscope itself can be used as a retractor. The width of the water sheath of the instrument as it pierces the fat pad is 6.5 mm. However, the width of the telescope and tungsten bulb (the latter in bayonette apposition) markedly increases the width. Traction on this instrument withdraws the fat pad, increasing the available room for removal of the loose body. This is not absolutely necessary, and fiber-optic telescopes can be used as well. However, it may be wise in this situation to resect the ligamentum mucosum to allow easier visualization. In the quadriceps bursa, the lateral pillar of the plica synovialis may

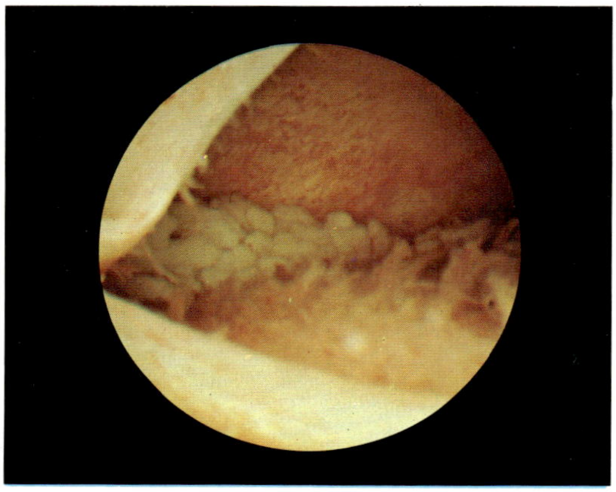

Fig. 7-7. Multiple cartilaginous loose bodies (approximately 300) of uniform size, many sequestered behind the plica synovialis.

obstruct the view of the loose body, and this structure may also have to be resected prior to grasping the loose body (Fig. 7-7).

Common Sites of Loose Bodies

In my experience, the common sites of osteocartilaginous loose bodies are: the intercondylar notch, suprapatellar recess and quadriceps bursa, and the medial and lateral gutters (Fig. 7-8). Cartilaginous loose bodies, however, show a disposition for the joint line, particularly the inferior aspect of the lateral joint line. They are usually found beneath the posterior third of the lateral meniscus, wedged between it and the tibia and sometimes between it and the lateral femoral condyle (Figs. 7-9, 7-10). They are generally visualized in the vicinity of the posterior third of the lateral meniscus, usually inferior to this structure, and they may be retrieved from beneath the lateral meniscus (Fig. 7-11). Digital pressure posterior to the popliteal space may bring the loose body to view from beneath the lateral meniscus and over the tibia.

In case a loose body is lost in this region, a small needle inserted in the joint and slid beneath the meniscus will sometimes bring it out from behind the tibia. Another useful trick is to palpate the lateral joint line posteriorly with the index finger while visualizing this area. If the loose body pops up over the tibia, it can be removed. These cartilaginous loose bodies have been found (rarely) in the medial joint line beneath the medial meniscus anteriorly, and on one occasion arthrotomy was necessary for successful removal.

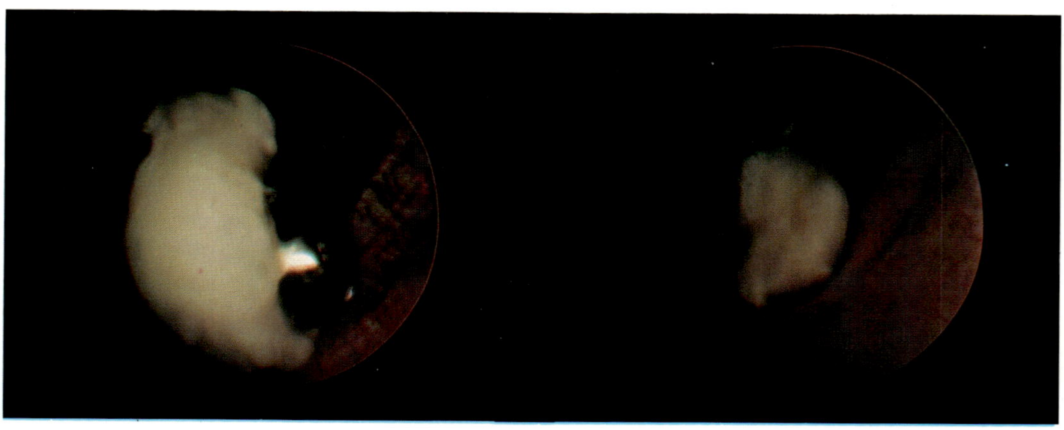

Fig. 7-8. Osteocartilaginous loose body in lateral gutter, being removed by double puncture technique. The grasping forceps were introduced through a stab wound lateral and superior to the patella.

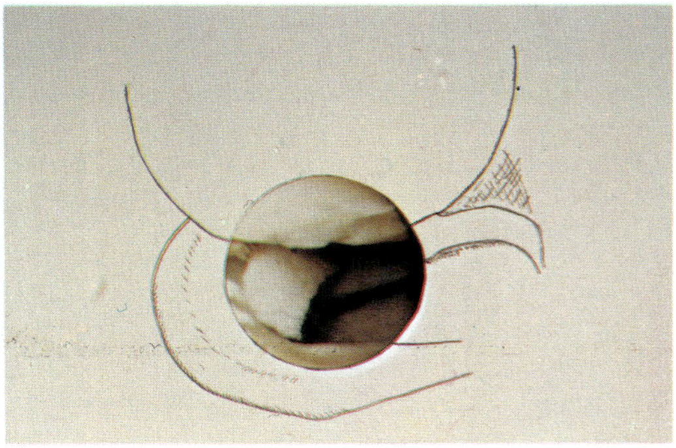

Fig. 7-9. Cartilaginous loose body trapped between the lateral femoral condyle and the lateral meniscus.

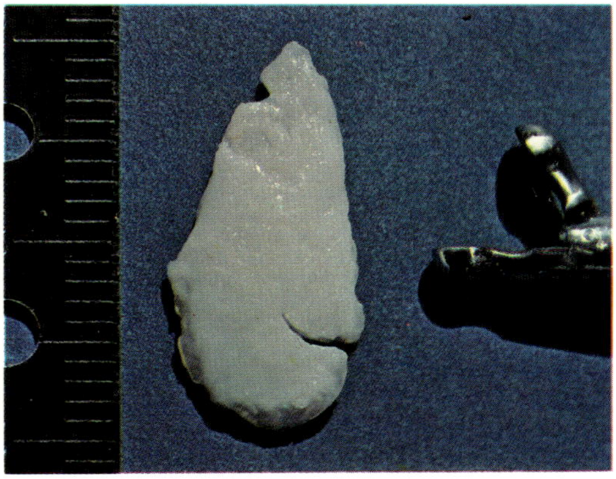

Fig. 7-10. Specimen: cartilaginous loose body from the knee in Fig. 7-9.

Failure of Removal

You can't remove what you can't see. This is axiomatic, but during the frustrating search the illusive loose body may vanish. It may be advanced by the telescope as the knee is fully investigated. In one patient with a locking knee, the preoperative roentgenograms revealed a loose body in the intercondylar notch. During the course of arthroscopy and after a one-hour search, it was never found. Roentgenograms were then obtained but failed to demonstrate this minimally ossified loose body. Arthrotomy was deferred. The next time the patient felt the loose body pop out of his joint so that he could palpate it, he placed his leg in an immobilizing splint. Arthroscopy was immediately repeated, and the loose body was successfully removed from the intercondylar notch.

Another error associated with ossific loose bodies is that of incorrect interpretation. Occasionally, ossification within the capsule may give the appearance of an intra-articular loose body.

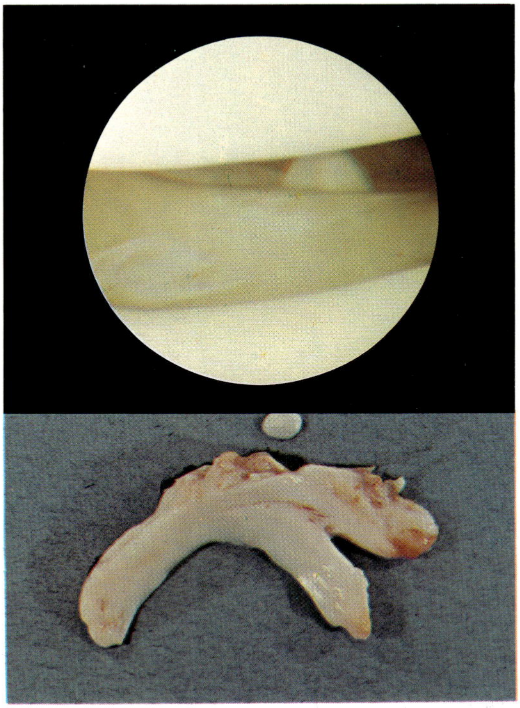

Fig. 7-11. Cartilaginous loose body trapped between the fragments of a longitudinal tear of the lateral meniscus: posterior third of the right knee.

Case 7-1. Ossification Within the Capsule of the Joint

A 40-year-old male was previously treated for a tear of his medial meniscus. No loose bodies were found at the time of surgery. Because of continuing symptoms one year postoperatively, roentgenograms were re-

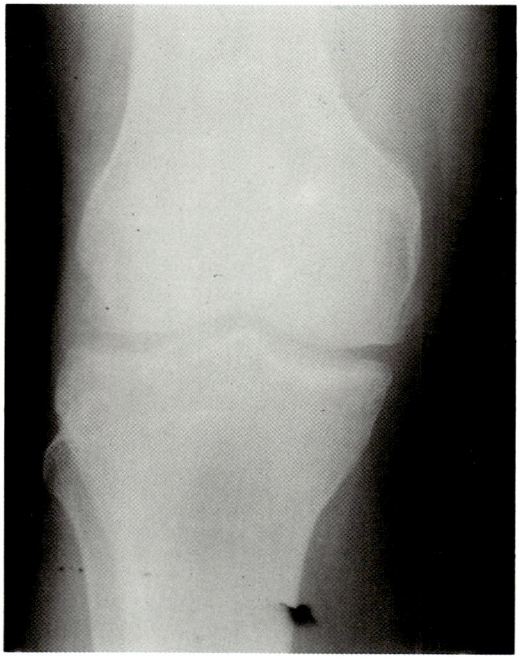

Fig. 7-12. Roentgenogram showing apparent ossified loose body. Another roentgenogram, taken with the joint distended, demonstrated that this was illusionary and was in fact ossification within the capsule.

peated. They showed an area of ossification apparently in the medial gutter (Fig. 7-12). After a diligent search during arthroscopy, roentgenograms were obtained with the joint distended with saline solution. The roentgenograms showed that the presumptive loose body actually represented an ossification within the capsule of the joint, not in an intra-articular location.

The popliteus recess, a not infrequent site of loose body entrapment, is an area that cannot be visualized. If this diagnosis is a definite possibility, this area should be searched and an accessory needle inserted to explore it. We have been able to recognize a loose body in this location arthroscopically only once.

Case 7-2. Mimic of Meniscal Tear by Loose Body

A 21-year-old male injured himself while jumping from a loading dock. He complained of intermittent locking of his knee thereafter and inability to extend the terminal 15 degrees. This was associated with mild effusion. There was tenderness to palpation over the posterior lateral joint line. An arthrogram was equivocal but suggested a tear of the medial meniscus. Arthroscopy was performed because of lack of correlation. Unfortunately, the pathology was misinterpreted. The slides showed in retrospect what was the obvious diagnosis: a loose body trapped beneath the posterior third of the lateral meniscus and the tibia (Fig. 7-13). Due to lack of experience with arthroscopy, this

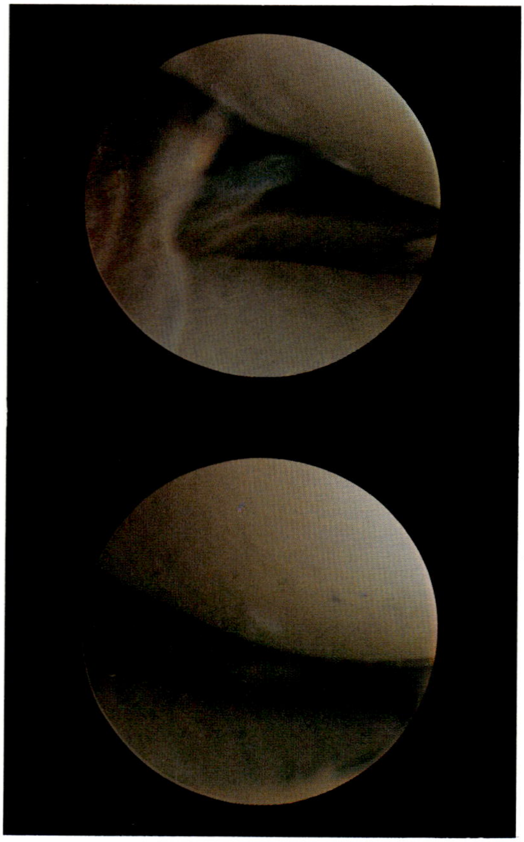

Fig. 7-13. Left knee: cartilaginous loose body tightly wedged between the lateral meniscus and the lateral tibial plateau. This was incorrectly interpreted as a tear of the lateral meniscus. To avoid a mistake such as this, the illuminating light should be lowered to allow visual differentiation of the colors, or the area should be probed with a needle or crochet hook.

misinterpretation resulted in excision of the lateral meniscus. Arthrotomy was performed, and a dissection of the anterior two-thirds of the meniscus was completed, when the sequestered loose body slipped out of the knee.

Multiple loose bodies may be present, and removing only the most offensive may be possible at one time. It may be desirable to do this rather than risk the morbidity associated with formal arthrotomy, as seen in the following case.

Case 7-3. Partial Removal of Loose Bodies

An 83-year-old female gave a 4-year history of locking in her knee produced just by sitting down. It sometimes took several days to unlock her knee, but she was able to do this herself by manipulation of the leg. Roentgenograms revealed 5 osteocartilaginous loose bodies, the main offender being in the intercondylar notch (see Fig. 7-2). Three loose bodies were removed from the joint (see Figs. 7-3, 7-4)—offending loose body in the intercondylar notch and two in the suprapatellar recess. Because of soft-tissue infiltration of the saline solution, the other two loose bodies were not removed. So far the other loose bodies have not caused any difficulty; the patient no longer complains of locking of her knees.

The importance of avoiding open surgery and arthrotomy and developing better arthroscopic technique of loose body removal is demonstrated by the following case:

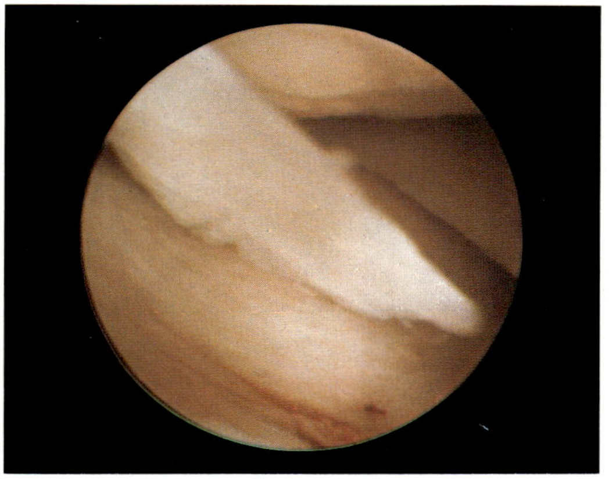

Fig. 7-14. A large osteocartilaginous loose body within the lateral joint line. The loose body mimicked a torn medial meniscus.

Case 7-4. The Importance of Arthroscopic Removal of Osteocartilaginous Loose Bodies

A 40-year-old male had a history of poliomyelitis with moderately severe involvement

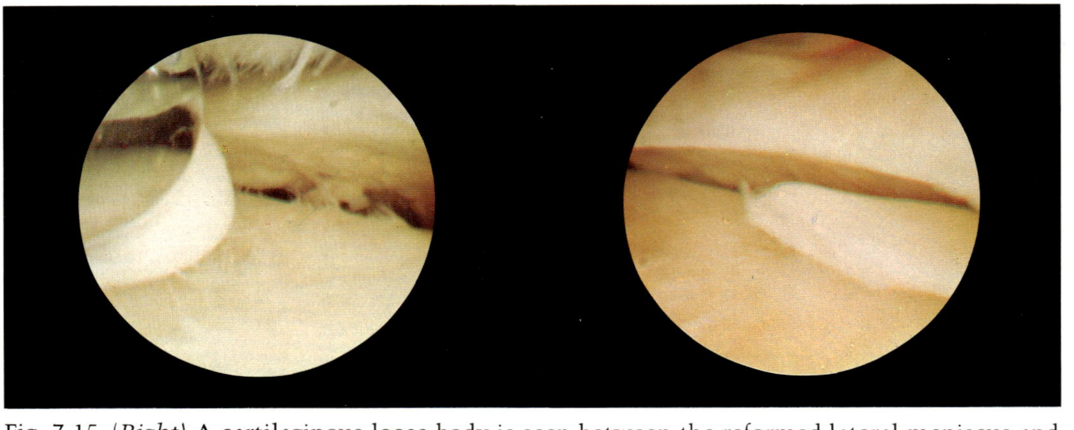

Fig. 7-15. (*Right*) A cartilaginous loose body is seen between the reformed lateral meniscus and tibia. (*Left*) A loose body forceps was used to extract it from the joint.

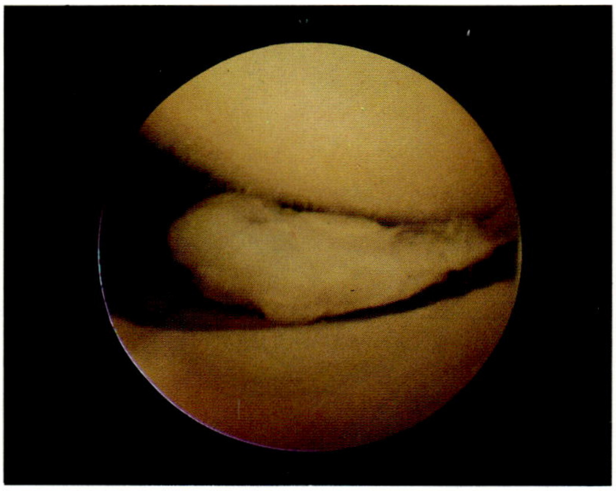

Fig. 7-16. A frequent source of loose bodies is the patella. This loose body was found still attached by a most precarious cartilaginous pedicle, which allowed it to flap to and fro. It was easily removed arthroscopically.

of the hamstrings and quadriceps as well as recurvatum of the knee. Due to severe neurological involvement, he was previously treated with a pantalar arthrodesis. This patient twisted his knee, incurring a hemarthrosis. An arthrogram was questionably positive for a medial meniscal tear. Arthroscopy was performed, which showed an osteocartilaginous fracture from the lateral femoral condyle trapped within the lateral joint line (Fig. 7-14). Considerable difficulty was experienced in grasping this object, as the proper instruments were not available. The loose body was finally removed from beneath the inferior surface of the posterior third of the lateral meniscus and the lateral tibial plateau, as it had slipped back into this recess. Arthrotomy had been avoided, with its resultant quadriceps wasting in a patient who could ill afford any further muscle weakness, albeit temporary.

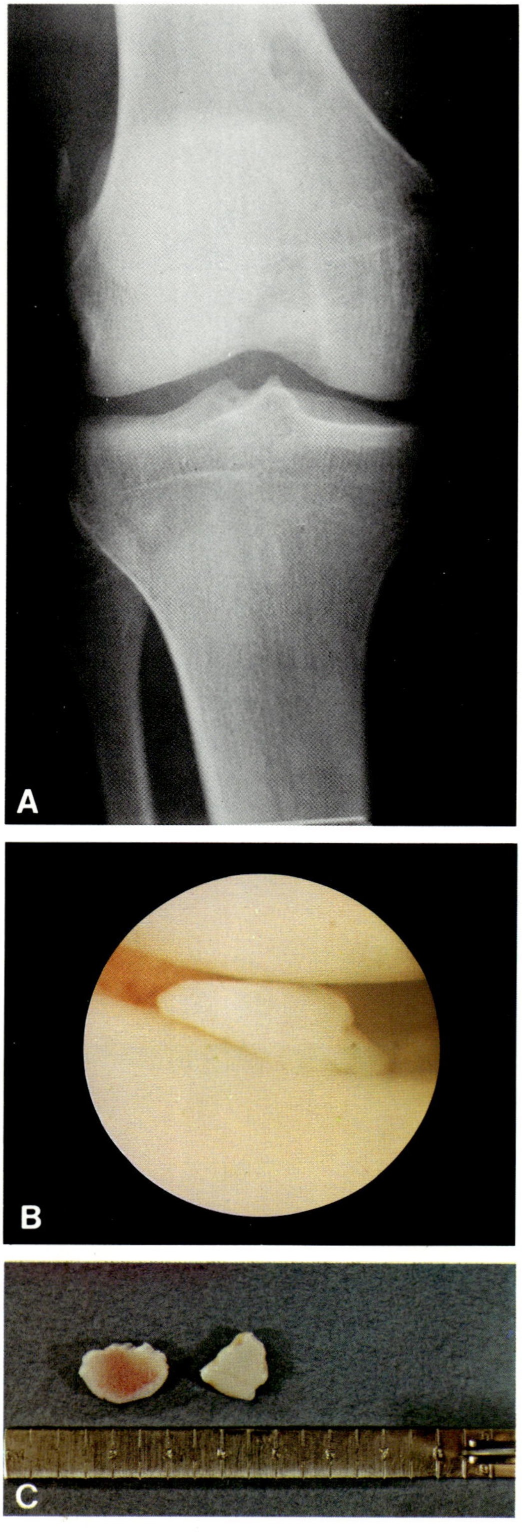

Fig. 7-17. (*A*) A 20-year-old football player dislocated his patella. Roentgenograms demonstrated a loose body. He was casted and 6 weeks later arthroscopy was undertaken. Two osteocartilaginous loose bodies were removed using the double-puncture technique. (*B*) Osteocartilaginous loose body between patella and femur. (*C*) Specimen: 2 osteocartilaginous loose bodies.

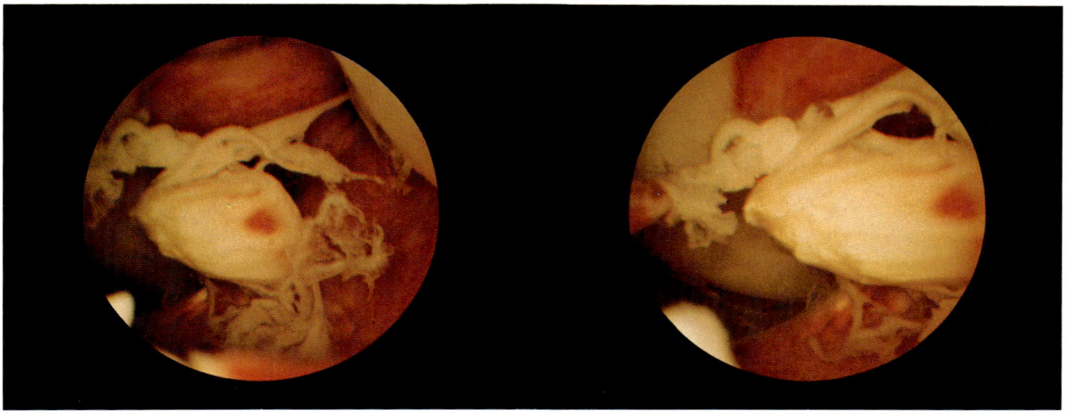

Fig. 7-18. A high school football player avulsed a fragment of meniscus, presenting what appeared to be a displaced knee cartilage. Arthroscopically the menisci appeared normal, but this loose body within the intercondylar notch, and responsible for his lack of full extension, was histologically identified as fibrocartilage. It was removed with the operating arthroscope and the single-puncture technique.

The possibility of a cartilaginous loose body must be kept on the list of diagnostic possibilities in order to allow quicker diagnosis and treatment.

Case 7-5. Removal of Cartilaginous Loose Body

An 18-year-old high school football player was treated in 1973 for a tear of the lateral meniscus. At that time, mild fragmentation of the lateral tibial plateau was noted, and a hypermobile medial meniscus was diagnosed arthroscopically. In 1974, while playing football, he reinjured his knee and presented with medial joint line pain and tenderness. Repeat arthroscopy revealed a cartilaginous loose body, which was found in the lateral aspect of the joint and removed (Fig. 7-15). The patient missed only five days of football practice.

Case 7-6. Pedunculated Loose Body

While cartilaginous loose bodies frequently arise from the patella, a pedunculated cartilaginous fragment is an infrequent finding and was the cause of retropatellar pain, crepitus, and giving way in this 55-year-old male (Fig. 7-16).

Case 7-7. Loose Bodies Resulting From Patellar Dislocation

A 20-year-old football player dislocated his patella. The dislocation was reduced on the playing field. Post-reduction roentgenograms demonstrated several osteocartilaginous loose bodies. Following 6 weeks of casting, arthroscopy was used to remove these loose bodies (Fig. 7-17).

Case 7-8. An Avulsed Fragment of Meniscus Mimicking a Hyaline Cartilage Loose Body

A high school football player presented with the clinical appearance of a displaced bucket handle tear of the medial meniscus. Arthroscopically no evidence of a meniscal tear was found, but a fragment of meniscus (histological examination demonstrated fibrocartilage) was found in the intercondylar notch. Removal with the operating arthroscope through a single puncture re-established full extension (Fig. 7-18).

REFERENCES

1. Eikilar, H.: Arthroscopy of the Knee. The Netherlands. Royal United Printers, Hoitsema B. V., 1975.
2. Nicholas, J. A., Freiberger, R. H., and Killbran, P. J.: Double contrast arthrography of the knee—its value in the management of two hundred and twenty-five knee derangements. J. Bone Joint Surg., *52A*:203, 1970.
3. Watanabe, M., Takeda, S., and Ikeuchi, H.: Atlas of Arthroscopy. ed. 2. Tokyo, Igaku Shoin Ltd., 1969.

8 Arthroscopy of the Acutely Injured Knee

DIAGNOSIS OF ACUTE INJURIES

In the acutely injured knee, arthroscopy is necessary to more accurately verify the pathology and determine the extent of the capsular laxity. Adequate visualization can be obtained if the joint is first aspirated of bloody fluid and irrigated with saline solution until the color of the effluent is a pale pink. This is rapidly accomplished with the Toomey syringe. When a clear irrigating flow has been established, insert the arthroscope. If necessary, the tourniquet may be inflated.

Rotational stresses that tear the medial capsule of the joint do not always leave the remaining compartments inviolate. Injury may include the menisci, cruciate ligaments or the articular cartilage of the femoral condyle, tibia, or patellofemoral articulation. The most frequent site of ligamentous injury within the knee is the anterior cruciate ligament, followed by the medial aspect and the posterior medial corner in particular.

Arthroscopy has been beneficial in most situations where laxity is borderline to either anteroposterior or valgus stress. The key to comprehension of the pathology resides in observation of the behavior of the medial meniscus while the leg is subjected to external rotational and valgus stress.[1] In severe tears of the medial capsular complex, the medial meniscus "bow-strings" across the medial tibial plateau proportionally to the degree of capsular involvement, and the capsular defect may be noted either superior or inferior to the meniscus. Only rarely is the meniscus itself torn. Integrity of the anterior cruciate ligament can be established by attempting the drawer test under direct vision. This is best done as soon after injury as possible before the synovium hypertrophies, obscuring visualization of the underlying cruciate ligament. If the synovium is not torn but is thin and the lesion is seen early, an interstitial tear of the ligament can be seen. In rotational stress, the lateral compartment does not always escape injury, and frequently one sees a tear of the lateral meniscus or a loose body. Despite reports to the contrary, visualization of the lateral compartment during the course of medial capsular repair or even during the course of medial meniscectomy is not as adequate as that obtainable by use of the arthroscope.

Case 8-1. "Unhappy Triad" and Tear of Lateral Meniscus

An 18-year-old football player hit from the side on a partially flexed knee was examined

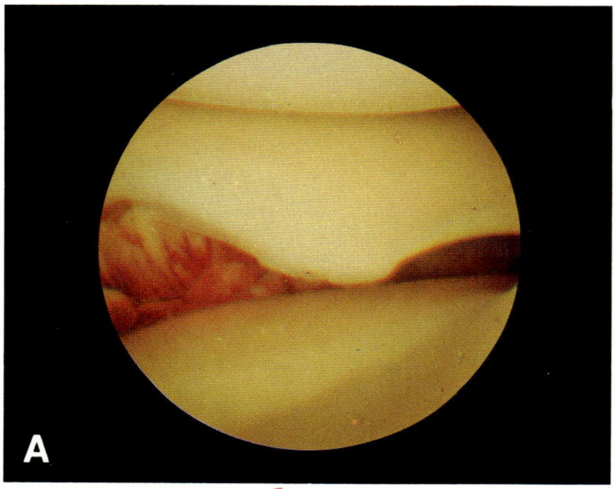

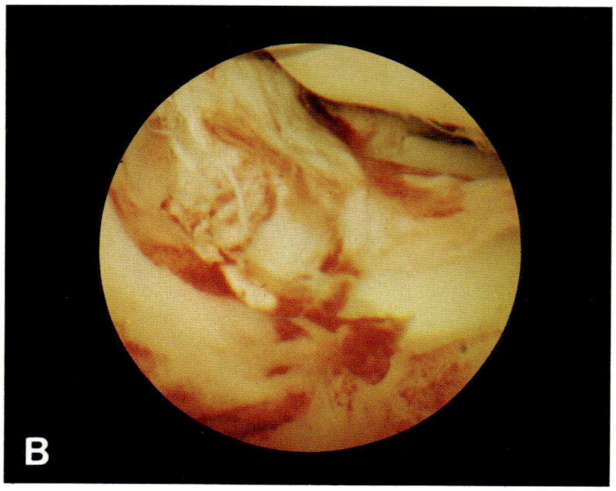

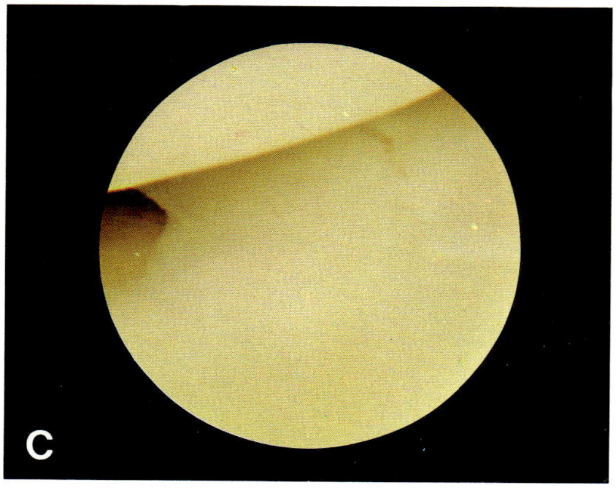

Fig. 8-1. Acute "unhappy triad" and torn lateral meniscus. (*A*) Medial joint line of the left knee. Note the separation between the medial femoral condyle and the tibia; the meniscus protrudes towards the intercondylar notch. Beneath the meniscus, the tear involving the menisco-tibial portion of the deep capsular ligament can be seen. (*B*) The partially torn anterior cruciate ligament protrudes into the lateral joint line. (*C*) The middle third of the lateral meniscus demonstrates the anterior extent of the tear. In addition, there was a hemorrhagic separation of the lateral meniscus from the capsule, that ran parallel to this tear.

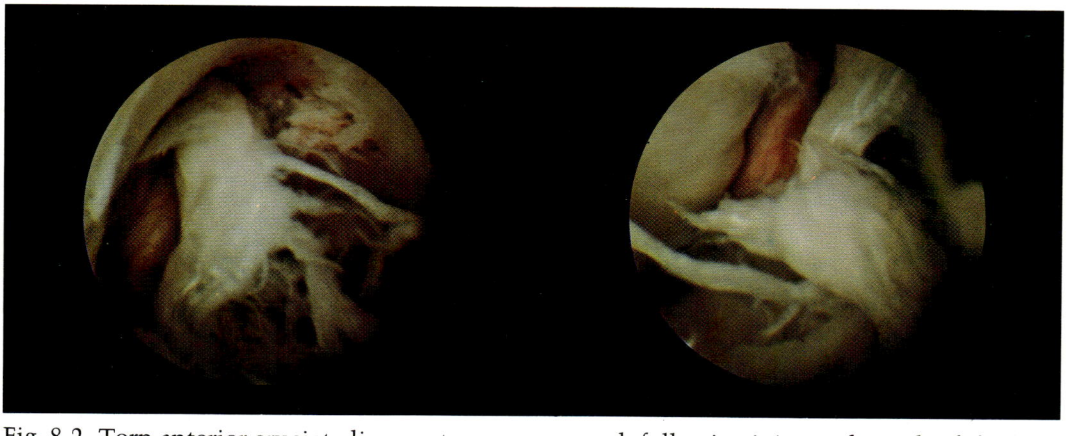

Fig. 8-2. Torn anterior cruciate ligament seen one month following injury. The ends of the ligament are resorbing, but still have not rounded off.

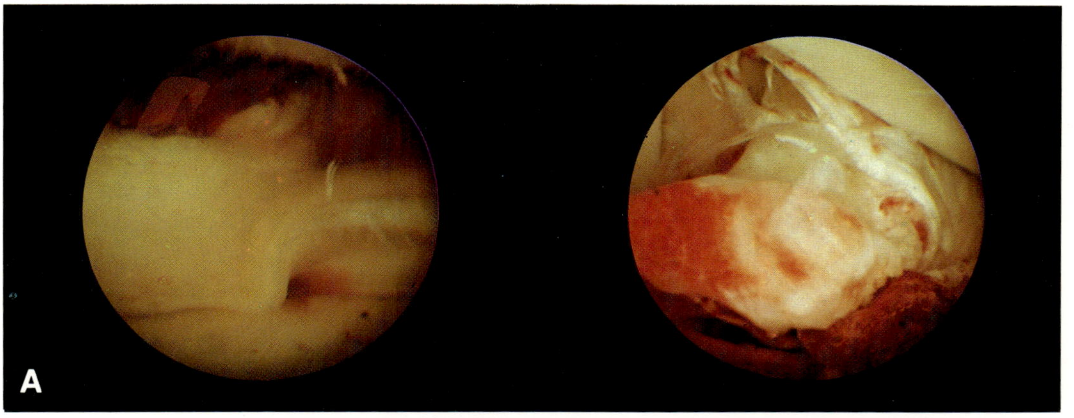

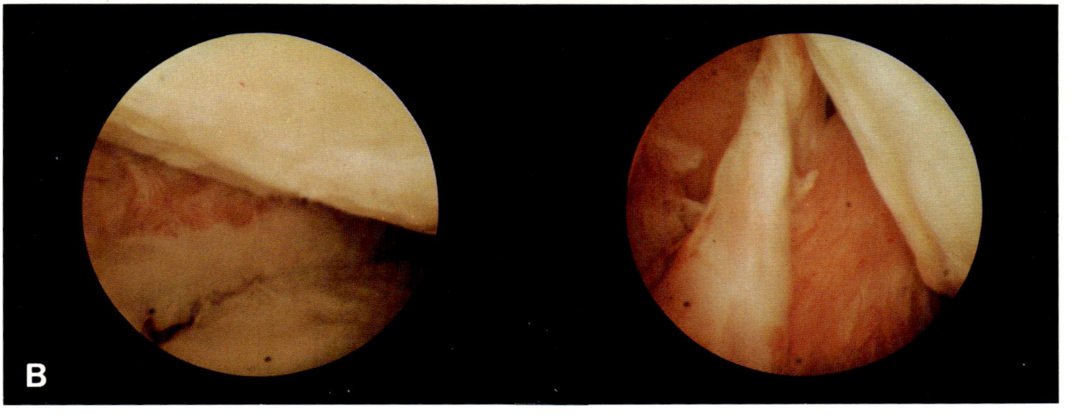

Fig. 8-3. (*A*) Acute tear of the medial capsule, and avulsion of the anterior cruciate ligament from the tibia. (*Left*) The tear of the menisco-femoral portion of the deep capsular ligament can be seen above the body of the meniscus. (*Right*) The cancellous base of the avulsed bone attached to the anterior cruciate ligament. (*B*) Three months later, repeat arthroscopy demonstrated a tight medial joint line and small "reformed" medial meniscus (*left*). The anterior cruciate ligament is solidly attached and functional. However, note the abundant synovial covering over the anterior cruciate ligament. (Courtesy of Dr. Robert Allen, Glendora, Calif.)

5 days after injury. He was unable to walk, and examination revealed a restricted range of motion and moderate laxity to anterior-posterior and valgus stress. These estimates of laxity were increased under anesthesia. Arthroscopy revealed a tear of the deep medial capsular ligament extending anterior to the medial collateral ligament (Fig. 8-1A). The anterior cruciate ligament was partially torn (Fig. 8-1B) the lateral meniscus was torn in its posterior half (Fig. 8-1C) and the peripheral margin was separated from the capsule.

Neither this meniscal tear nor the peripheral attachment separation could have been diagnosed with certitude without arthroscopy.

Arthroscopy obtains its greatest diagnostic yield in patients with a twisting injury, a hemarthrosis, and either absent or minimal instability to valgus stress. The diagnostic benefits are twofold. The joint can be adequately examined clinically under general anesthetic, and assess-

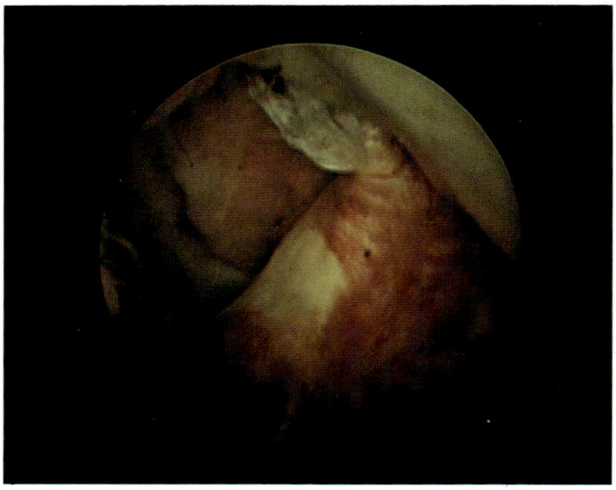

Fig. 8-4. Tear of a single fasciculus of the anterior cruciate ligament resulted in massive hemarthrosis and pseudolocking.

ment of the problem can be completed reliably by arthroscopy. The following case exemplifies this.

Case 8-2. Mop-End Tear of the Anterior Cruciate Ligament

A 58-year-old fireman jumped over a fence, incurring a valgus strain of the knee. He felt a sharp snap; an effusion started soon afterwards. When he was seen one month following the injury, the effusion was subsiding and no instability to anterior-posterior or valgus stress was noted. There was tenderness to palpation of the medial capsule, and the patient could momentarily lock his knee by attempting to hyperextend it. An arthrogram revealed a small hole in the posterior medial capsule. Arthroscopy was performed, which showed a mop-end tear of the anterior cruciate ligament from its femoral origin (Fig. 8-2) protrusion of the medial meniscus into the joint, and posterior capsular laxity. Along with the medial meniscectomy that had been contemplated, repair of the posterior capsule and pes anserinus transplantation was performed.

In the following case, conventional methods of diagnosis did not fully assess the situation.

Case 8-3. Avulsion of the Anterior Cruciate Insertion

A 55-year-old male was hit by a car, incurring anteromedial instability of the left knee and a tear of the medial meniscus of the right knee. Roentgenograms revealed a fracture through the anterior tibial spine of the left knee. Arthroscopy, however, showed bow-stringing of the medial meniscus over the medial tibial plateau and a large capsular defect superior to the meniscus (Fig. 8-3A). The anterior cruciate ligament was found attached to a corticocancellous fragment avulsed from the tibial plateau. The patient was treated by reattachment of the anterior cruciate fragment to the medial tibial plateau and posterior medial capsular repair. Three months later the medial capsule was found to be completely healed and stable, and the cruciate ligament was without evidence of laxity (Fig. 8-3B).

Case 8-4. Fascicular Tear of the Anterior Cruciate Ligament

A 16-year-old female suffered a twisting injury while water skiing at high speed. A hemarthrosis was present, but there was no joint instability. Arthroscopy revealed a tear of one fasciculus of the anterior cruciate ligament (Fig. 8-4); the rest of the ligament was normal. After arthroscopy, her pseudolocking disappeared, and after quadriceps exercises she was able to return to her sport.

Occasionally visualization of the intercondylar notch is difficult, due to the overlying ligamentum mucosum, fat pad, and hemorrhage. The following is an example of this situation.

Case 8-5. Excision of the Anterior Cruciate Ligament Insertion

A 28-year-old male incurred a twisting injury with resulting hemarthrosis but an apparently stable joint. Examination under anesthesia revealed laxity to valgus stress, and roentgenograms showed an osteocartilaginous loose body beneath the kneecap. The anterior cruciate ligament appeared to be torn, but the

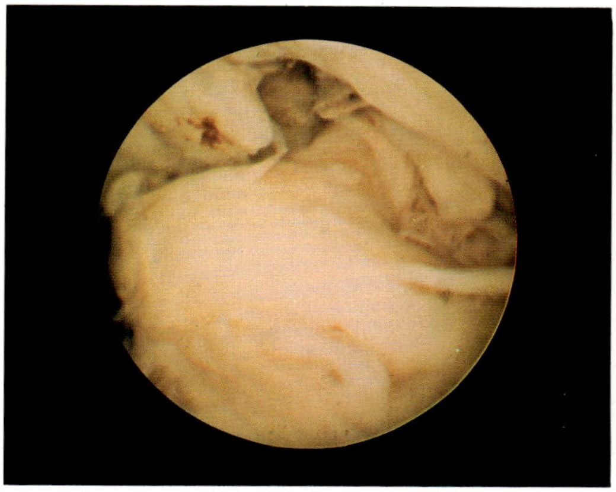

Fig. 8-5. This large bony mass has become rounded, and has increased in size. The anterior cruciate ligament has been replaced with lax fibrous tissue. (Courtesy of Dr. Robert Allen, Glendora, Calif.)

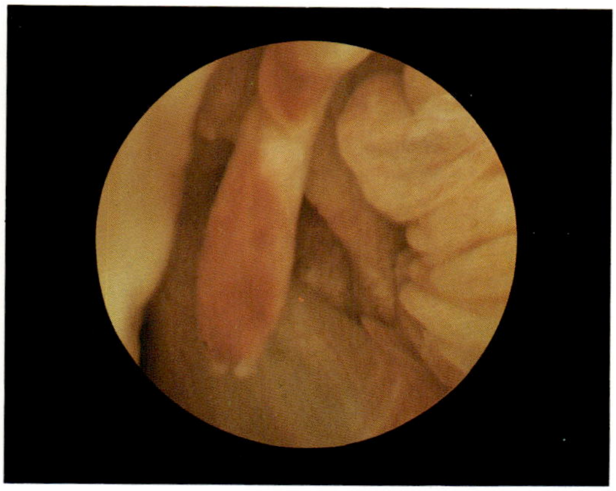

Fig. 8-6. Not all stable hemarthritic knees following a twisting injury, result from "isolated tears of the anterior cruciate ligament." This patient's symptoms are due to an "isolated" (i.e., no other causitive agent identified) tear of the ligamentum mucosum. Note the normal anterior cruciate ligament and posterior cruciate ligament.

loose body could not be found. The behavior of the medial meniscus to valgus stress and external rotary laxity was marked, and it was felt that an operation was indicated. The patient wished surgery done in a hospital closer to his home. A ligamentous repair was performed elsewhere and the patient did amazingly well, considering that he was unable to extend the terminal 15 degrees. Following another twisting injury and hemarthrosis, he was seen again. Roentgenograms of the knee showed the osteocartilaginous mass still present inferior to the patella. Arthroscopy was

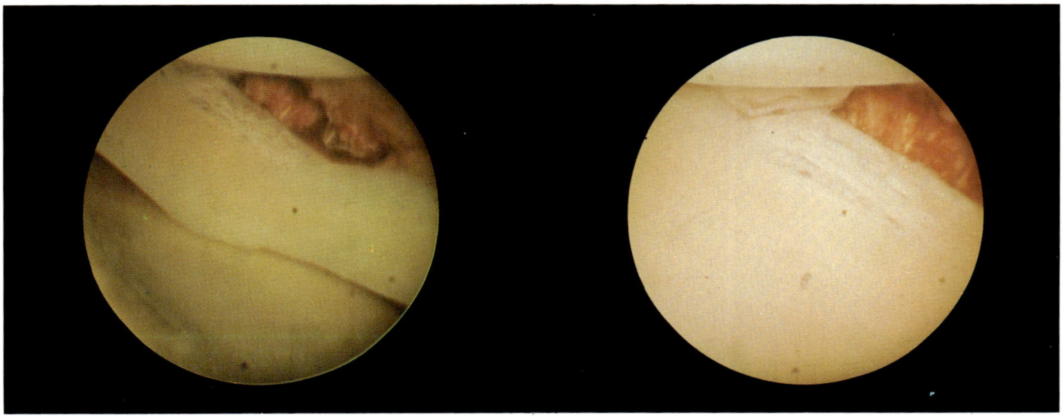

Fig. 8-7. Tear of medial capsule and medial meniscus. Generally with a severe medial ligamentous injury, only the mooring of the meniscus is torn, not the meniscus itself. In this patient, however, the deep capsular ligament, as well as the medial meniscus, was torn. At the time of ligament repair, meniscal excision became manditory (*right*). The tear in the periphery of the meniscus is quite obvious.

performed, revealing that the loose body was still attached to fibrous tissue from the lateral femoral condyle, which represented the remnants of the anterior cruciate ligament (Fig. 8-5). The block to extension of his knee was due to hypertrophy of the overlying cartilage of the osteochrondral fragment. This was excised, resulting in full extension.

Since performing arthroscopy is slightly more difficult in the acute knee, sufficient experience should be gained with arthroscopy with the chronic problems before tackling a patient with an acute injury. Until one is reasonably sure that the meniscal reaction to valgus stress in external tibial rotation is deviant, observations of abnormal meniscal behavior may only tend to cause confusion. Two more cases are discussed with Figs. 8-6 and 8-7.

REFERENCE

1. O'Connor, R. L.: Arthroscopy in the diagnosis and treatment of acute ligament injures of the knee. J. Bone Joint Surg., *56A:* 333, 1974.

9 The Septic Knee

DIAGNOSIS AND MANAGEMENT

Fortunately, my experience with the septic knee has been minimal. However, arthroscopy appears to have a definite role in the diagnosis and management of septic knee problems.* If the infection occurs postoperatively, involving the wound, the standard techniques of opening the wound and debridement are indicated. However, there are occasions when the wound appears to be healing well and the infection is not predominantly at the surgical site or the wound may have completely closed and the joint infection becomes obvious several weeks later. These cases, as well as those of hematogenously incurred sepsis, can be effectively treated with the arthroscope.

The postoperative onset of knee sepsis is usually heralded by an elevated temperature and white count, quadriceps inhibition, and severe pain. These findings certainly raise the index of suspicion. Absolute proof of joint infection depends on a positive bacterial culture of the synovial fluid, but such a finding occasionally is lacking. Arthroscopy allows inspection of the postoperative joint suspected of infection and allows another chance for culture of the synovial fluid and for biopsy of the synovium under direct vision. The synovial tissue may be minced for culture. If after arthroscopy the clinician is still suspicious or the bacterial culture positive, closed-circuit irrigation may be installed through the arthroscope. Arthroscopy also has a place in the management of the septic knee after clinical abortion of the infectious process.

Case 9-1. Hematogenous Septic Arthritis

A 31-year-old male was involved in an industrial accident in which he incurred a contusion of his left knee. Several weeks later, the knee became painful and swollen. Roentgenograms were negative. Aspiration of the knee yielded an increased white cell count of the synovial fluid and a positive culture for *Staphylococcus aureus* coagulase-positive. Irrigation tubes were inserted in the knee blindly. Forty-eight hours later, after malfunction of the tubes, the patient was referred for arthroscopy. The culture remained positive. Arthroscopy was performed, which revealed whitish placques scattered within the synovium. Normal cartilaginous surfaces of the femoral condyles, tibia, and patella were noted. Irrigation tubes were placed through the arthroscope using a medium-sized Hemovac to exit medially in the suprapatellar pouch and laterally through the posterolateral joint line. The joint

* Jackson, R. W.: Personal communication, 1974.

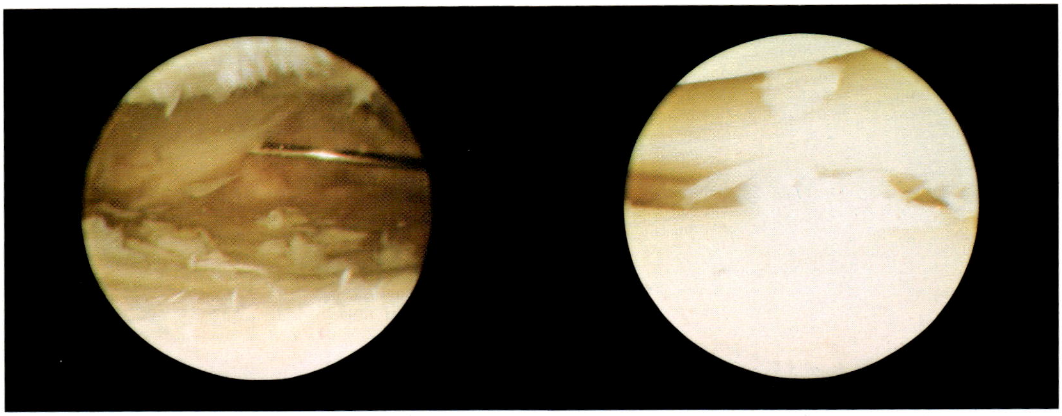

Fig. 9-1. (*Left*) Quadriceps bursa: fibrillation of the retropatellar surface is now evident. The synovium is becoming increasingly fibrotic, and synovial slough is present in both the quadriceps bursa and the lateral joint line (*right*).

was perfused with antibiotics for a 5-day period and after two negative cultures, the tubes were withdrawn. The patient's white count rapidly returned to normal, although his quadriceps inhibition persisted and his range of motion was slow to return. The patient returned to work in 2 months. Six months later, however, when the patient was seen prior to discharge, marked crepitus was noted on flexion and extension of the knee, although the patient's effusion had subsided many months ago and his range of motion had returned. On examination, very minimal quadriceps atrophy was noted with no increase in the girth of the knee. Repeat arthroscopy revealed evidence of necrotic synovium that had been sloughed into the joint proper (Fig. 9-1). The villous contour of the synovium had been replaced by increased fibrosis, and the undersurface of the cartilage of the patella showed marked evidence of chondromalacia, as well as some cartilaginous degeneration of the medial femoral condyle. The necrotic tissue was removed by lavage.

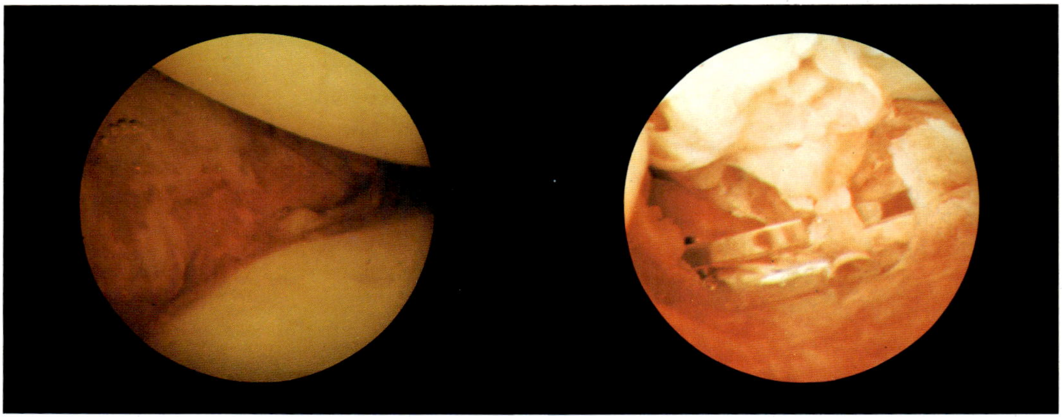

Fig. 9-2. Septic arthritis 6 days following medial meniscectomy. (*Left*) Medial joint line. (*Right*) Medium-sized drainage tube has been installed in lateral joint line.

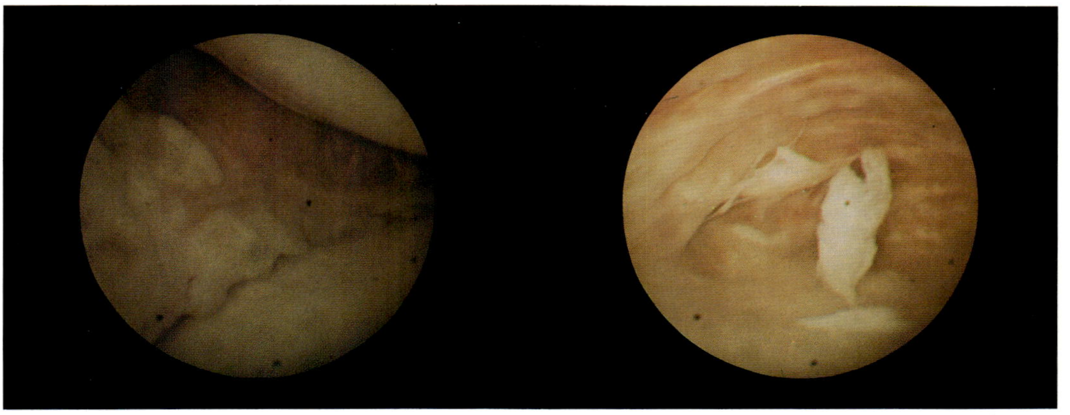

Fig. 9-3. The same knee as in Fig. 9-2, 3 months following irrigation-drainage. (*Left*) Medial joint line: compare with Fig. 9-2, *left*. (*Right*) Quadriceps bursa: note the synovial debris and the increasing fibrosis of the synovium.

Case 9-2. Postoperative Joint Sepsis

A 48-year-old fireman had been disabled for several years, owing to an industrial accident. Because of continuing complaints following a lateral meniscectomy 6 years previously, arthroscopy was performed, and it showed a tear of the posterior third of the medial meniscus with moderate degeneration of both medial and lateral compartments. Due to Workmen's Compensation problems, a medial meniscectomy was delayed for a month, but, when performed, was relatively atraumatic. He was capable of straight leg raising on the first postoperative day, but thereafter quadriceps strength decreased and his pain significantly increased in the knee. The white count remained normal, and on the third postoperative day the patient was discharged home.

Several days later a tense effusion was present. A specimen was taken for culture, and tests revealed a hemolytic *Staphylococcus aureus*, coagulase-positive. There was a small amount of redness at the operative site. Arthroscopy was performed on the sixth postoperative day (Fig. 9-2). The synovium appeared reddened, inflamed, and edematous. Only scattered opaque placques in the synovium were noted. Two tubes were inserted for continuous irrigation, and the medial knee incision was opened down to the capsule. The drainage from the exit tube was cultured 48 hours following arthroscopy, and the culture grew out *Pseudomonas* instead of *Staphylococcus aureus*. The antibiotics were switched, and the tubes were kept in place for another 5 days, at which time the effluent tube culture was negative. The tubes were withdrawn from the joint, and mobilization of the knee was started. The effusion decreased rapidly, but the quadriceps strength was slow to return.

Three months following arthroscopy, the patient returned with a swollen, warm knee. Aspiration of the effusion revealed cloudy synovial fluid containing whitish particulate matter. A white count was normal and the culture yielded no growth. Arthroscopy was performed, and multiple necrotic bodies were irrigated from the joint (Fig. 9-3). Following this, the effusion decreased dramatically, and the patient has had little disability since, and he has redeveloped his quadriceps to a good degree.

Arthroscopy is contraindicated when there is a recent abrasion of the skin or an abscess involving the region of the knee.[1] I do not feel that arthroscopy and closed-circuit irrigation is contraindicated unless the particulate matter within the joint is so heavy and thick that good drainage cannot be established. In the postoperative infection, this technique is not a substitute for adequate wound care, it may be instituted concurrently. If the particulate matter within the knee is of large diameter and cloggage of the tubes is a possibility, the joint should be opened immediately in the conventional manner.

REFERENCE

1. Casscells, S. W.: American Academy of Orthopaedic Surgeons Instructional Course: Arthroscopy and Arthrography of the Knee. Boston, 1975.

10 *Postoperative Joint Assessment*

AREAS OF POSTOPERATIVE CHANGE

Complaints following surgery of the knee continue to plague both the patient and the physician. The clinical tests, supplemented by the arthrogram, do not always yield useful information. However, arthroscopy provides information that has been otherwise unavailable.[1]

Synovium

Synovial changes may well persist after arthrotomy. Subacute synovitis is manifested by edematous villi, increased vascularity, and occasional fibrotic change. This synovitis may be secondary to continuing or increased hyaline cartilaginous degeneration and, if so, may well respond to irrigation of the joint at the time of arthroscopy. Follow-up studies of the regenerated synovium, following synovectomy, has recently been found to be of benefit.[2]

Patella

Arthroscopy may also permit study of the results of operations on the patella,* such as shaving or drilling (Fig. 10-1).

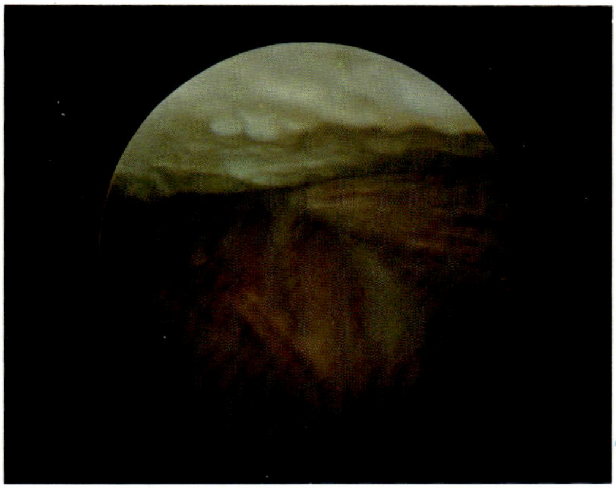

Fig. 10-1. The retropatellar surface 6 months following patelloplasty in a patient still symptomatic. The surface is studied with magnification, yet appears relatively smooth. Can this be the cause of this patient's continuing complaints?

Case 10-1. Fragmented Articular Cartilage

A 31-year-old female incurred an industrial injury. Her surgeon performed arthrotomy on the knee, at which time he performed a patellar shaving. The suspected meniscal tear was not found. Because of continuing complaints and markedly limited range of motion, arthroscopy was repeated, and it showed swollen fragmented articular cartilage of the undersurface of the patella (Fig. 10-2). This was widespread

* Joyce, J.: Personal communication, 1974.

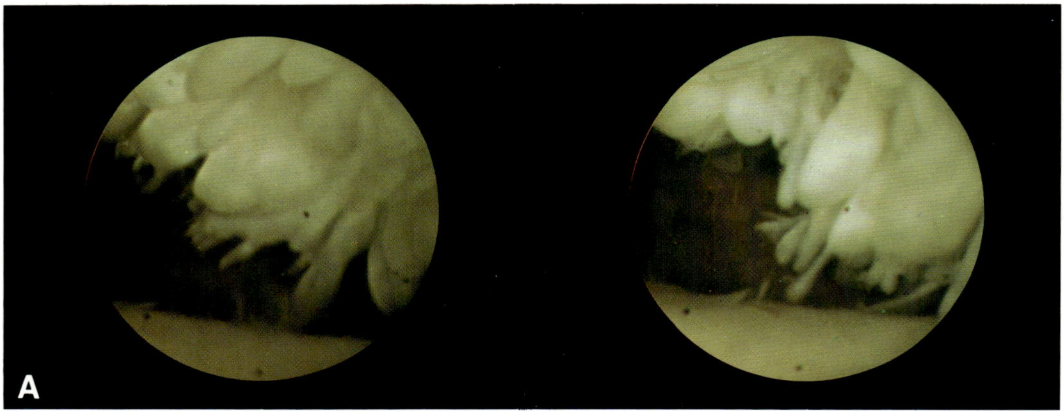

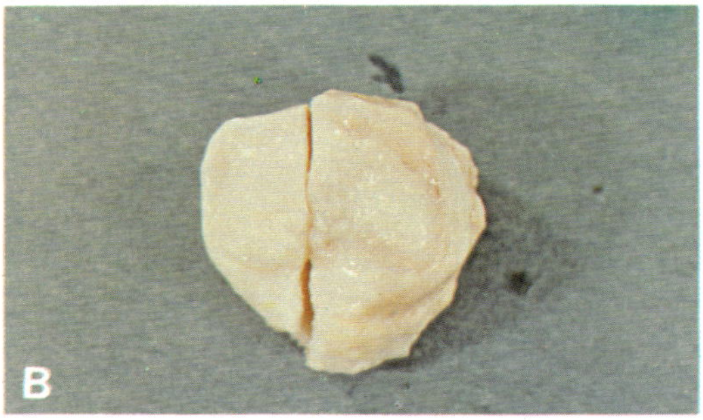

Fig. 10-2. (*A*) Fragmentation of the patellar cartilage. (*Right*) Note the globular appearance. (*B*) Surgical specimen.

throughout the patella, so the patient was treated by patellectomy.

Articular Cartilage

Arthroscopic findings can be important in assessing the damage of the articular cartilage, whether it be an osteochondritis dissecans or a crater defect of the condyle or tibial plateau following meniscal tears (see Chap. 6).

Anterior Cruciate Ligament

Following repair of the anterior cruciate ligament, arthroscopic assessment can be made of the stability of the joint or laxity of the repaired ligament.* I have had no experience examining either transplanted or reconstructed anterior cruciate ligaments or anterior cruciate ligament prosthetic replacements, but such investigation is presently being carried out by others.

* Marshall, J.: Personal communication, 1975.

Posterior Medial Capsular Tear

Assessment of medial capsular laxity following reconstruction of a posterior medial capsular tear allows assessment of the general stability of the posterior medial corner. When excessive rotary laxity persists, there is an increased space posterior to the medial femoral condyle, as has been noted by Nicholas[3] during arthrographic assessment of the knee with posterior capsular laxity. The arthroscope can be passed behind the femoral condyle, and in this region one has a good view of the posterior cruciate ligament (see Fig. 3-14).

Case 10-2. Posterior Capsular Defect

A 33-year-old policeman suffered an injury to his knee and was treated by medial meniscectomy. However, he was unable to return to duty. Following another twist of his knee, he complained of increased instability with inability to pivot, and stated that he could not run. Arthroscopy revealed a retained fragment

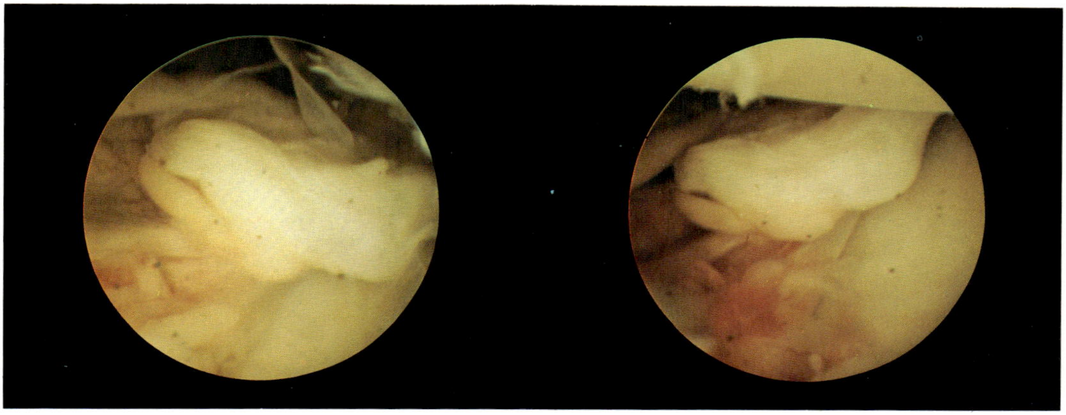

Fig. 10-3. Retained fragment of medial meniscus of the right knee. (*Left*) Note the large space posterior to the medial femoral condyle, due to medial capsular and external rotatory laxity. Normally a large-diameter arthroscope cannot pass into this area by the anterior approach.

in the posterior medial corner of the joint, which had large capsular space posterior to the medial femoral condyle (Fig. 10-3). The patient was treated by repair of the posterior capsular defect and pes anserinus transplant. He was then able to go back to work.

Retained Versus Reformed Meniscus

For clinical as well as medicolegal reasons, postoperative assessment of the meniscus is occasionally necessary. Many patients complain postoperatively of giving way of their knee. Usually this is due to persistent quadriceps weakness and failure to completely rehabilitate the knee, but it may also be due to such other factors as loose bodies, catilaginous incongruity of the joint surfaces, or a retained fragment of the meniscus (Fig. 10-4). Arthrography may well demonstrate the presence of a triangular or wedge-shaped mass lying in the place usually occupied by the meniscus. Often, evaluating the actual size of the fragment and declaring it to be a retained or reformed meniscus is out of the realm of competence of the arthrographer; however, the arthroscope can reveal not only the relative size of the structure, but also its integrity and whether it displaces within the joint to cause obstruction of motion (Fig. 10-5).

After reviewing many of these reformed menisci, I find it difficult to agree with

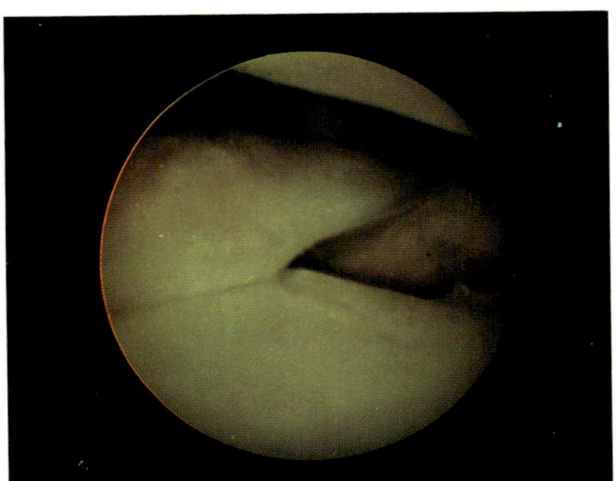

Fig. 10-4. Small retained fragment of posterior lateral meniscus. It is doubtful that this fragment is causing symptoms. It is small, rounded, and has a firm attachment to the tibia; I believe it would be erroneous to ascribe symptoms to this finding.

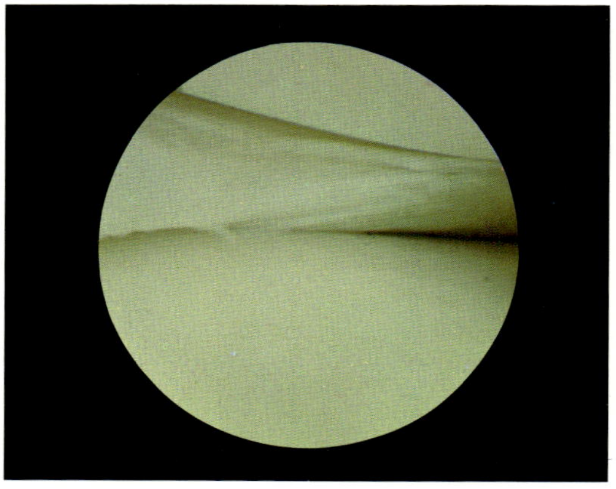

Fig. 10-5. Retained posterior third of the lateral meniscus of the right knee. Note the tear within its substance. This tear caused locking, and its mobility could be demonstrated dynamically at arthroscopy. The patient's symptoms abated following arthrotomy and meniscal excision.

Smillie's contention that they are structures of any importance besides possibly their lubricating function.[4] Certainly they do not add stability to the joint, as they are, in my experience, usually very thin (Fig. 10-6). Recently Iseaki reported his findings on over 100 reformed menisci.[2] He found no correlation between the degree of regeneration of the menisci and protection of the hyaline cartilage of the tibia and femur. When arthroscopically viewing these knees in 90 degrees of flexion, marked incongruity was noted between the femur and tibia, indicating that this structure assumes little function in integrating the complex movements of the knee. A retained piece of meniscus may cause symptoms if it is capable of protruding between the tibia and the femur; however, the majority of retained meniscal fragments are attached peripherally to the capsule and cannot protrude beneath the condyle to catch within the joint. If the retained fragment of the meniscus has a peripheral attachment, it seems to blend into the reformed meniscus (Fig. 10-7). The reformed meniscus may serve a practical function as a landmark during arthroscopy: when assessing the stability of a deep capsular ligament on the medial aspect, if one can see the entire peripheral margin of the reformed meniscus, this indicates that considerable laxity to valgus stress and external rotatory stress is present (Fig. 10-7). In one case a reformed meniscus was surrounded by intra-articular adhesions (Figs. 10-8, 10-9).

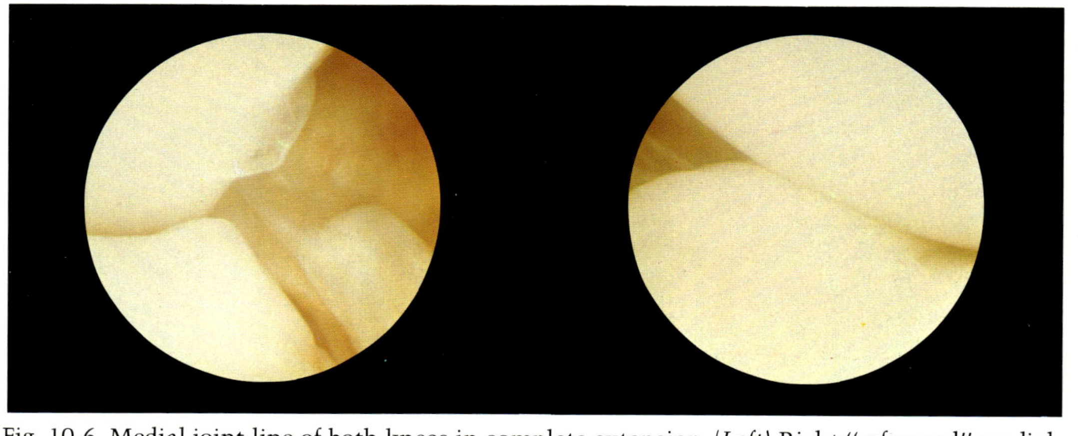

Fig. 10-6. Medial joint line of both knees in complete extension. (*Left*) Right "reformed" medial meniscus does not articulate with the femur or tibia. (*Right*) Left medial meniscus articulates with both the medial femoral condyle and the medial tibial plateau.

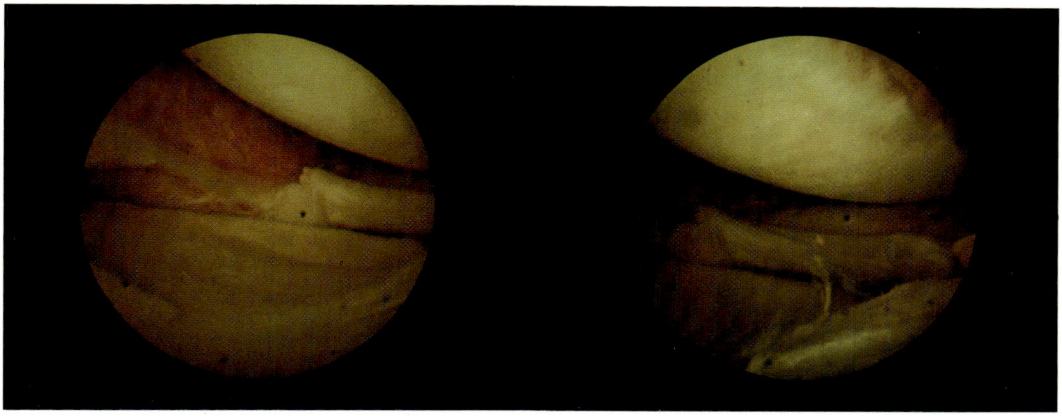

Fig. 10-7. Reformed and retained medial meniscus of the left knee. A small "reformed meniscus" has gained attachment to the retained peripheral rim posterior. Note the wide separation between the medial femoral condyle and the medial tibial plateau. Excision of this meniscus will not alleviate the patient's symptoms, which are due to postoperative capsular laxity—not to meniscal mobility.

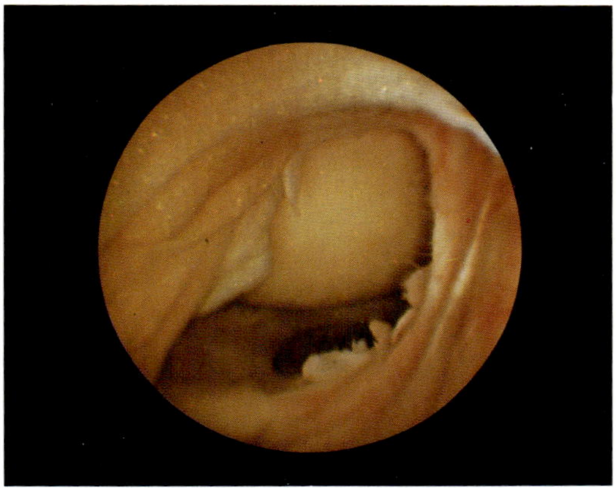

Fig. 10-8. A "reformed" lateral meniscus is seen surrounded by intra-articular adhesions.

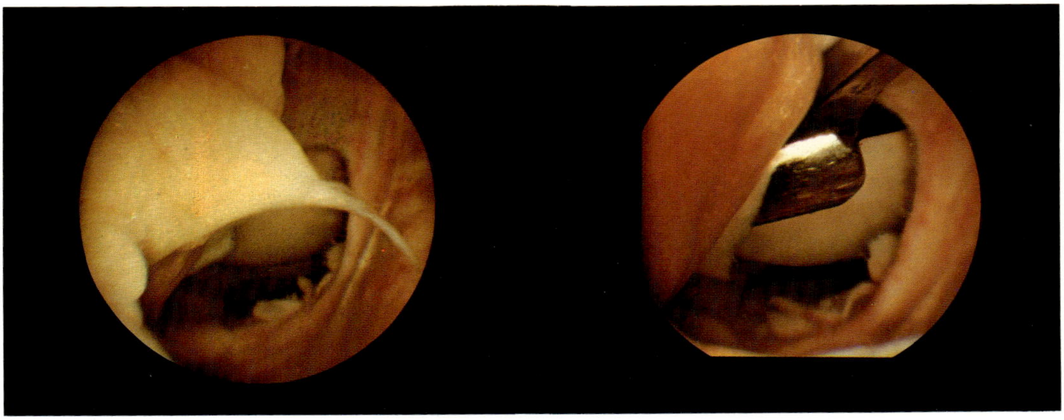

Fig. 10-9. Same knee as in Fig. 10-8. The patient's symptoms were ameliorated by surgical lysis of these thick adhesive bands.

Loose Bodies

Frequently, cartilaginous loose bodies are found postoperatively and may cause considerable complaints. Dandy and Jackson state that condylar degeneration and loose bodies, rather than the retained posterior horn of the meniscus, are responsible for the majority of post-meniscectomy complaints (see Chap. 7).[1]

REFERENCES

1. Dandy, D. J., and Jackson, R. W.: The diagnosis of problems after meniscectomy. J. Bone Joint Surg., *57B*:349, 1975.
2. Iseaki, F.: The Regenerated Meniscus with Special Reference to Functional Anatomy. Second Congress, Interantional Arthroscopy Association Meeting. Copenhagen, Denmark, July, 1975.
3. Nicholas, J. A.: The five-one reconstruction for anteromedial instability of the knee. Indications, technique, and the results in fifty-two patients. J. Bone Joint Surg., *55A*:901, 1973.
4. Smillie, I. S.: Injuries of the Knee Joint. Baltimore, Williams & Wilkins, 1974.
5. Watanabe, M., Takeda, S., and Ikeuchi, H.: Atlas of Arthroscopy. ed. 2. Tokyo, Igaku Shoin, 1969.

11 *Other Intra-articular Problems*

In the preceding chapters, I have described the use of the arthroscope for more than diagnostic purposes. As with any endoscopic procedure, familiarization with the instrumentation and learning to properly interpret the information it reveals initially take precedence over treatment. As the arthroscopist develops more confidence in technique and becomes able to maneuver the instrument within the joint, surgical possibilities arise. The limiting factor is experience, confidence, and—even with the experienced arthroscopist—ingenuity. It is hoped from this discussion, which attempts to summarize the current status of intra-articular arthroscopic surgery, the horizon will be broadened so that new ideas will supercede present ones.

The ability to remove loose bodies is well established; the procedure is performed by many arthroscopists at this time. Synovial biopsy is of particular interest to the rheumatologist, but also on occasion to the orthopaedic surgeon. Excision of synovial tags is occasionally per-

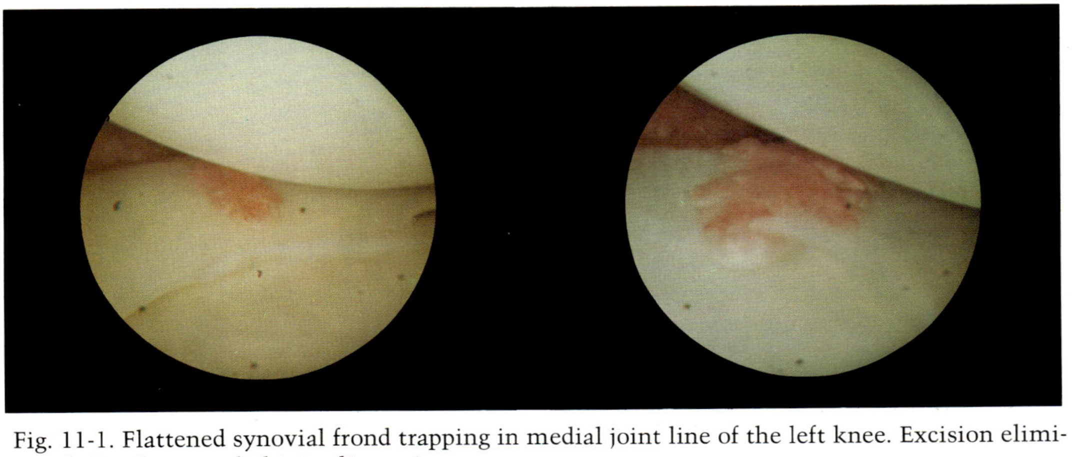

Fig. 11-1. Flattened synovial frond trapping in medial joint line of the left knee. Excision eliminated the sharp medial joint line pain.

formed arthroscopically if there is evidence of significant hypertrophy of an area of synovium that may be trapped within the joint, causing pain (Fig. 11-1). R. W. Jackson has told me (1973) of arthroscopic excision of meniscal tags trapped within the joint in several cases.

HYPERTROPHY OF THE MEDIAL INTRA-ARTICULAR BAND

Occasional hypertrophy of the medial intra-articular band causes symptoms mimicking internal derangement of the knee; resection of this band alleviates the problem. Others have found this band to be the sole cause of their patients' symptoms.*

Survey of Results of Surgery

Excision of the alar ligament or shelf on the medial aspect of the joint may be performed arthroscopically. This is a tough synovial band that arises from the medial side wall and passes between the medial femoral condyle and medial facet of the patella to attach to the fat pad. I have excised this band in 18 patients whose clinical history and physical examination suggested this diagnostic possibility. Fourteen of the patients showed definite improvement. One patient was lost to follow-up. In one patient, while improved, the cause of the improvement was felt to be removal of two large cartilaginous loose bodies rather than the excision of the shelf. Two patients were definitely not improved. Later, it was found in both of these patients that subluxation of the patella occurred repeatedly. Interestingly, 14 of the 18 knees showed evidence of fibrillation of varying degrees of the medial facet of the patella and, in several cases, involvement of the trochlear groove of the femur. A normal patellofemoral joint was noted in only four of these knees. The overlap of symptoms makes for difficulty in the diagnosis of this problem. A tear of the medial transverse patellar ligament, associated with subluxation of the patella, hypertrophy of the shelf, a tear of the medial meniscus, and even chondromalacia of the patella may all give rise to similar symptoms and may well cause erroneous interpretation. Nonetheless, when clinical suspicion is high enough, the patient may be improved by excision of this band.

Case 11-1. Resection of a Fibrotic Shelf

A 24-year-old college football player complained of pain over the medial patellar border, aching of the knee during flexion, and extension and inability to comfortably assume the squatting position necessary for football. He also complained of pain at the superior lateral pole of the patella when driving off from his right leg. Roentgenograms demonstrated irregularity of the retropatellar surface.

Arthroscopy demonstrated a huge fibrotic shelf (Fig. 11-2) and chondromalacia of the lateral patellar facet. The shelf was resected, and a lateral capsular release was performed using the arthroscope and several quarter-inch ancillary incisions. Six hours postoperatively the patient was able to assume a crouching position and drive off his right leg. After the appropriate rehabilitation, he was able to resume playing football.

UNUSUAL PROBLEMS

Case 11-2. Arthroscopic Discovery of a Bilobular Mass

A 13-year-old male was admitted to the hospital with a diagnosis of a displaced bucket-handle tear of the lateral meniscus. Arthrography failed to reveal a tear of the lateral meniscus and seemed to incriminate the medial meniscus. Later, however, arthroscopy revealed a bilobular mass that arose from the lateral aspect of the anterior cruciate ligament (Fig. 11-3). It was flattened, indicating that it

* Watanabe, M.: personal communication, 1972; Andrews, J., Goldner, J. L., and Hughston, J.: personal communications, 1976.

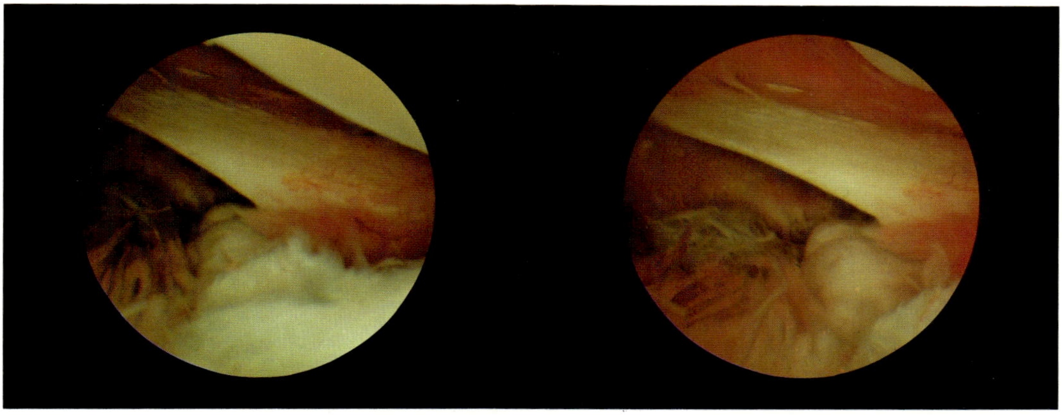

Fig. 11-2. Superior lateral approach: the broad shelf is seen between the patella superior and the medial femoral condyle. Inferior approach: distally it inserts into the medial pole of the fat pad. Its origin is always along the medial side wall of the quadriceps bursa; if a plica synovialis is present, this acts as the proximal origin. Note the broad expanse of this band.

had been trapped between the femoral condyle and tibia, and it also had evidence of hemosiderin deposition on the surface. The histology was interpreted by the pathologist as compatible with that of a ganglion cyst. Treatment was extirpation through an arthrotomy approach; however, this can be accomplished arthroscopically.

CYSTIC DEGENERATION OF THE MENISCUS

Occasionally cystic degeneration is found within the lateral meniscus. Watanabe describes a case with a bulge of the meniscus secondary to the underlying cystic degeneration in the middle half of the lateral meniscus.[2] The patient in the following case had cystic replacement of the posterior portion of the posterior third of the lateral meniscus.

Case 11-3. Arthroscopic Diagnosis of Cystic Degeneration of the Lateral Meniscus

A 24-year-old male presented with a history of an industrial accident and pain in the posterior lateral aspect of the knee for over a year. Arthrograms were equivocal and were repeated, but failed to yield a concrete conclusion from the participating arthrographers. Arthroscopy (see Fig. 5-29) showed considerable alteration from the normal appearance of the lateral meniscus, with the posterior inner meniscal edge rotated slightly and lifted off the tibial plateau and the undersurface showing a lobular defect. With the source of the pathology identified, the patient was sent back

(*Text continues on p. 109.*)

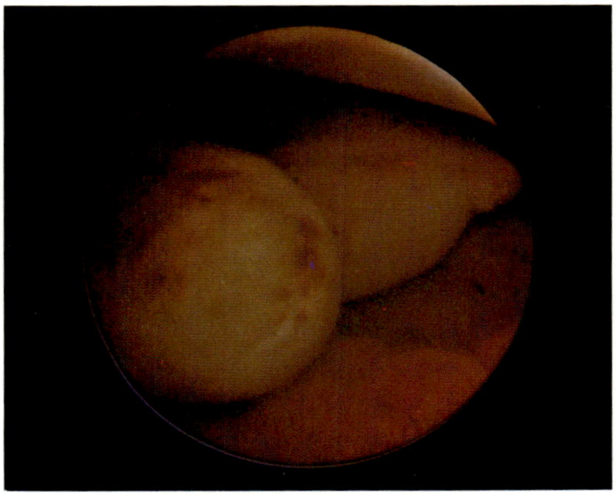

Fig. 11-3. This bilobular mass, histologically identified as a ganglion cyst, was responsible for loss of 12 degrees of knee extension. It rose from the lateral aspect of the anterior cruciate ligament.

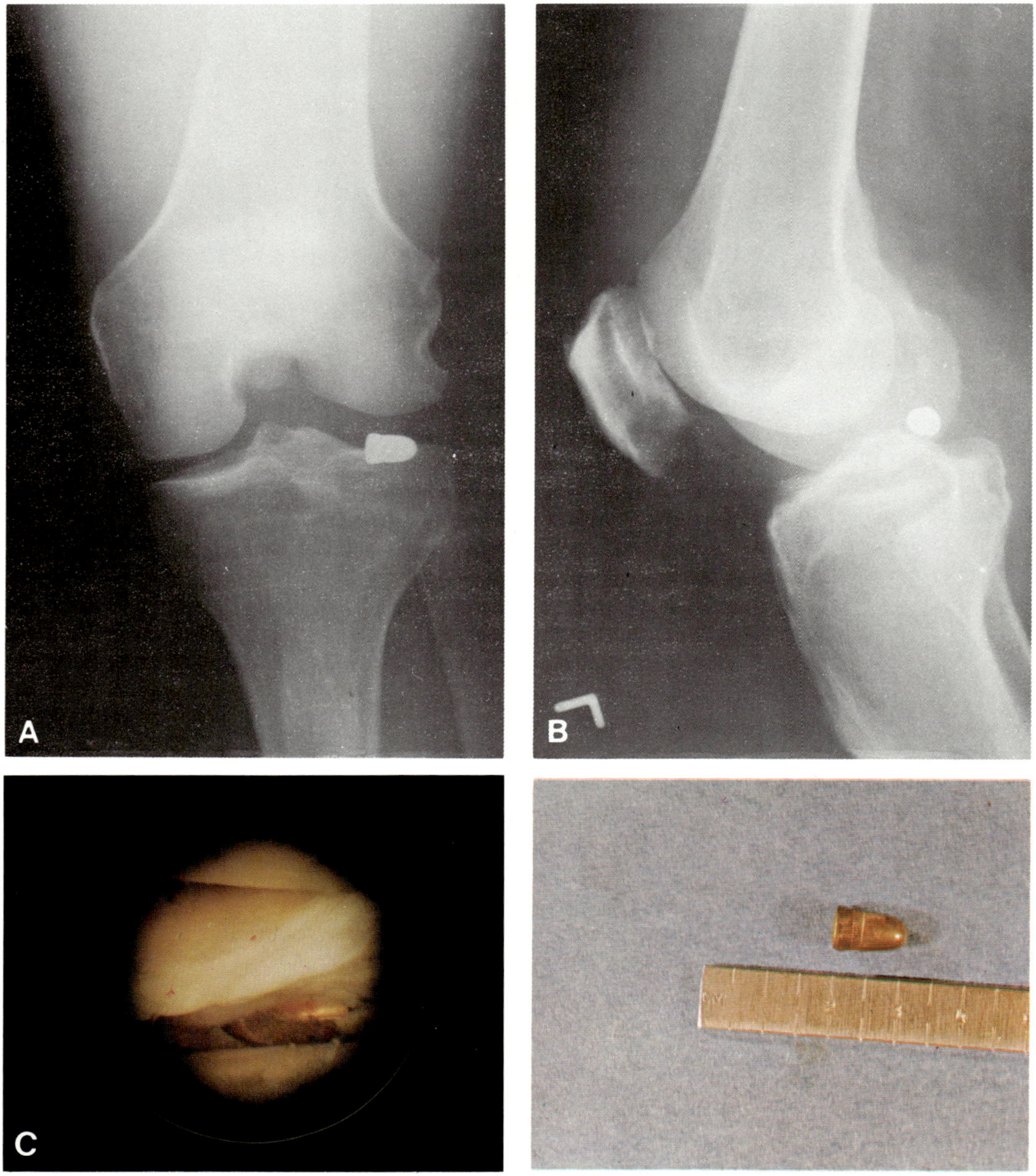

Fig. 11-4. (*A*) Tunnel view of the left knee. A .25 caliber bullet lies at joint line level. (*B*) Lateral view demonstrates its posterior location. (*C*) The brass-clad bullet is seen beneath the lateral meniscus (*right*). Removal under arthroscopic control was accomplished by the double-puncture technique, using a 5 mm. biopsy forceps. (*Left*) The specimen.

→

Fig. 11-5. (*A*) Diagrammatic demonstration of the arthroscopic finding when the popliteus tendon has avulsed a fragment of lateral femoral condylar cortex, and a thin sliver of articular cartilage of the right knee. The pedunculated mass may slip beneath the lateral femoral condyle and ride superior to the lateral meniscus, as seen in the following. (*B*) A similar lesion was seen

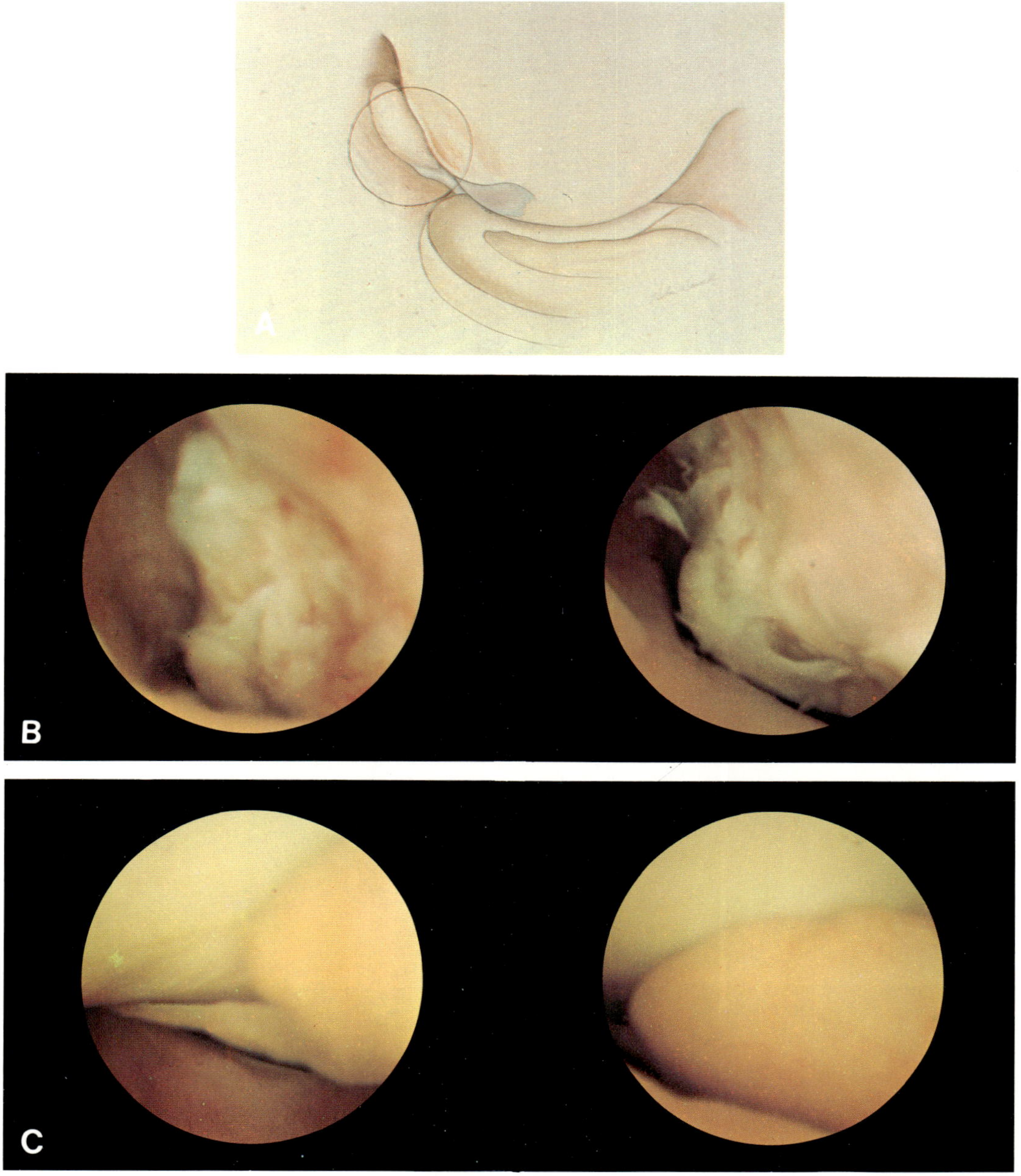

in a 15-year-old male. Defect in the lateral femoral condyle was secondary to avulsion of the cartilage of the lateral face of the lateral femoral condyle; the insertion of the popliteus tendon. (*Left*) Close-up of defect of the lateral femoral condyle's articular cartilage. (*Right*) The defect extended from the lateral face of the lateral femoral condyle to the weight-bearing surface. A portion of the middle third of the lateral meniscus is seen. (*C*) The hyaline cartilage fragment is attached by a slender fibrous pedicle and lies superior to the lateral meniscus. This fragment was retracted medially and was then removed arthroscopically.

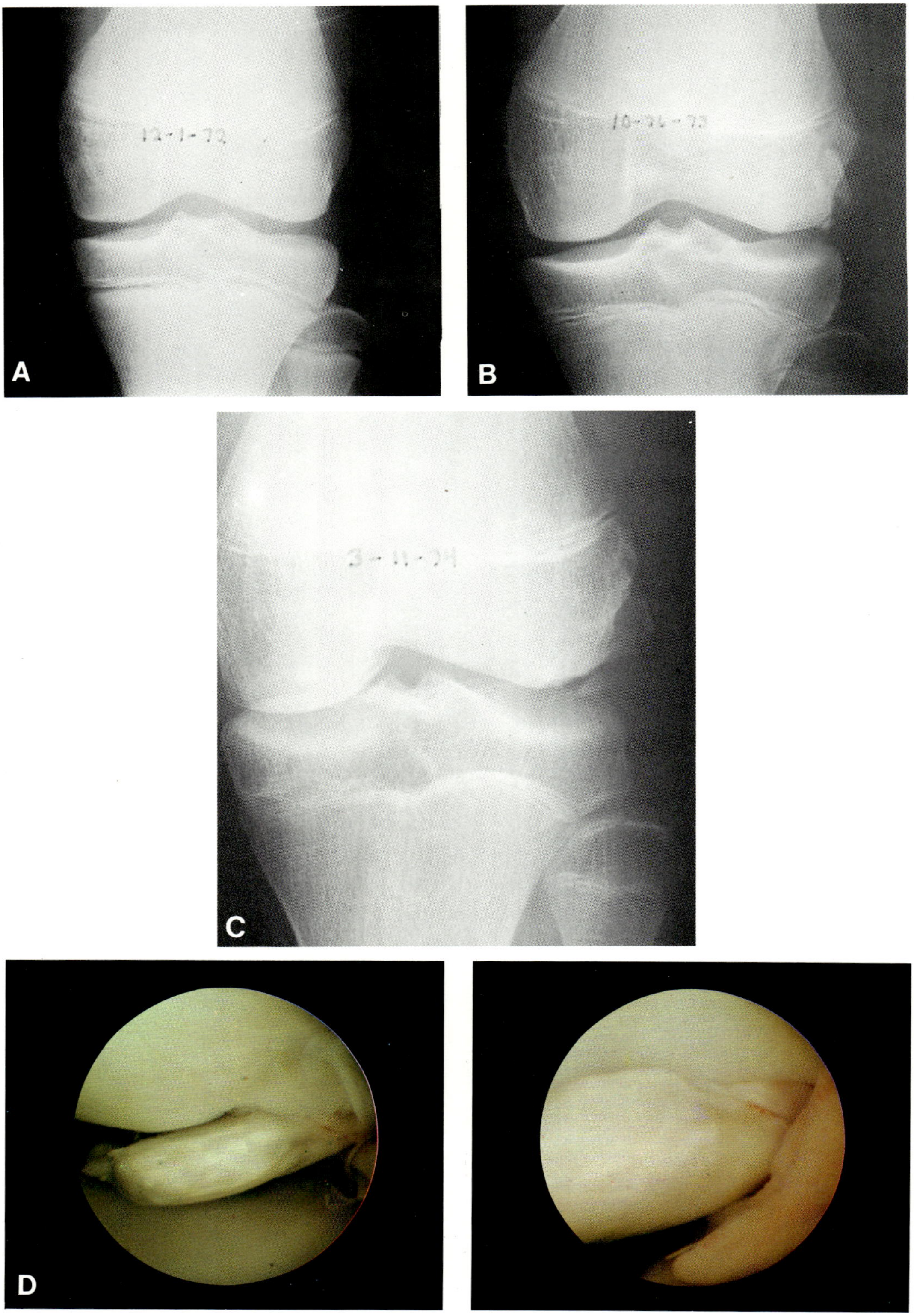
12-1-72
A
10-26-73
B
3-11-74
C
D

←

Fig. 11-6. Avulsion of the insertion of the popliteus tendon. (*A*) Posterior-anterior roentgenogram of the left knee at time of lateral meniscectomy: normal lateral femoral condyle contour. (*B*) Roentgenogram of the left knee following bicycle injury: two bony fragments lie parallel to the lateral femoral condyle. (*C*) Five months later one fragment has healed, resulting in an abnormal appearance of the lateral femoral condyle: one loose fragment is visible. (*D*) The arthroscopic appearance of the lateral joint line. The osteocartilaginous fragment has retained its attachment to the popliteus tendon. (*Right*) Traction at this junction during arthrotomy produced motion in the popliteus tendon behind the "reformed" lateral meniscus. Interestingly, in our small series this avulsion injury occurred only in 14- and 15-year-old males, and in all three the mechanism of injury was external rotation of the tibia. In two of these cases, the injury was associated with a lateral dislocation of the patella.

to his referring orthopaedic surgeon, who states that when he performed the lateral meniscectomy and reached the posterior third of the meniscus, he encountered considerable cystic material.

METALLIC FOREIGN BODIES

On different occasions, two children presented with basically the same history: while they had been crawling on a rug a needle had penetrated their knee. In one case, the needle migrated posteriorly in the posterior capsule and could not be detected either arthroscopically or at arthrotomy. In the other, the needle perforated the medial femoral condyle, causing discoloration of the articular cartilage. When the foreign body protrudes from the cartilage, there is a chance that this may be retrieved with special equipment. In the latter patient, the needle was removed through a very small incision.

Another infrequently seen metallic body is a bullet within the knee (Fig. 11-4).

INTRA-ARTICULAR AVULSION INJURIES

Jackson has recently described two cases of unusual fractures of the popliteus tendon insertion on the lateral femoral condyle.[1] Both patients were adolescents. In one case, the surgeon was able to replace the avulsed fragment; the other required resection of the osteocartilaginous fragment. I have had three similar cases.

Case 11-4. Loose Body Attached to the Popliteus Tendon

A 14-year-old boy suffered a twisting injury while roughhousing, resulting in a dislocation of his patella. He was treated by his family doctor and referred for consultation. Roentgenograms that accompanied the patient showed a small sliver of bone in the vicinity of the lateral joint line. Oblique views showed it more distinctly. After he was treated in a cast

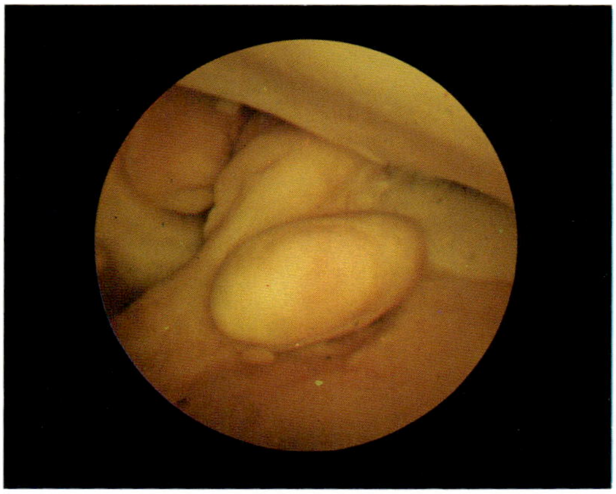

Fig. 11-7. A large pedunculated cyst of the anterior cruciate ligament. The lesion was not associated with trauma, and produced only vague knee discomfort and occasional radiation of pain down the anterolateral aspect of the leg. Removal was achieved by using the double-puncture technique. (Patient of Dr. Robert Allen, Glendora, Calif.)

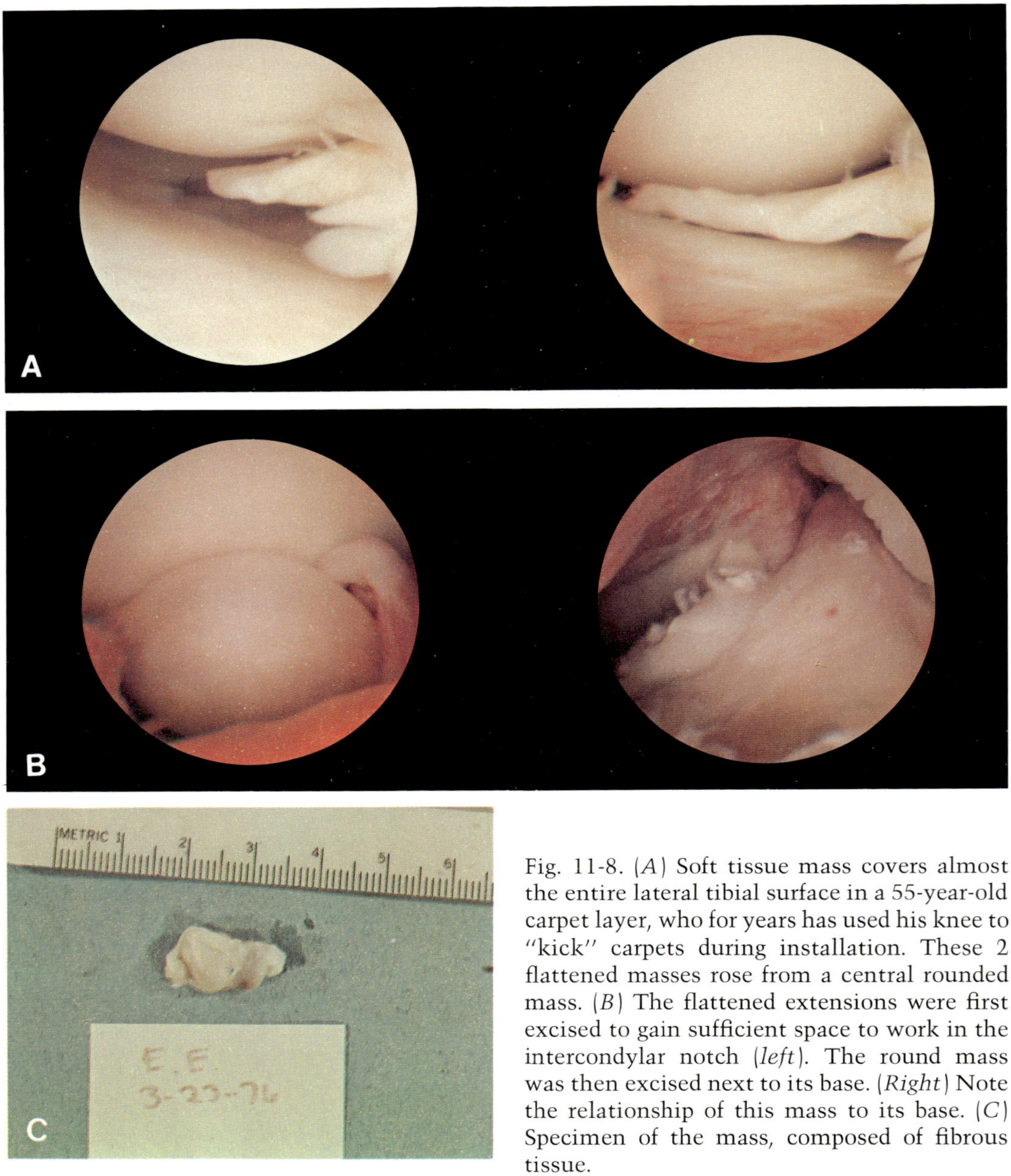

Fig. 11-8. (*A*) Soft tissue mass covers almost the entire lateral tibial surface in a 55-year-old carpet layer, who for years has used his knee to "kick" carpets during installation. These 2 flattened masses rose from a central rounded mass. (*B*) The flattened extensions were first excised to gain sufficient space to work in the intercondylar notch (*left*). The round mass was then excised next to its base. (*Right*) Note the relationship of this mass to its base. (*C*) Specimen of the mass, composed of fibrous tissue.

for 6 weeks, arthroscopy was performed in an attempt to remove the loose body. It was found to be attached to the popliteus tendon (Fig. 11-5). An attempt was made to remove this through the arthroscope, which failed because the loose body was connected posteriorly. However, upon opening the joint, one could see that the fragment had been significantly loosened by prior manipulation and now floated free. A defect was noted on the lateral femoral condyle where the bony fragments had avulsed, carrying with them a portion of articular cartilage. It appears that this was an external rotation injury.

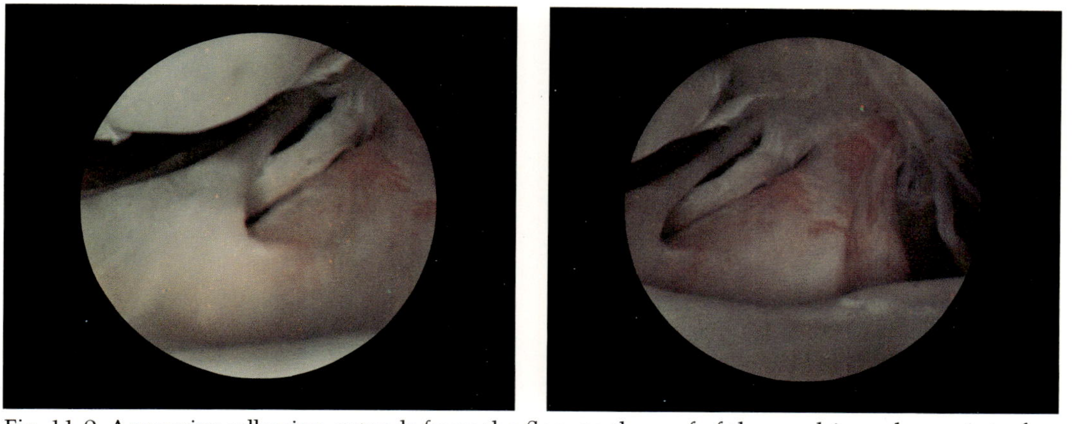

Fig. 11-9. A massive adhesion extends from the floor to the roof of the quadriceps bursa, interfering with the excursion of the patella in this patient 2 years following a meniscectomy. The patient's complaints suggested a diagnosis of chondromalacia patella; he was referred for arthroscopy to determine if the patella was salvageable or whether a patellectomy should be performed. Resection of these adhesions decreased his symptoms and avoided patellectomy.

Case 11-5. Resection of a Pedunculated Fragment

A 15-year-old boy was involved in a twisting accident, incurring a tear of the lateral meniscus. A lateral meniscectomy was performed, and the patient's postoperative course was uneventful (Fig. 11-6). Approximately one year later, he was involved in a bicycle injury in which he incurred an external rotary force and developed a hemarthrosis. Roentgenograms (*Text continues on page 115*)

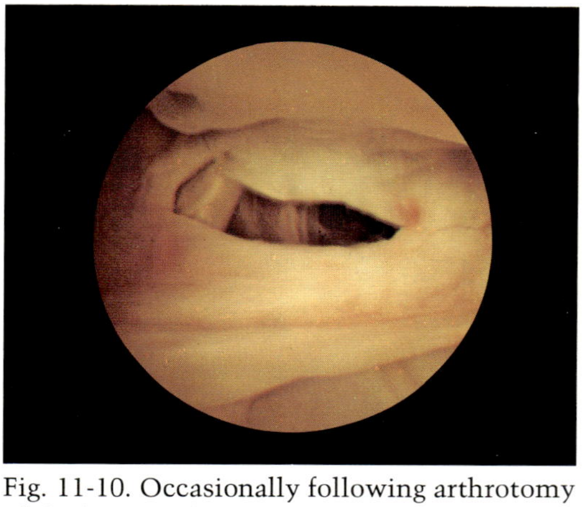

Fig. 11-10. Occasionally following arthrotomy of the knee, and more commonly following patellectomy, significant joint motion is lost. In these cases, arthroscopy can be a valuable aid in determining the cause and treatment. Using arthroscopy, I have found that the condition is due to a thick fibrous transverse band at the superior pole of the patella. The first hint the arthroscopist has in confirming this diagnosis is a severely limited acceptance of saline solution when he attempts to distend the joint. Normally the capacity is between 80 and 150 ml., but in this condition is limited to 40 to 60 ml. This figure shows this dense band with the patella above. The arthroscope was inserted from a lateral infrapatellar approach, creating a hole in the band. Preoperatively this patient lacked 15 degrees of complete extension and 20 degrees of complete flexion. Arthroscopic scissors placed on either side of this defect provides a plane to dissect medially and laterally. Manipulation of this knee under anaesthesia did not result in any increase in motion. However, following division of this band, manipulation was accompanied by the crepitant sound of lysis of adhesions. Range of motion approached normal, which, with postoperative effort, the patient was able to secure actively.

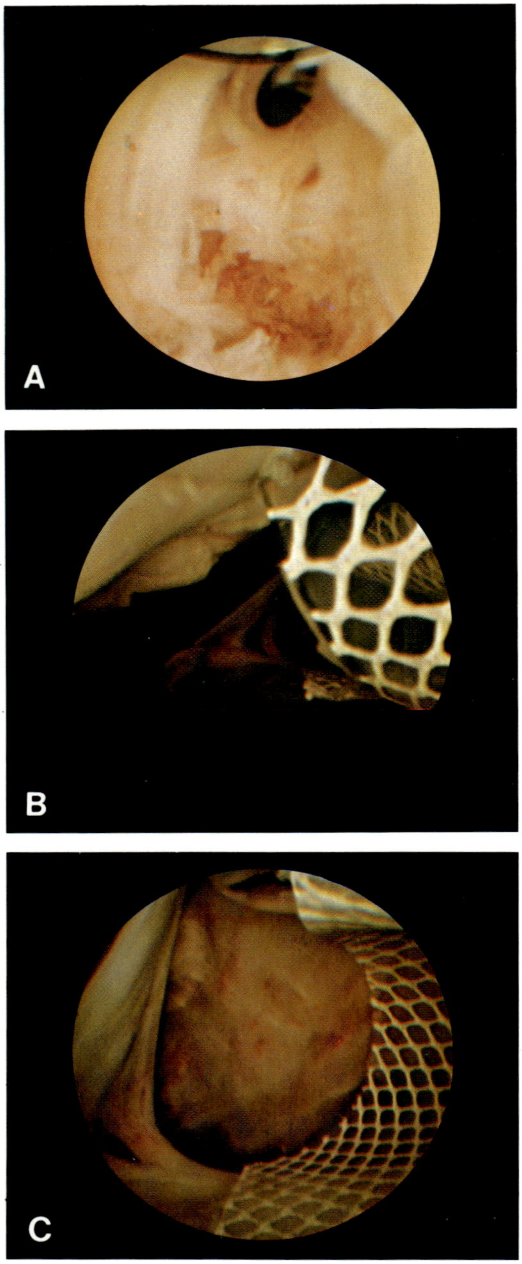

Fig. 11-11. (*A*) Fibrous ankylosis allowing less than 50 degrees of motion may require quadricepsplasty. This was taken in the quadriceps bursa in a 21-year-old patient, one year following a synovectomy and six weeks' casting. Passive range of motion was between 0 and 40 degrees of flexion. The quadriceps bursa was completely replaced with scar tissue. Note the needle hole at the top. Little increase of motion followed partial resection of this dense mass. Eventually a quadricepsplasty was performed, and a silastic interpositional membrane was inserted. Six months later this membrane was removed arthroscopically. (*B*) A panoramic view showing a fibrous cord, the patella, and the silastic membrane (*top*). A close-up of the fibrous band and side wall. The patient has 105 degrees of active flexion (*bottom*).

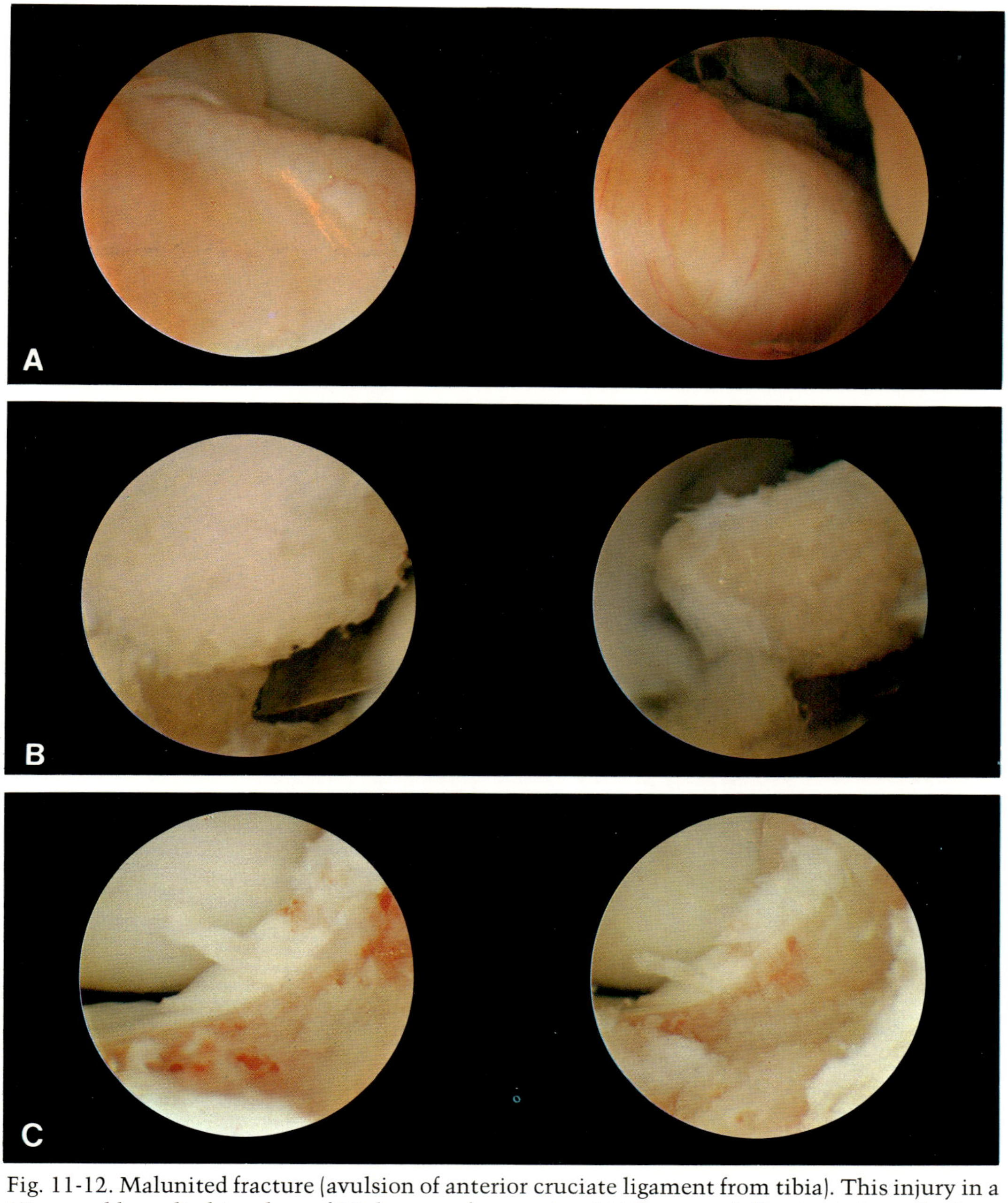

Fig. 11-12. Malunited fracture (avulsion of anterior cruciate ligament from tibia). This injury in a 17-year-old resulted in a loss of 12 degrees of extension. (*A*) One year following injury, the fracture healed in a malunited position. The fragment was attached to a lax fibrous cord resembling the anterior cruciate ligament but nonfunctional. The proximity of the fat pad (*right*) interferes with visualization. (*B*) A small osteotome introduced through a second puncture is used to elevate the malunited fragment. The fragment was removed from the joint in several pieces. (*C*) The postoperative appearance of the osteotomy site. Ten degrees of extension was gained by this procedure.

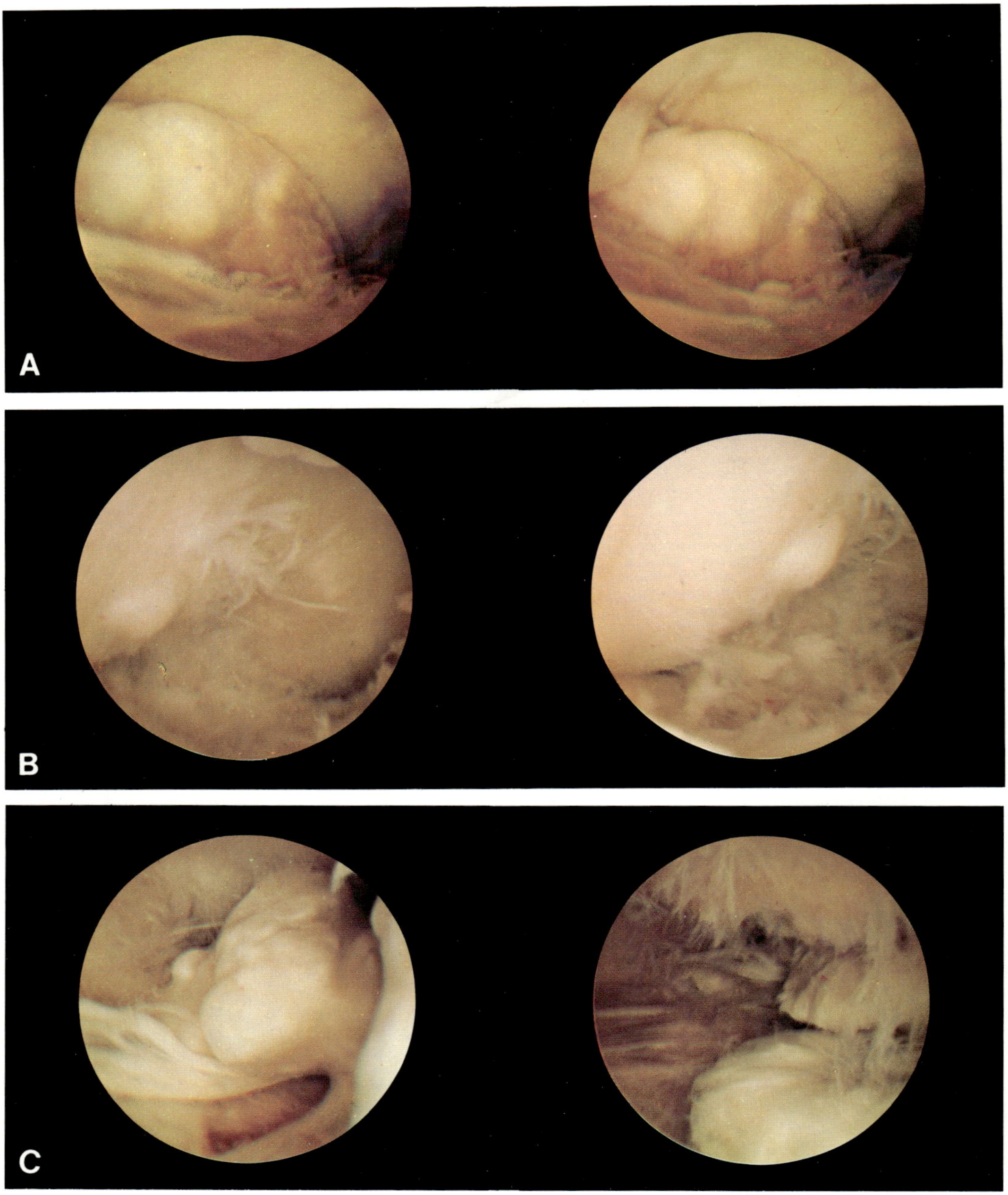
A
B
C

←

Fig. 11-13. Intra-articular osteophytes. Perhaps one of the most challenging ideas in knee surgery is to relieve the degenerative knee without resorting to a Magnusson debridement or prosthetic replacement methods. (*A*) A bony excrescence on the medial tibial plateau (right knee) of a 55-year-old former professional football kicker who has lost his terminal 26 degrees of extension. An avid handball player, the patient has declined both the general joint debridement and total joint replacement. An osteotome introduced through a medial stab wound was used to excise this mass at its base. (*B*) The immediate postoperative appearance. The patient gained 12 degrees of extension in spite of numerous other bony excrescences. (*C*) The patellofemoral joint seen from the superolateral approach is degenerated, with massive osteophytes, but was not attacked surgically. The patient states that his knee is somewhat improved, but he has not returned for work on the contralateral knee. Nevertheless, with improved equipment, including small power-driven burrs, some avenues may open to the treatment of the degenerative knee in the future.

demonstrated several loose bodies lateral and superior to the joint line. Several months later, roentgenograms were repeated and showed an unusual cortex of lateral femoral condyle and one loose body still present. Because of continuing complaints, particularly those of locking, arthroscopy was performed which showed a large pedunculated fragment protruding into the lateral joint line. This was resected at the area of its base. By applying traction on this area, I was able to demonstrate that traction caused the popliteus tendon to ride back and forth. This was easily seen in the absence of the lateral meniscus.

REFERENCES

1. Jackson, R. W.: Arthroscopy Instructional Course. American Academy of Orthopaedic Surgeons Meeting, Dallas, 1974.
2. Watanabe, M., Takeda, S., and Ikeuchi, H.: Atlas of Arthroscopy. ed. 2. Tokyo, Igaku Shoin, 1969.

Arguments from authority are invalid; the proof of a theory is in its reasoning, not in its sponsorship; and with all due respect for the masters, it must be said that they have not justified their position very thoroughly in this matter.

Ludwig Von Mises

12 *Partial Meniscectomy*

ARTHROSCOPIC DIAGNOSIS AND EVALUATION OF TEARS

Many physicians, such as O'Malley,[14] still cling to the view that the diagnosis of a meniscal tear can be made from the patient's history and physical examination alone. Recent evidence that the majority of orthopaedic surgeons are skeptical of total reliance on clinical findings in deciding on operative treatment is provided by the resurgence of interest in arthrography and, more recently, in arthroscopy. A logical extension of arthroscopic study of meniscal tears is the search for improved methods of treatment. Correlation of the history, physical examination, roentgenograms and special studies with arthroscopic views allows improved prognostic appraisal. With increasing experience, the arthroscopist recognizes patterns of meniscal tears and becomes able to correlate with each type a general classification of signs and symptoms. Instead of relying on arthroscopy only to determine compartment localization and the presence or absence of a meniscal tear, arthroscopic input can also introduce other factors that may affect the eventual surgical result. For example, arthroscopic study of the dynamics of meniscal tears allows them to be classified with those capable or not capable of mechanically obstructing joint motion. Certain tears are always associated with localized progressive chondromalacia of the overlying medial femoral condyle, secondary to mechanical pressure. Postoperative study of the specimen, while important for correlative purposes, fails to convey the dynamics of the in vivo state and truly is anticlimatic following arthroscopic study.

I have already discussed other factors involving or affecting the prognosis: (1) the status of the synovium; (2) chondromalacia of the femoral condyles and tibia; and (3) chondromalacia of the patella. Obviously additional factors are involved, such as ligamentous stability, general body build of the patient, the presence or absence of angular deformities about the knee joint, age, and such metabolic conditions as gout or pseudogout.

This concept that meniscectomy is not an innocuous procedure and that it may well hasten localized degenerative changes was supported by Fairbank in 1948.[4] He described roentgenographic changes occurring as early as 5 months following meniscectomy. In 1965 Huckell[6] warned, "the surgeon should not be extravagant in his promise that a normal knee will result from this operation." Clearly the meniscus is not the atavistic structure the appendix is.

FUNCTION OF THE MENISCI

Generally four functions are ascribed to the menisci:

Nutrition

It is generally accepted that the menisci function to spread synovial fluid over the articular surfaces, nourishing the hyaline cartilage of both the tibia and femur. The wedge-shaped configuration of the meniscus facilitates this function.[13] Theoretically, with the excision of the meniscus and the development of adequate reformed meniscus, this function could be retained postoperatively.

Weight Distribution

It has been stated that the menisci act as shock absorbers[11] and, with increasing weight loads, act to distribute this weight throughout the tibial and femoral portion of the joint.[4] It appears that, with the increasing load, more of the meniscus assumes an increased amount of weight acceptance.[17]

Stabilization

The menisci also function as peripheral stabilizers. As the pressure inside the joint increases, much of the excess energy is dissipated through the peripheral portions of the meniscus and to the joint capsule of the knee.

Knee Movement

The menisci facilitate rapid and complex movement of the knee, involving abduction adduction, and rotation during flexion and extension.[15] Recent arthroscopic evidence suggests that when the meniscus is totally excised, even in the presence of a reformed meniscus, this particular function, as well as weight acceptance, is lost.[9]

During weight-bearing, compressive forces occurring between the femur and tibia are absorbed by the hyaline cartilage, and excessive force is dissipated through the intact meniscus by alteration of its elastic tension. If the peripheral (capsular) attachments and the tibia anchors remain intact, theoretically the compressive forces generated in the center of the joint may still be partially dissipated by the remaining meniscal rim following partial meniscectomy.

THE LOSS OF THE MENISCUS AND ITS EFFECT ON JOINT FUNCTION

Experimental Evidence

King,[11] in his experimental excision of the menisci in dogs in 1936, noted that after extirpation of the medial semilunar cartilage, the resulting defect is filled by ingrowth of fibrous tissue. In spite of this, he concluded that considerable roughening and degeneration of the articular cartilage occurs. He believed that the amount of degenerative cartilaginous change was dependent on the size of the segment removed, and was greater with complete meniscectomy. He concluded that a semilunar meniscus served to protect the articular hyaline cartilage and that operative excision should probably be limited to removal of the mobile portion. A recent report[2] supports King's findings regarding the degenerative changes occurring in the hyaline cartilage and the finding that the more extensive the excision, the greater the degeneration.

Review of the Literature

Conflicting opinions still exist in the literature, however, regarding the effect of meniscectomy in the human being. Various authors have attributed the unsatisfactory results following meniscectomy to excision of too much meniscus, too little meniscus, early excision of the meniscus, late excision of the meniscus, and poor operative technique. Disagreement also exists regarding the significance of the postoperative radiographic changes and their relation to the clinical result.

In an early study (1923) Love[12] reported that 70 per cent of the patients treated by meniscectomy had a good result. The same year, however, a more critical report from a military depot[13] demonstrated continuing difficulties during a 6- to 12-month period following discharge. The authors attributed this to minor degrees of instability of the knee, possibly due to laxity of the anterior cruciate ligament. Fairbanks,[4] in his oft-quoted report of 1948, described the roentgenographic changes that follow meniscectomy, but concluded there was no correlation between those cases with positive radiographic changes and those with clinical findings. He attributed these changes to loss of the weight-bearing function of the meniscus. In 1965 Gear[5] noted that in patients followed for more than 10 years there were severe symptoms in 37 per cent, and he further noted the correlation between symptoms and roentgenographic changes. He also stated that if the meniscectomy was performed within a few weeks following injury, there was a good prognosis. Huckell[6] also noted correlation of the roentgenographic changes and increased clinical symptoms. Ominously, he also found that the highest percentage of unsatisfactory results (80%) were in those patients in which a normal meniscus was excised. Moreover, only 50 per cent of the patients in his study had a satisfactory result. Of those patients he was able to examine, 50 per cent had mild to moderate ligamentous laxity (cruciate laxity 45%, collateral laxity 10%); and he also noted a generally better result in those patients who had the operation less than a year after the onset of symptoms.

Jackson[10] found degenerative changes in 23 per cent of 448 knees followed for between 5 to 40 years. He felt that the timing of the operation either before or after 6 months following injury made little difference in the long-term result and concluded, "changes of the joint were more likely due to the meniscectomy than to the original injury." Tapper and Hoover,[16] in a study of patients examined longer than 10 years after meniscectomy (excluding ligamentous injuries), were able to determine the site of operation in 85 per cent of the roentgenograms examined. They found the incidence of normal knees was only 40 per cent following meniscectomy, but offered the first ray of hope that better results might be obtained in the future. Of the patients they studied, 83 per cent of those that were treated by excision of the bucket handle had a good or excellent result by their criteria. Unfortunately this was a small group of patients. Recently a similar report was issued by Cargill and Jackson on removing only the bucket handle of the medial meniscus.[1]

Definition of a Meniscal Tear

Just as it is unwise and inaccurate to compare apples and oranges because of their relatively equal size, it is also erroneous to use the phrase *meniscal tear* to describe any alteration in meniscal continuity. Better than any other technique, arthroscopy allows differentiations to be made in such situations. The loss of continuity of the meniscus seen arthroscopically may take many forms. The fracture line may be complete or incomplete. A complete vertical tear along the long axis of the meniscus will cause complete displacement and locking. This may be preceded, however, by an incomplete tear, frequently seen on the posterior inferior or superior surface of the lateral meniscus. The depth and extent of the tear, in the absence of displacement, cannot always be ascertained by manipulation of

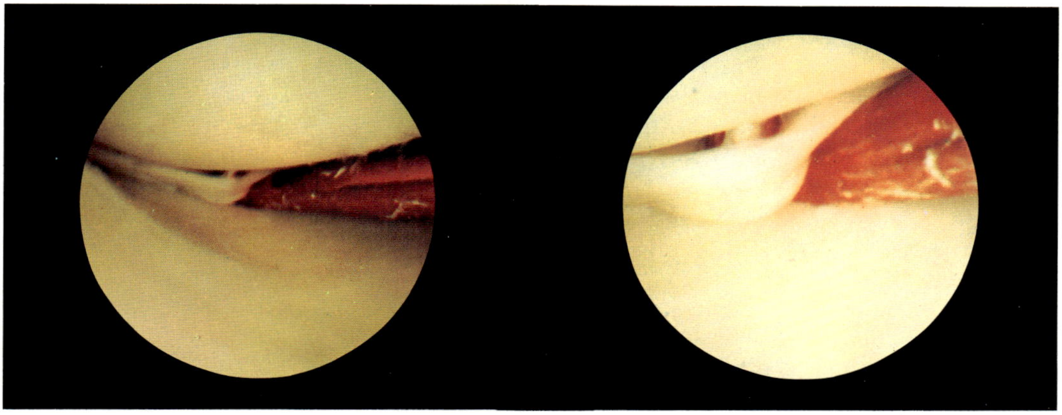

Fig. 12-1. Medical joint line of the right knee: A crochet hook has been slid between the two leaves of a vertical, or longitudinal, tear of the medial meniscus. Traction on the hook will allow displacement of the mobile fragment.

the leg and rotation of the tibia. The insertion of a probe can be used to ascertain the depth of the tear by attempting to place the probe within the fracture (Fig. 12-1). A small biopsy forceps may be used to exert traction on the inner edge of the fragment with an attempt to displace it. An incomplete tear is found to still have numerous fibrous attachments across the rupture. The incompletely ruptured surface separates during complex joint motion when the joint is loaded, and this separation is responsible for the clinical complaints of giving way. True locking is always associated with a complete vertical separation, usually originating in the posterior segment of the meniscus. Occasionally this may result from anteromedial or anterolateral separation of the meniscus from the capsule.

Tears may also originate in either the anterior or posterior tibial attachments; however, secondary tears will occur with the passage of time, due to the increased mobility of the meniscus. These tears are usually incomplete and are not clinically disabling, and delay of meniscectomy is in order unless excessive mobility can be demonstrated at the time of arthroscopy.

Other types of tears are common as well. The horizontal cleavage tear may result in a flap or, as the Japanese refer to it, an "L-shaped tear"[18] extending at an angle to the long axis of the meniscus. I have not found these to be associated with symptoms other than pain, tenderness over the joint line, and occasional complaints of giving way. I have not recorded any locking episodes with this type of tear and, as Smillie has indicated, it is usually seen in the patient over 40 years of age.

The common tear of the lateral meniscus begins as a transverse slit perpendicular to the long axis of the meniscus. With continued trauma, it then extends anteriorly and posteriorly, as has been previously described. This tear is associated with symptoms of joint instability and localized lateral joint line pain.

In the elderly, multiple areas of tear may be present. The fragments have lost most of their matrix and appear as fibrous bands at an angle to the long axis of the meniscus. They are usually associated with severe underlying changes of the femoral condyles and tibia. Obviously these tears do not belong in the classification of dislocating meniscal tears.

Attritional tears also occur on the inferior surface of the meniscus. If this results in increased width of the posterior horn, it may cause dislocation of the meniscus into the intercondylar notch with external tibial rotation, such as pivoting. Such tears may be found in patients with relatively normal femoral hyaline cartilage, and give rise to symptoms of instability and (occasionally) of locking.

TYPES OF MENISCECTOMY

Total Meniscectomy

This requires complete detachment of the meniscus from the capsule and also severance of the meniscal attachments to the tibial head. The reason given to perform a total meniscectomy is that, theoretically, maximal regrowth of a meniscal substitute follows complete removal.

Subtotal Meniscectomy

The surgical cleavage allows a small peripheral rim, 1 to 2 mm. in width, of the meniscus to remain attached to the capsule. The advantages of subtotal meniscectomy are that this (1) allows excision of the meniscus in an avascular plane to minimize postoperative hemarthrosis, and (2) allows increased joint stability.

Partial Meniscectomy

This involves the removal of the dislocating flap or fragment, leaving behind a stable intact peripheral rim. Theoretical disadvantages of partial meniscectomy are (1) failure of regrowth of re-formed meniscus (from existing evidence, this appears to be inconsequential, inasmuch as the form may be retained but the function is lost), and (2) the possibility that a secondary attritionary tear exists in the peripheral segment and may be missed at the time of removal of the dislocating flap. This latter situation tends to occur more frequently in those patients with multiple injuries and with a long history of locking of the knee. Usually at arthroscopy a hint that a secondary longitudinal tear exists in the periphery can be ascertained by abnormal movement of the meniscus and, on many occasions, the secondary tear is seen in the peripheral segment (Fig. 12-2). After completion of partial meniscectomy, the policy of repeated examination of the meniscus with valgus stress on the leg and external rotation of the tibia tends to eliminate or at least diminish this potential. Following meniscal excision, either meniscus can be probed with a crochet hook.

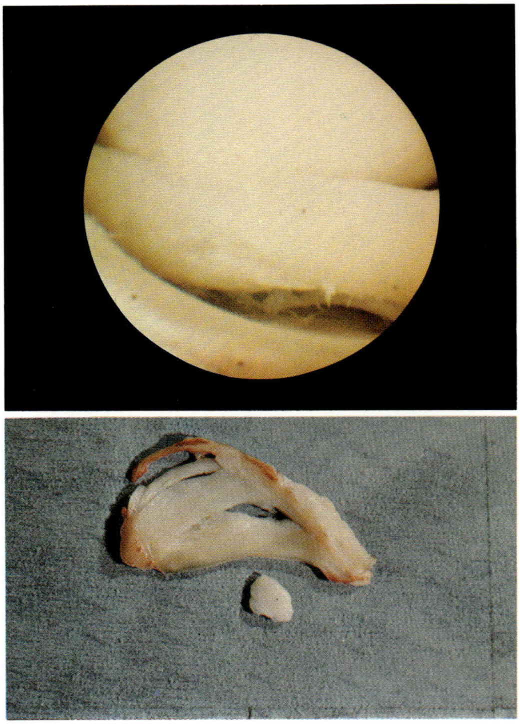

Fig. 12-2. Beneath the displaced bucket handle tear of this right medial meniscus is another longitudinal tear. Total meniscectomy was clearly the indicated treatment. Three longitudinal tears of the medial meniscus and a cartilaginous loose body are demonstrated in the specimen.

Advantages of the partial meniscectomy include (1) lower operative morbidity;* (2) the maintenance of the integrity of the posterior capsular mechanism, increasing postoperative joint stability; (3) limited evidence suggests lesser future

---

* Ikeuchi, H.: Personal communication, 1972.

arthritic changes in both femoral and tibial articular cartilage following partial meniscectomy than with a total meniscectomy (Tapper and Hoover's study at the Mayo Clinic support this view); (4) only partial loss of weight acceptance; and (4) only partial loss of the facility of the meniscus to participate in the complex joint movements required in normal joint motion. Obviously, the last two advantages must be directly dependent upon the amount of functional normal meniscus remaining.

I have found that many tears are amenable to partial meniscectomy under arthroscopic control (the technique is given below). The advantages of partial meniscectomy done with this technique are: lack of quadriceps inhibition, decreased hemarthrosis, rapid rehabilitation, and the ability to inspect the remaining peripheral rim following removal of the torn tissue.

INDICATIONS FOR MENISCECTOMY IN GENERAL

Pain

This is a prominent feature in certain types of tears.

Parrot-beak or horizontal cleavage tears of the medial meniscus with dislocation of a flap cause great pain. Usually this is an intermittent aching type of complaint localized at the joint level with tenderness to palpation noted either beneath the medial collateral ligament or slightly anterior to it. The pain usually is described as throbbing, but occasionally as a sharp stabbing. Often the patient complains that to rest at night he must place a pillow between his knees.

Longitudinal tears. These may be painfree, but usually a sharp pain is associated with partial displacement of the meniscus momentarily. The displaced bucket handle usually is painful at the time of the initial displacement. However, as time passes, the pain is markedly decreased, and I have found a few patients walking with a displaced bucket handle tear of the meniscus for up to 8 years. The pain in the displaced bucket handle tear probably results from tension on the capsular attachments. Pain is, of itself, not an absolute indication for meniscectomy.

Buckling or Giving Way

This is a difficult symptom to evaluate. It may be related to quadriceps weakness, patellar instability, cartilaginous intra-articular cartilaginous loose bodies, or impingement of synovial tags in the joint line. Occasionally cartilaginous incongruity of the patellofemoral or tibiofemoral joint may also be associated with all types of meniscal tears. This symptom cannot be used preoperatively to attempt to determine the type of tear present. But, when repetitive episodes occur, there is indication for meniscectomy if a tear can be demonstrated.

Locking and Unlocking

True locking of the knee is due to a displaced meniscal fragment that prevents complete extension and terminal external tibial rotation. It is enhanced by associated hamstring spasm. This may be imitated by a cartilaginous or osteocartilaginous loose body, hypertrophied medial intra-articular band (alar ligament or shelf), an effusion, a torn anterior cruciate ligament with stump caught in the joint line, a trapped fat pad, or even patellofemoral instability. The history of unlocking helps eliminate the other diagnostic possibilities. This is the prime clinical reason for meniscectomy, and usually a longitudinal tear originating in the posterior segment of the meniscus is found.

Arthrographic Demonstration

An arthrographic shadow of air and dye in the area of the meniscus may demonstrate an abnormality of the meniscus, but it is not in itself an indication for a meniscectomy. This information must be correlated with clinical complaints of pain, buckling, and locking.

Arthroscopic Evidence

The demonstration of either a displaced flap or dislocating fragment or a tear altering the elastic tension of the meniscus, is an indication for surgical treatment, in the absence of gross joint destruction.

Arthroscopy used in conjunction with clinical evidence (and with the arthrogram to evaluate the posterior medial corner) allows determination of the type of meniscal tear and estimation of the alteration of the hyaline cartilage above and below the rupture. This evidence is much better evaluated under low-powered magnification than at arthrotomy. Preoperative, postoperative and long-term follow-up photographs add much useful information in determining the rapidity of the arthrotic process following meniscectomy, either subtotal or partial.

The use of arthroscopy in evaluating meniscal tears allows three possible conclusions regarding each tear: (1) the tear is amenable to partial excision under arthroscopic control; (2) the tear is not amenable to partial excision, requiring subtotal meniscectomy; or (3) the tear does not require surgical attention (those tears which are very minor and not interfering with joint mechanics or a degenerative tear found associated with severe compartmental degeneration).

ANALYSIS OF ARTHROSCOPIC EXAMINATION RESULTS

Over a 53-week period, 400 arthroscopies were performed. In 92 patients, a meniscal tear was encountered that fulfilled the previously mentioned criteria for meniscal excision. 59.7 per cent of the patients had a tear of the medial meniscus. 31.5 per cent had a tear of the lateral meniscus and 8.7 per cent had significant tears of both menisci. Of these 100 meniscal tears, 28 per cent were successfully treated by partial excision under arthroscopic control. Partial excision failed in 3 patients, owing to the inexperience of the surgeon, and arthrotomy was required to perform a subtotal meniscectomy on these patients.

Since this time, 10 additional patients were treated by partial meniscal excision under arthroscopic control, making a total of 40 meniscal tears: 28 tears involving the medial meniscus, 9 involving the lateral meniscus, and 3 patients having tears of both medial and lateral menisci.

After completion of arthroscopy and correlation of the history, clinical examination, and arthroscopic features of the meniscal rupture, the decision was made to proceed with its arthroscopic removal.

TECHNIQUE OF ARTHROSCOPIC MENISCECTOMY

Basic Principles

The details of excision varied from tear to tear. However, I conform to certain basic principles that I feel to be necessary in this type of surgery: (1) The peripheral rim left in must be nonmobile; that is, it must have an anchorage to the periperhal capsule. (2) The instruments for removal of the tear are inserted at an angle to the telescope (medial telescope, lateral operative instrument). (3) The flap or displaced rim must be retracted away from the intact peripheral rim and placed on a "stretch" if at all possible. This has been accomplished by insertion of a 15-gauge needle retractor to place the meniscal flap under tension. In one instance a Kocher forceps was introduced on the same side as the arthroscope to aid in this maneuver. (4) If bleeding occurs, the tourniquet should be inflated immediately. At the termination of the procedure the joint line should be inspected for the adequacy of removal of the meniscal tissue and to check the femoral condyles and tibial plateau for cartilaginous damage. The tourniquet is then deflated, and, if bleeding starts, the joint should be distended with saline solution in order to tamponade the hemorrhage.

Technique of Excision

In the course of excision, it may be necessary to switch the telescope from lateral to medial aspect and then back again several times to gain the necessary visual vantage. The meniscal scissors should be the type that cut at the point rather than at the base of the scissors so that they may be used as a retractor, pulling the meniscal tissue towards the operator before severing the meniscal rim of flap. To gain the best mechanical advantage from the scissors, the blades should be perpendicular to the area of the meniscus being cut, rather than oblique to it, although this is not always possible. One should have an assistant to manipulate the leg and check the irrigating outflow and occasionally to pull on the meniscal retractor. (Prior to attempting to perform partial meniscectomy under arthroscopic control, the operator should have considerable experience in the arthroscopic evaluation of meniscal tears. A good learning technique is the use of a probe or crochet hook to probe the menisci as routine arthroscopy is performed. It is quite difficult at times to line up the area of meniscal tear, introduce an operating instrument, and position the telescope within the same small area.)

As experience is gained, it is often possible to remove the entire flap or displaced inner rim in one segment rather than in multiple pieces; however, if any fragment remains and is likely to dislocate, this should be removed as well.

If it is felt that during the procedure, contamination has occurred, an antibiotic solution may be added to each bottle of irrigant. In my experience, no infections have been directly attributable to arthroscopy, and the only complications have been a severe postoperative hemarthrosis in 2 patients and some mild cartilaginous scuffing due to movement of the arthroscopic instruments.

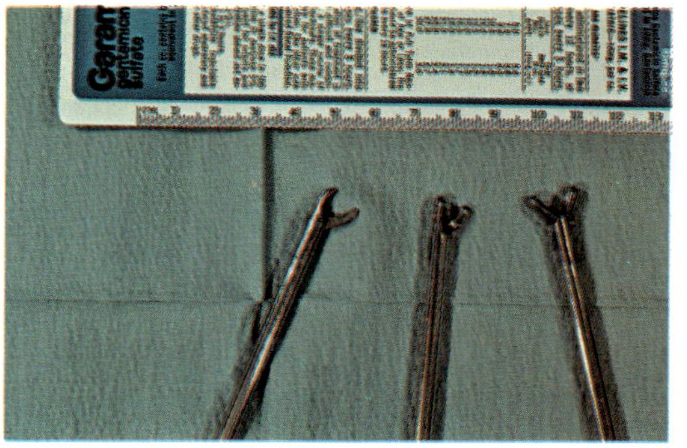

Fig. 12-3. Three essential instruments for partial meniscectomy. (*Left*) A 5 mm. arthroscopic scissors with jaws that "bite" at the point, and can be used to retract the fragment. (*Center*) A serrated edge basket biopsy forceps for contouring the meniscal margin. (*Right*) A hooked biopsy forceps to withdraw the fragment from the joint.

Instrumentation

As the design of the operating instruments improves, a more artistic postoperative result will surely follow. The peripheral edges may be more smoothly contoured. The instruments used for this type of technique have included arthroscopic biopsy forceps with and without serrated edges, meniscal scissors with end biting tips, and 3 mm. Cushing pituitary rongeurs with upward, downward, and straight ahead biting tips. Occasionally a Smillie meniscal knife and, on one occasion, a Kocher clamp have been used as well (Figs. 12-3–12-10). Initially the introduction of the operating instrument is done by using a trocar within the water sleeve and, once the water sleeve is properly placed in the joint line, the trocar is

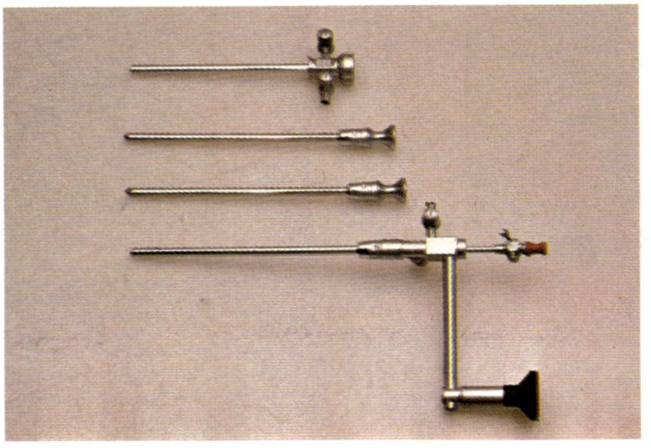

Fig. 12-4. Recently an operating arthroscope has been developed which facilitates meniscal excision. The advantage is that the secondary portal can be used to insert a meniscal retractor. The operating arthroscope is introduced into the joint with either a trocar or an obturator and water sheath. The operating channel (covered with a sealing cap) accommodates 3 mm. accessory operating instruments.

removed. A sealing cap is applied to the water sleeve and the operating instrument inserted. In some instances it may be necessary to remove the water sleeve and introduce the instrument directly through the established opening in the fat pad.

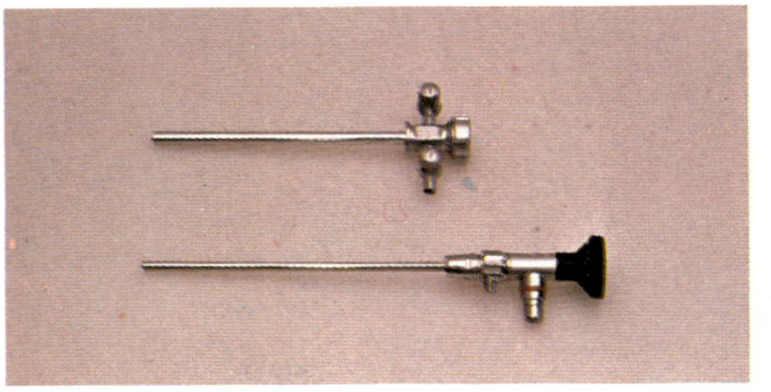

Fig. 12-5. The operating arthroscope may be replaced in the water sleeve with the standard diagnostic arthroscope for photography.

Postoperative Care

Following partial meniscectomy, arthroscopically performed, the patient is encouraged to start straight-leg raising immediately upon awakening, and is allowed to be ambulatory. The only dressing is a soft pressure dressing of cotton and Ace bandages covering the sterile dressing previously applied, extending from the ankle to groin. The knee should be checked within 24 hours for the presence of effusion. If present, this is aspirated and weight bearing is discontinued until the effusion is under control.

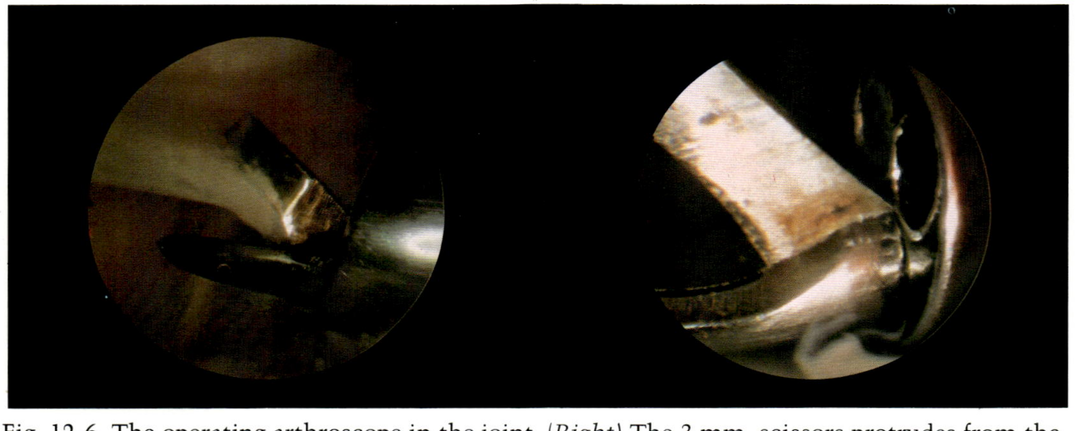

Fig. 12-6. The operating arthroscope in the joint. (*Right*) The 3 mm. scissors protrudes from the inferior channel. The telescope is superior to the operating channel and several water channels are at each side. The light fiber bundles are dispersed around these orifices. (*Left*) The shelf is being severed.

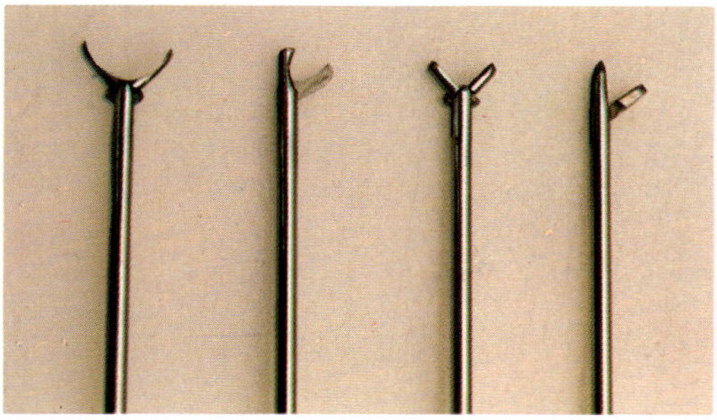

Fig. 12-7. Various 3 mm. operating accessories (*left* to *right*). A loose body forceps, meniscal scissors, biopsy forceps, and the serrated-edged biopsy forceps.

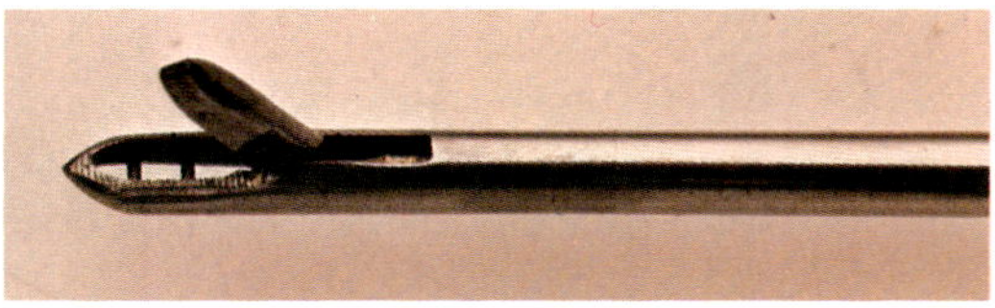

Fig. 12-8. Extremely valuable in partial meniscectomy and for excision of "the shelf" is the basket biopsy forceps with serrated edges. This instrument stores the cut fragments, eliminating the need for withdrawal of the forceps after each bite.

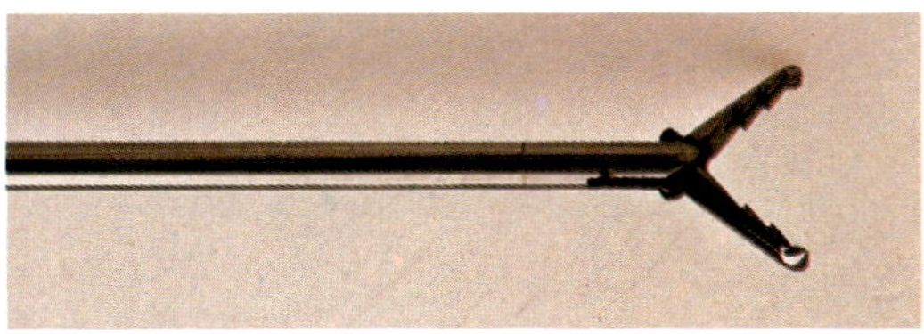

Fig. 12-9. A small meniscal retractor greatly facilitates clean meniscal excision by placing tension on the tissue to be severed. This instrument is usually introduced through a separate portal.

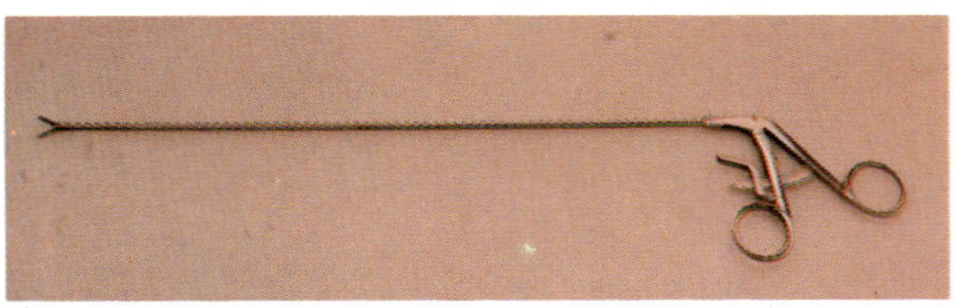

Fig. 12-10. A locking mechanism on the handle of the meniscal forceps aids in retracting, thus relieving finger fatigue.

TYPES OF TEARS AMENABLE TO PARTIAL MENISCECTOMY PERFORMED WITH THE ARTHROSCOPE

DIAGRAMMATIC ILLUSTRATIONS OF TECHNIQUE

Medial Meniscal Tears

Oblique Tear of the Posterior Third of the Left Medial Meniscus

This tear can be seen on the inner edge of the medial meniscus (Fig. 12-11, *left*). It runs obliquely anterior and towards the periphery, and is associated with articular cartilage degeneration of the medial femoral condyle and the medial tibial plateau. Rotation of the tibia opens the torn surfaces (Fig. 12-11, *right*). Excision is started with an oblique cut through the lateral portal, anterior to the tear. The operating arthroscope is removed and reinserted through the medial portal. A small retractor is inserted laterally, retracting the fragment. The torn flap can be excised with a small meniscal scissors placed through the operating arthroscope.

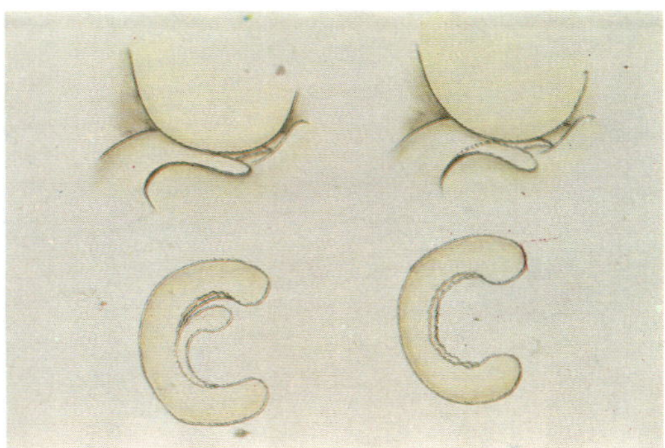

Fig. 12-11. (*Left*) Oblique tear of the posterior third of the medial meniscus. (*Right*) External tibial rotation separating the torn fragments allows an estimation of where the anterior incision in the meniscus must be placed to remove this tear.

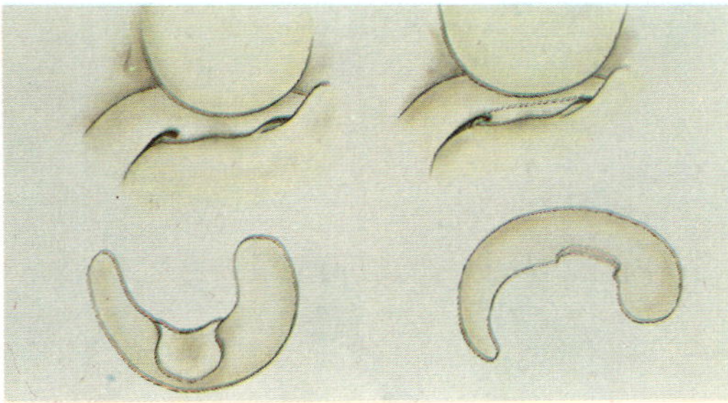

Fig. 12-12. Flap tear of the posterior third of the medial meniscus lodged beneath the peripheral rim.

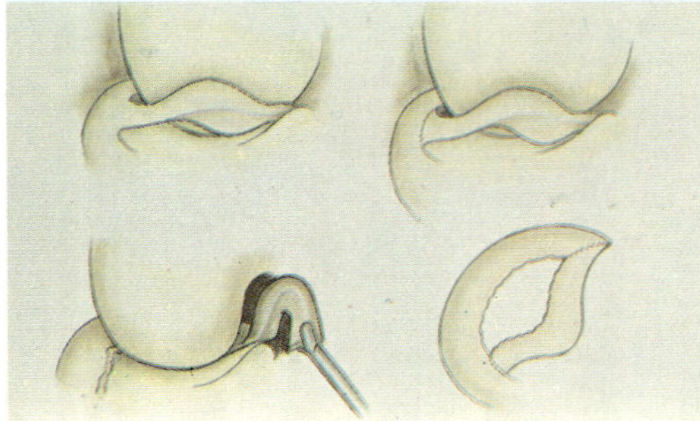

Fig. 12-13. Displaced bucket handle tear of the medial meniscus.

Flap Tear of the Left Medial Meniscus Displaced Beneath the Meniscus

This common degenerative tear passes from the posterior third of the medial meniscus and is trapped beneath the anterior medial meniscus (Fig. 12-12, *left*). For verification it may be dislodged with a crochet hook; however, ignoring the displaced position facilitates its excision (Fig. 12-12, *right*). Through the lateral portal, using the operating arthroscope, a small meniscus scissors is placed at the base of the fold of the tear, and cuts the flap at its base. The rest of the inner edge of the meniscus is trimmed with a basket forceps.

Bucket Handle Tear of the Medial Meniscus

The anterior horn of the displaced inner rim of the bucket is resected first. The operating arthroscope is inserted laterally, and the small fold of fat pad overlying the anterior medial meniscus is coaxed anterior with the barrel of the arthroscope. A small meniscal scissors is used to cut the meniscus as close to its base as possible. The operating arthroscope is removed from the lateral portal and reinserted through the medial portal, the direct viewing telescope replacing the operating unit in the water sleeve. A retractor is then placed through the lateral portal, and, under direct vision, the anterior fragment of the medial meniscus is grasped and retracted superiorly and laterally. The direct telescope is then replaced with the operating arthroscope, through which the scissors is directed beneath the free fragment that has been placed on a stretch. The fragment is then severed at its base. An area of obstruction, the medial tibial spine, partially obscures the area to be cut. After the large inner fragment is removed from the joint, the peripheral rim is studied as well. A small pituitary rongeur (downward biting) has been most useful in working around the posterior medial tibial spine.

Lateral Meniscal Tears

Longitudinal Tear of the Posterior Third of the Lateral Meniscus

This is a common tear, which extends from the posterior tibial attachment of the lateral meniscus to the level of the popliteus tendon (Fig. 12-14, *left*). This tear is often associated with locking. To excise this torn inner fragment, the operating arthroscope is inserted from the lateral portal and the inner edge is connected to the torn surface (Fig. 12-14, *right*). This allows complete mobility of the fragment. A retractor is inserted from the medial portal; the fragment is grasped and rotated on its intact posterior attach

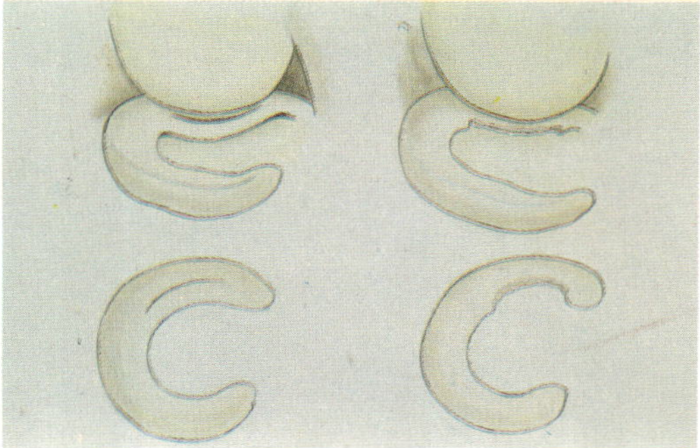

Fig. 12-14. Longitudinal tear of the posterior third of the lateral meniscus.

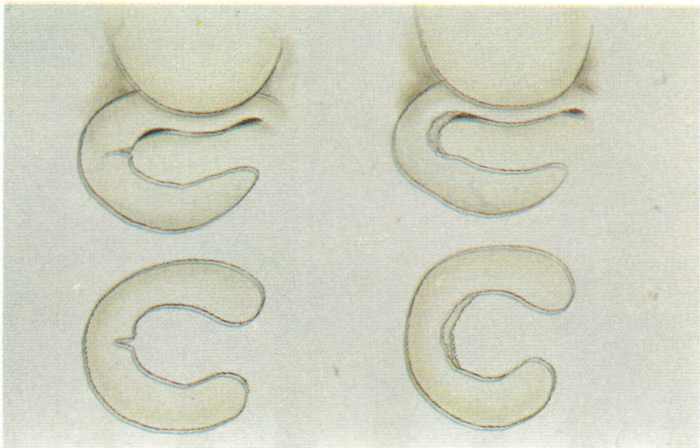

Fig. 12-15. (*Left*) Transverse tear of the lateral meniscus of the right knee. (*Right*) The edges must be saucerized to prevent extension of this tear.

ment. With the small meniscal scissors, the posterior attachment is severed and the fragment removed through the medial portal. The edges are trimmed with a basket biopsy forceps.

Transverse Tear of the Lateral Meniscus (Right Knee)

A transverse split running from the inner edge a variable distance through the body of the meniscus is another frequent tear of the lateral meniscus (Fig. 12-15, *left*). Experience shows that this tear has a propensity for spreading anterior and posterior to form the so-called parrot beak. To excise this tear in its localized state, the operating arthroscope is introduced medially, and the edges anterior and posterior are trimmed and saucerized to prevent the tear from spreading (Fig. 12-15, *right*).

SPECIFIC TEARS AMENABLE TO PARTIAL MENISCECTOMY AND THEIR PREOPERATIVE AND POSTOPERATIVE APPEARANCE

The orthopaedic surgeon faced with the possibility of performing a partial meniscectomy may fear that he might make an inadequate excision, removing either too much or too little. He may be justly concerned that the edges of excision are thick or ragged. For this reason, the following tears will be shown with the immediate postoperative appearance and, where possible, the appearance months later.

Medial Meniscal Tears

Degenerative Tear of the Posterior Third of the Medial Meniscus

This injury kept a 63-year-old orthopaedic surgeon awake at night and interferred with his leisure activities of skiing and tennis. Retropatellar grating and a positive patellar compression test were found in addition to a positive Apley compression test. Arthroscopy demonstrated hyaline cartilage degeneration of the patella, medial femoral condyle, and the tear of the medial meniscus (Fig. 12-16). Note the flap beneath the medial meniscus in the left view.

Figure 12-17 was taken immediately after partial resection of the medial meniscus. Note the ragged border of the medial meniscus (magnified). Medial infrapatellar approach.

The patient continued heavy activity of tennis, Racquet ball, and bicycle riding, and continued to complain of knee swelling following these activities. Repeat arthroscopy 2½ months later demonstrated that the medial meniscus has rounded off (Fig. 12-18). Lateral infrapatellar approach.

The cause of the patient's complaints

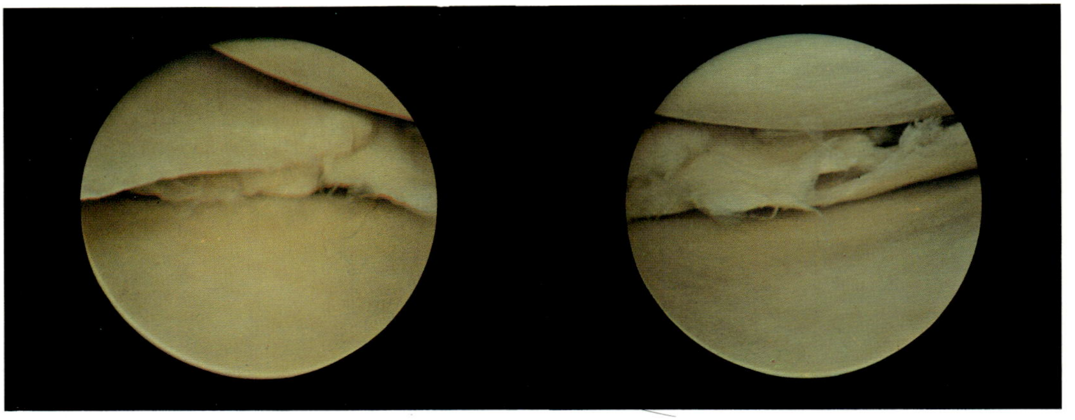

Fig. 12-16. Degenerative flap tear of the posterior third of the medial meniscus of the left knee with fragment caught between meniscus and tibia. There is moderate degeneration of the articular cartilage of the medial femoral condyle.

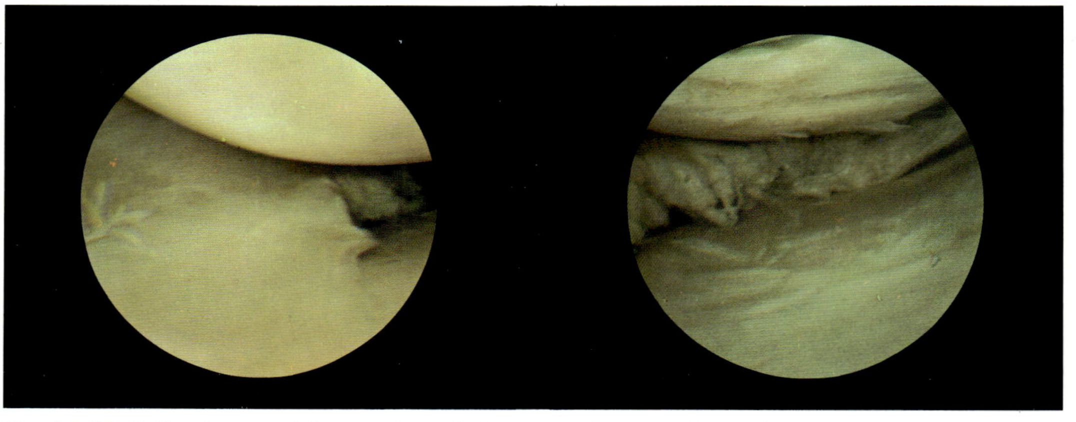

Fig. 12-17. Following partial resection of this tear, the ragged peripheral rim is seen from the medial infrapatellar approach.

was chronic synovitis. These edematous villi contain several areas of fibrosis (Fig. 12-19, *right*). A close-up of the medial joint line demonstrates the smoothness of the fibrocartilage (Fig. 12-19, *left*).

Bucket Handle Tear of the Medial Meniscus

This injury, present for 4 months, was found to be this 18-year-old's cause of symptoms (Fig. 12-20). The peripheral rim seen in the background is studied in Fig. 12-21. In 4 months this rim has become smooth, reassuring to both surgeon and patient. The inner rim of the bucket handle tear was excised. The joint line is seen in Fig. 12-22. The specimen excised with the operating arthroscope is seen in Fig. 12-23. This extensive mass of fibrocartilage will easily pass through the arthroscopy portal by virtue of its elasticity and, to a lesser degree, the elasticity of the anterior capsule.

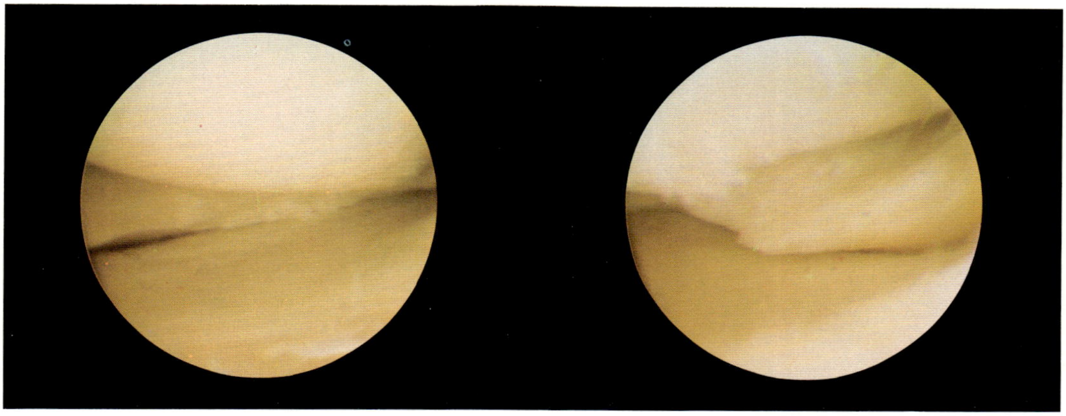

Fig. 12-18. (*Left*) Arthroscopy through the lateral infrapatellar approach demonstrates the rounding off of the peripheral rim 2½ months after partial excision of the medial meniscus. (*Right*) Postoperative view of the resected meniscus at its posterior tibial attachment.

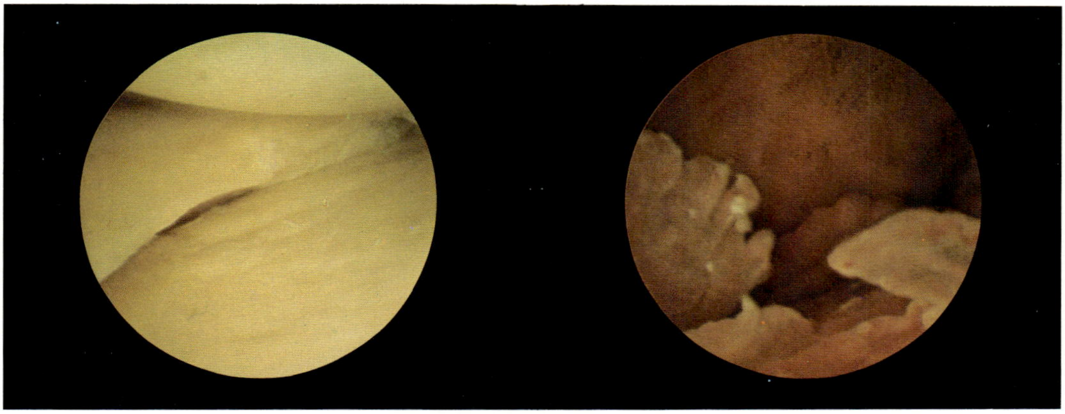

Fig. 12-19. (*Right*) The recurrent effusion in this patient was found to be due to chronic synovitis. Note the edematous villi, which contain several areas of fibrosis. (*Left*) This view of the medial joint line demonstrates the smoothing of the peripheral rim.

Nondisplaced Tear of the Medial Meniscus

An abnormality of the peripheral rim of the left medial meniscus is seen in Fig. 12-24, *left.* In Fig. 12-24, *right,* the medial meniscus protrudes abnormally into the joint. In order to find the anterior and posterior ends of the tear, a crochet hook has been introduced into the joint from a medial portal and the tear is dislocated (Fig. 12-25). The anterior cut is made, diagrammatically demonstrating that this tight tear has disappeared behind the medial femoral condyle to lie perpendicular to the peripheral rim of the meniscus and parallel to the posterior cruciate ligament (Fig. 12-26). If not forewarned of this possibility, the surgeon will search to find the fragment. The arthroscope must be placed medially and the knee manipulated in such a manner that it can be passed posteriorly between the medial femoral condyle and medial tibial spine.

(*Text continues on page 132*)

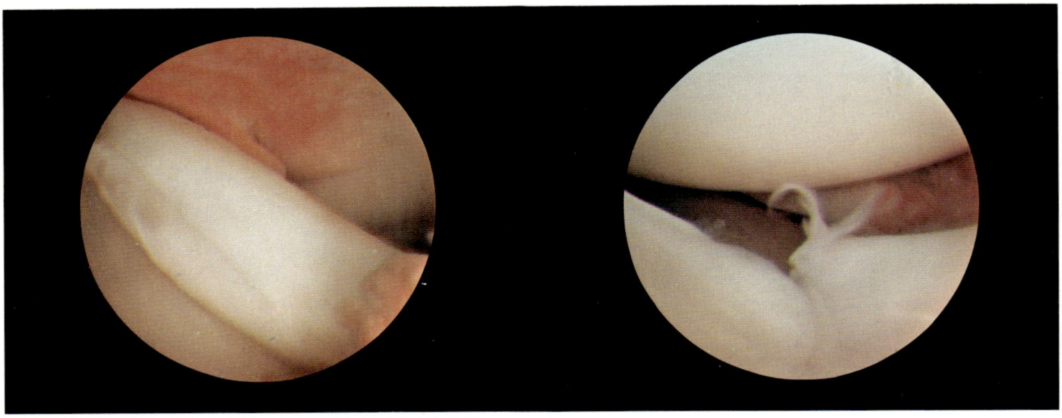

Fig. 12-20. Displaced bucket handle tear of the medial meniscus. (*Left*) The displaced fragment. (*Right*) The anterior attachment of the displaced bucket and the peripheral rim.

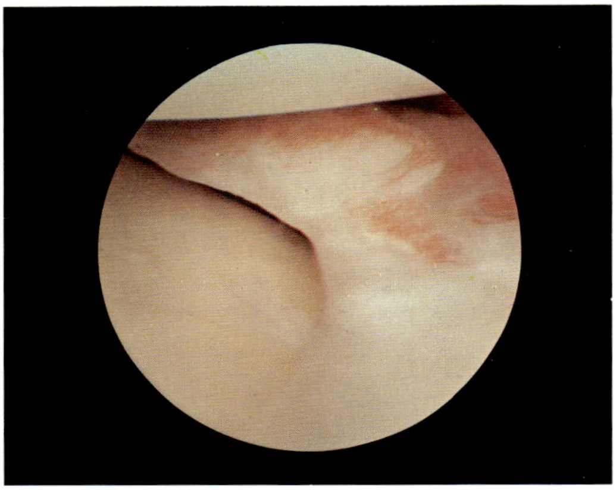

Fig. 12-21. The peripheral rim has become smooth over the intervening 4 months since injury, demonstrating again how the ragged fibrocartilage will become smooth.

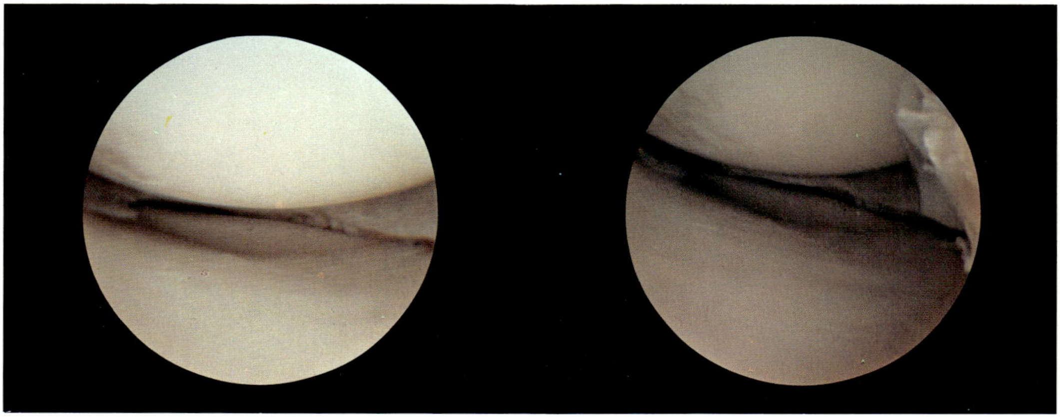

Fig. 12-22. The appearance of the medial joint line following excision of the displaced bucket handle tear of the medial meniscus.

Fig. 12-23. The specimen is the displaced inner rim of the bucket handle seen in Fig. 12-20.

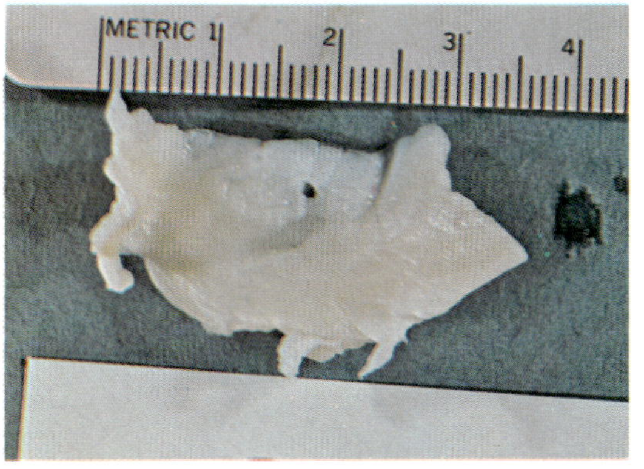

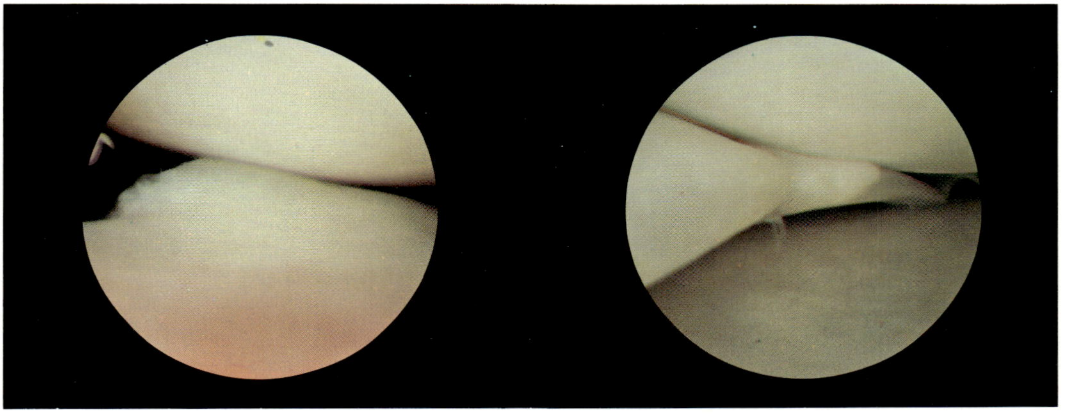

Fig. 12-24. (*Left*) A tear through the peripheral rim of the medial meniscus of the left knee is evident. (*Right*) Abnormal rotation of the inner edge of the medial meniscus.

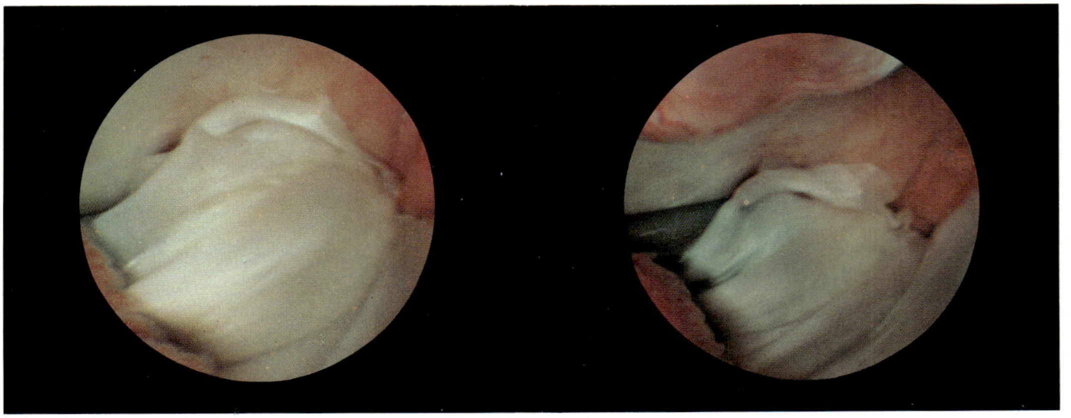

Fig. 12-25. A crochet hook is used to displace the mobile fragment centrally.

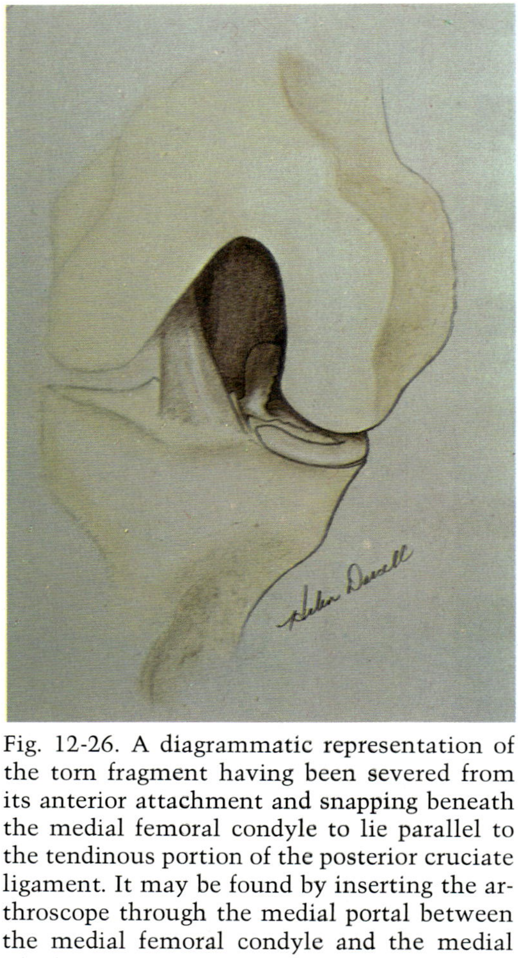

Fig. 12-26. A diagrammatic representation of the torn fragment having been severed from its anterior attachment and snapping beneath the medial femoral condyle to lie parallel to the tendinous portion of the posterior cruciate ligament. It may be found by inserting the arthroscope through the medial portal between the medial femoral condyle and the medial tibial spine.

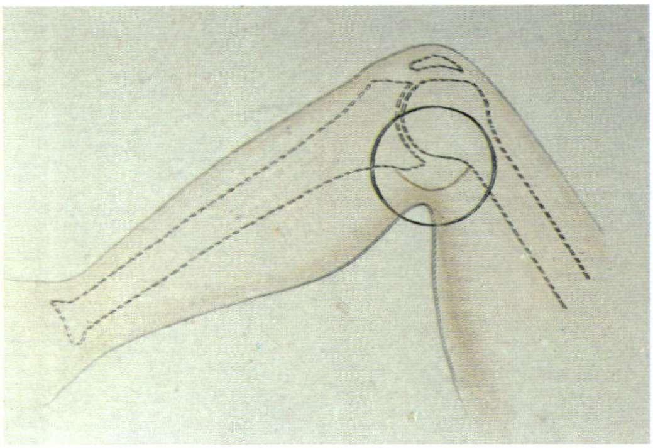

Fig. 12-27. Posterior approach to medial compartment.

The operating arthroscope must be used in order to cut the meniscal flap at its base.

If difficulty is encountered passing the arthroscope between the medial femoral condyle and the medial tibial spine, it may be introduced posterior to the medial femoral condyle and slightly above joint line level (Fig. 12-27). This approach is used as a last resort and probably should be used more often. On several occasions, excision of the flap was accomplished through the posteriorly inserted operating arthroscope.

This patient had a torn anterior cruciate ligament and, because of continuing complaints, his knee was reexamined arthroscopically 5 months following meniscal excision. The unreabsorbed anterior cruciate ligament was found to be "catching" in the joint line. This offered an excellent opportunity to view the medial joint line (Fig. 12-28). In Fig. 12-29, *left,* the medial joint line is viewed from the medial infrapatellar approach. Note how the peripheral rim has smoothed out. In Fig. 12-29, *right,* the arthroscope has been inserted posterior to the medial femoral condyle, and the peripheral meniscal rim can be seen as rounded off. The medial tibial plateau is inferior and a small portion of the medial femoral condyle is superior.

Injuries of the Peripheral Rim Following Partial Meniscectomy

If doubt exists concerning the integrity of the peripheral rim following partial meniscectomy, the medial meniscus should be investigated through the anterior and posterior medial portals. The lesion in Fig. 12-30 was an extensive flap of the posterior medial meniscus rotated and displaced beneath the medial meniscus anterior (lateral portal). The magnitude of the tear suggested possible involvement of the posterior peripheral segment. A similar postoperative situa-

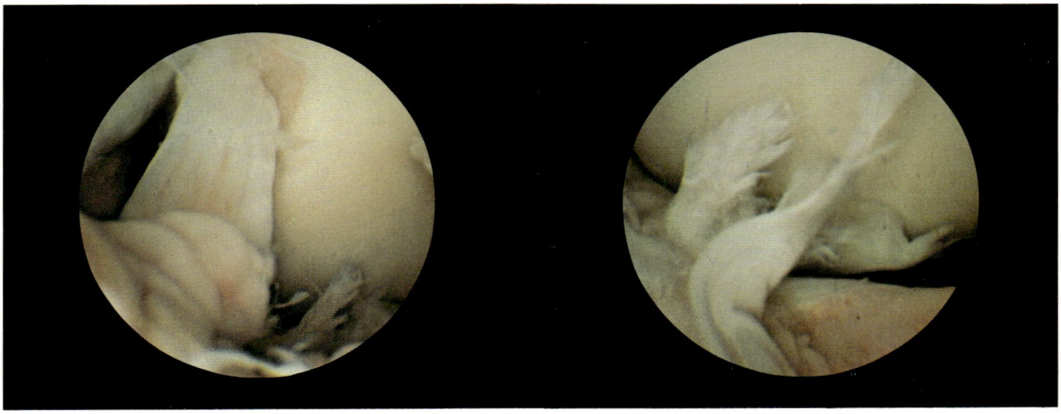

Fig. 12-28. Medial meniscus 5 months following partial medial meniscectomy. Arthroscopy demonstrated an unresorbed tear of the anterior cruciate ligament.

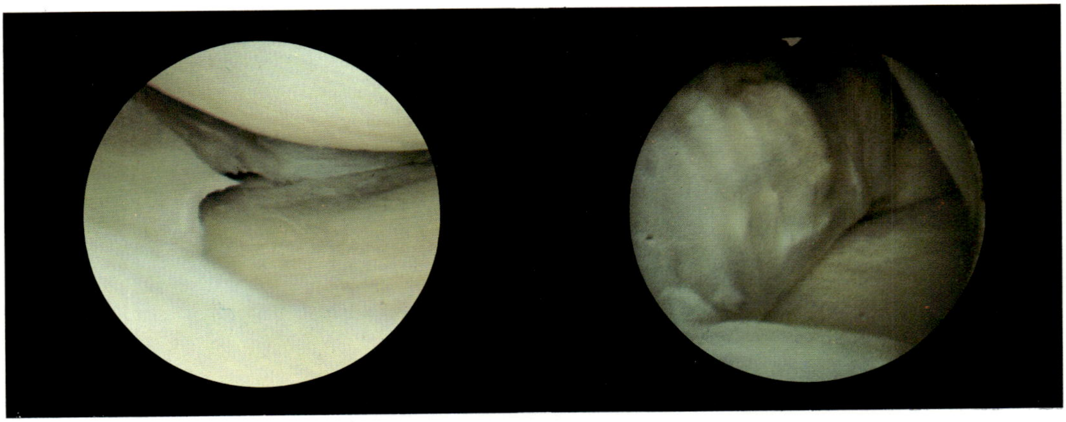

Fig. 12-29. (*Left*) Medial joint line from medial intrapatellar approach. (*Right*) The peripheral posterior margin of the medial meniscus is seen through a posterior medial approach. The peripheral attachments are intact.

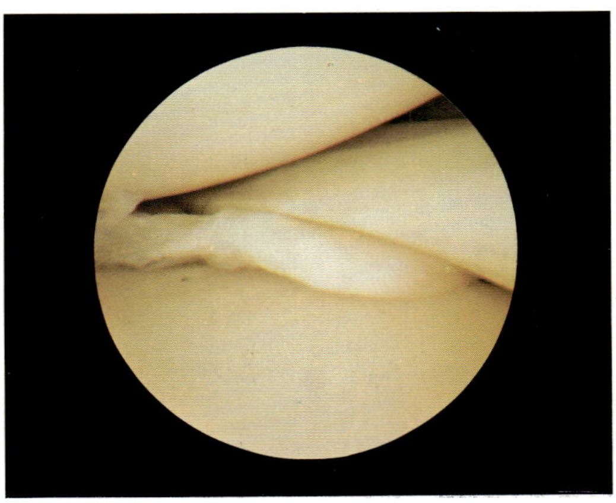

Fig. 12-30. Flap tear originating from the posterior third of the medial meniscus, which has rotated anteriorly and been trapped beneath the intact medial meniscus.

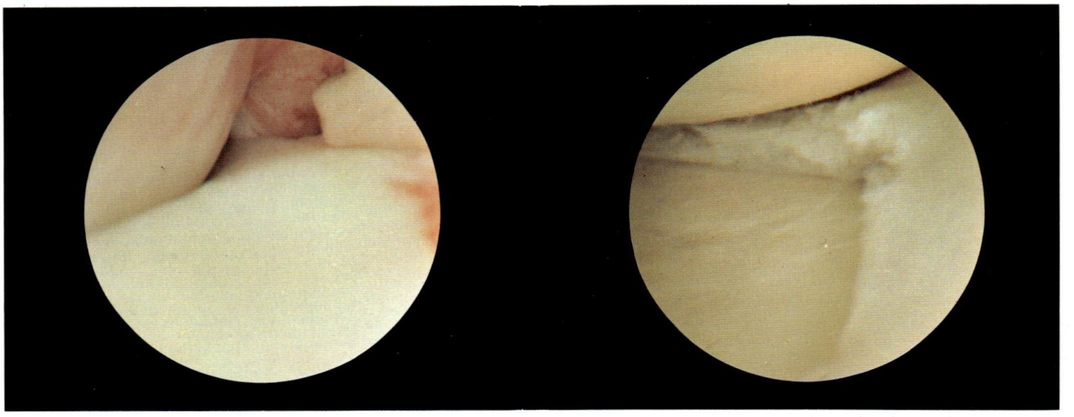

Fig. 12-31. View, after a partial medial meniscectomy, through the anteromedial portal on the right; the posterior margin of the medial meniscus has a firm capsular attachment, as seen through the posteromedial portal.

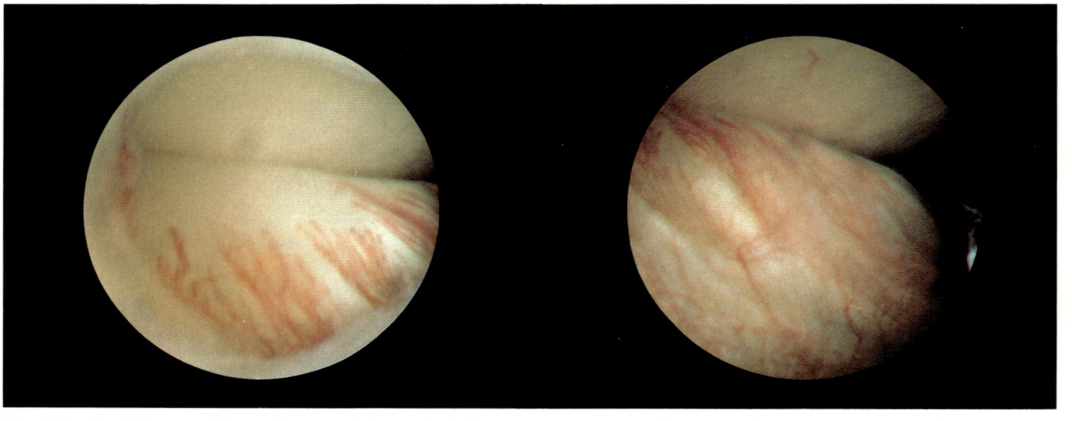

Fig. 12-32. The peripheral rim of the medial meniscus seen through the posteromedial approach.

tion is seen in Fig. 12-31: The anterior medial approach demonstrates the level of resection of the flap following partial excision (*right*); the posterior segment of the medial meniscus has a firm capsular attachment (*left*). Blood vessels indicate the peripheral extent of the meniscus. The medial femoral condyle is seen on the left. The peripheral margin can be studied as well (Fig. 12-32): the peripheral vascular pattern (*left*) confirms the integrity of this segment of the meniscus beneath the medial collateral ligament; (*right*) area posterior to the medial collateral ligament.

Meniscal Tear With Irreversible Damage to the Articular Cartilage

An ideal indication for partial meniscec-

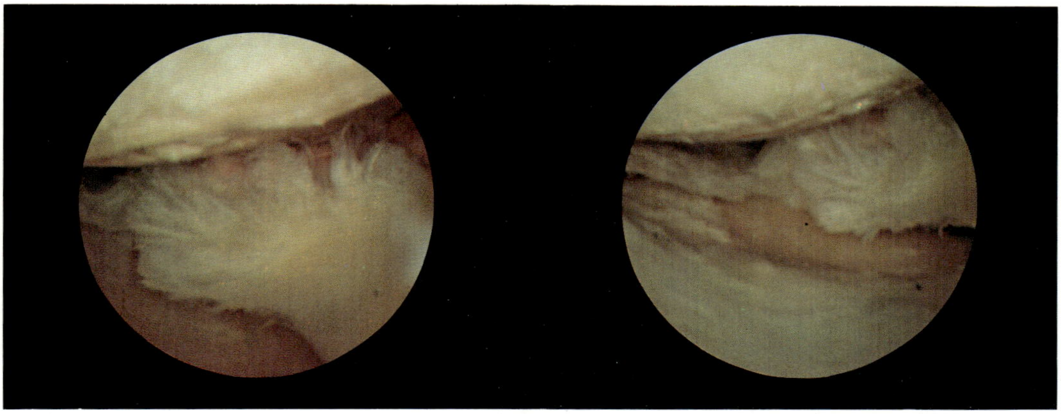

Fig. 12-33. A degenerative tear of the posterior third of the medial meniscus is associated with degeneration of the medial femoral condyle and the medial tibial plateau.

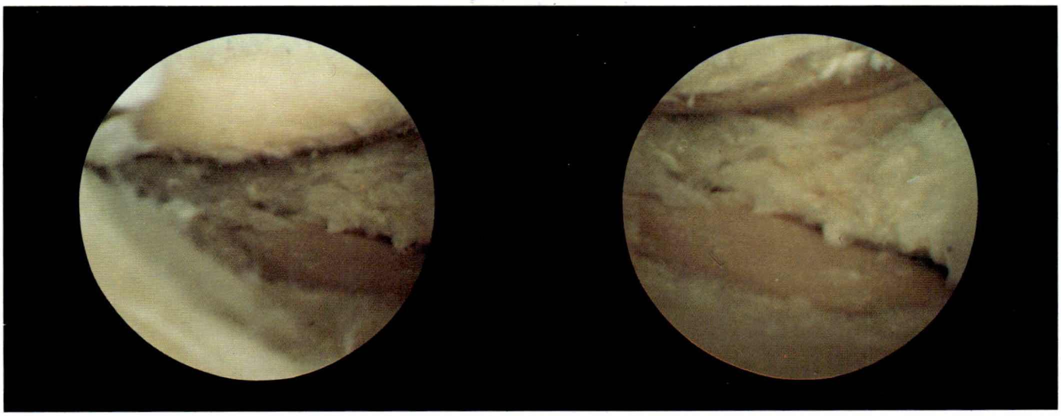

Fig. 12-34. The postoperative appearance of the meniscus (see Fig. 12-33).

tomy is a tear of the meniscus in the presence of irreversible damage to the articular cartilage of the medial femoral condyle and the medial tibial plateau, as illustrated in this 40-year-old professional dancer. Eburnation of the medial tibial plateau accompanies articular cartilage degeneration of the medial femoral condyle and a degenerative tear of the posterior medial meniscus (Fig. 12-33).

Despite the ragged appearance of the meniscal margin after partial excision (Fig. 12-34), the patient's joint line pain was greatly relieved, allowing him to continue limited professional activities.

Complex tears of the meniscus occur when a torn meniscus is allowed to remain over a number of years and reinjury occurs.

In Fig. 12-35, separate tears are appar-

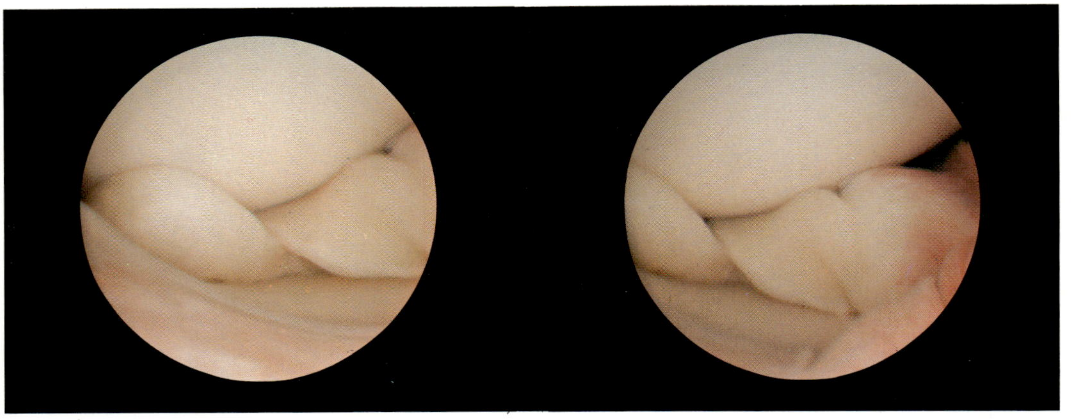

Fig. 12-35. Complex tear of right medial meniscus, consisting of a bulbous pedunculated fragment, and a longitudinal tear. After excision of both fragments a third tear (longitudinal) was found in the peripheral rim.

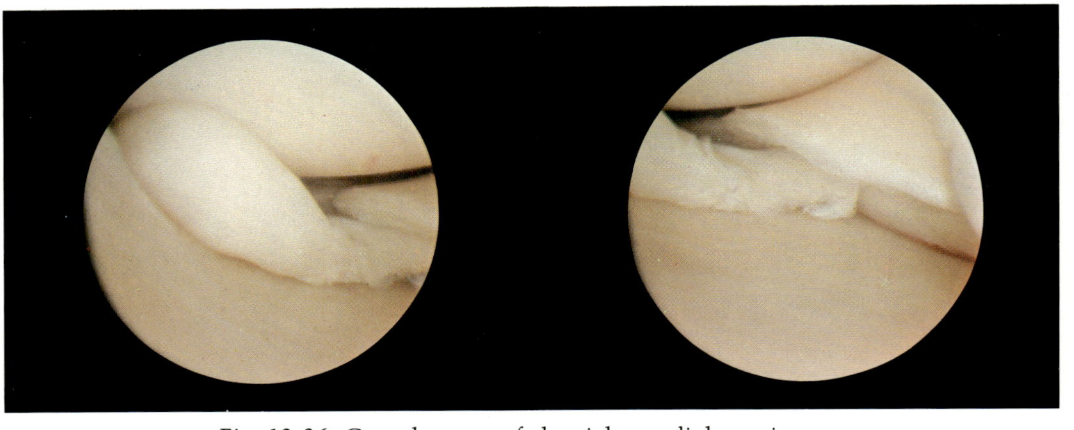

Fig. 12-36. Complex tear of the right medial meniscus.

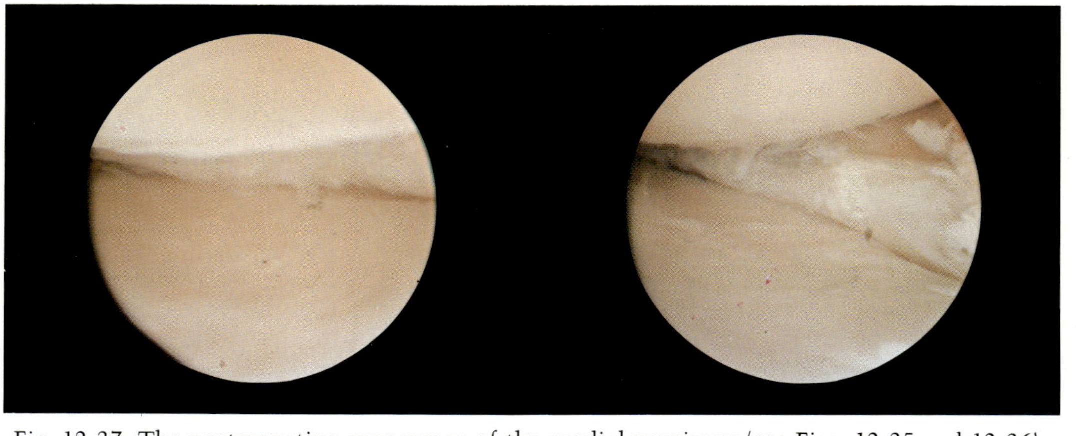

Fig. 12-37. The postoperative appearance of the medial meniscus (see Figs. 12-35 and 12-36).

ent, one a rounded flap; another a longitudinal tear cover; still another, a short longitudinal tear of the peripheral rim. Accurate preoperative assessment of the situation allowed partial meniscectomy. "Working room" was increased by resection first of the pedunculated flap, then of the large longitudinal tear, and finally of the short longitudinal tear in the peripheral rim (Fig. 12-36). Figure 12-37 depicts the postoperative appearance.

LATERAL MENISCAL TEARS

Lateral Displaced Bucket Handle Tear

This injury may be surprisingly silent. This 25-year-old basketball player gave a history of repeated injuries to his left knee over a 5-year period. However, examination showed his knee (aside from vague lateral joint line symptoms) as being remarkably normal, and arthroscopy was postponed for an inordinately prolonged period. Arthroscopy (Fig. 12-38) revealed that a large displaced bucket handle tear occupied the intercondylar notch, supplanting a resorbing torn anterior cruciate ligment. Considerable laxity of the fragment was due to the anterior extent of the tear. Resection was accomplished by using the double puncture technique, inserting a 5 mm. meniscal scissors through the medial portal and detaching the anterior horn of the lateral meniscus while viewing through a lateral portal. A meniscal retractor replaced the scissors, and the meniscal fragment was drawn towards the medial joint line. The operating arthroscope was inserted through the lateral portal to allow detachment of the posterior horn from its base. Figure 12-39 shows both the anterior and posterior sites of detachment.

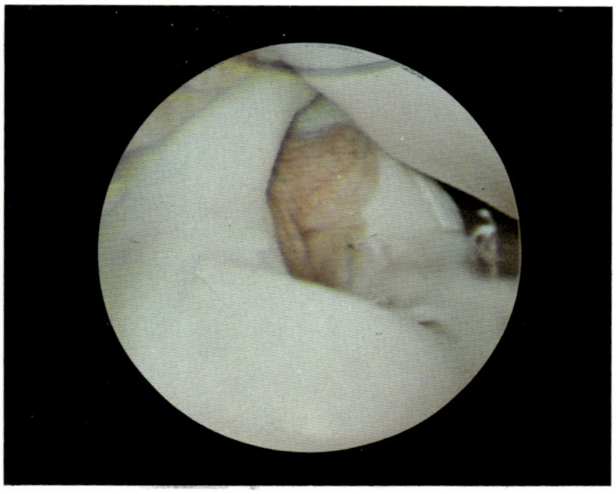

Fig. 12-38. A large, widely displaced bucket handle tear of the lateral meniscus in a left knee.

Longitudinal Tear of the Lateral Meniscus

Occasionally the wrong meniscus is removed, or a combination medial and lateral meniscal tear is present and only the medial meniscus is excised. This embarrassing situation occurred in a 24-year-old male who could lock his knee following his medial meniscectomy. After reviewing the patient's laterally negative arthrogram, the surgeon referred the patient for arthroscopy. Predictably, based on this patient's history, a longitudinal tear of the lateral meniscus confined to the posterior third was found (Fig. 12-40) and dealt with in the following manner.

The operating arthroscope was inserted laterally, and a small meniscal retractor

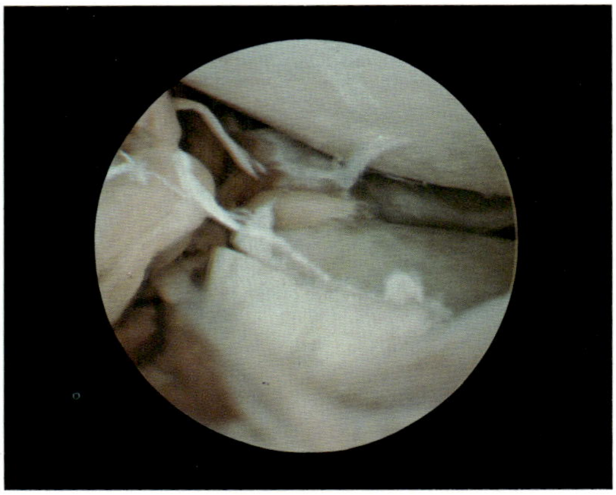

Fig. 12-39. Areas of surgical cleavage between the attachments of the anterior and posterior horns and the inner rim (compare with Fig. 12-38).

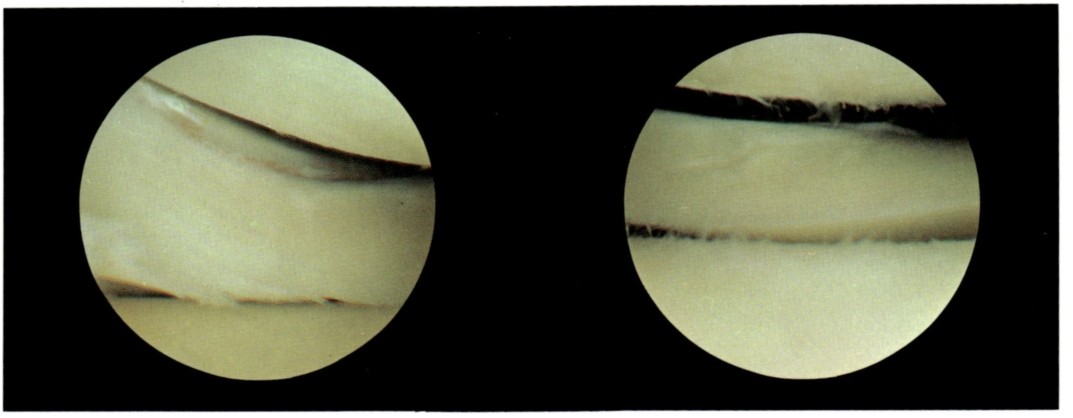

Fig. 12-40. Longitudinal tear of the posterior third of the lateral meniscus.

was inserted medially to grasp the torn inner fragment (Fig. 12-41). The lateral edge of the tear was cut, the cut running from the inner margin of the meniscus to the tear proper (thus permitting the tear to be mobilized), and retracting the fragment toward the medial compartment. The posterior attachment was then severed and the fragment removed from the joint. Failure to grasp the torn inner margin of the meniscus results in the situation depicted in Fig. 12-42: After the fragment is detached laterally, it sweeps beneath the lateral femoral condyle to lie posterior to this condyle, and disappears from view. Even this situation may be salvaged by inserting a meniscal retractor through the medial portal, sliding it between the anterior cruciate ligament and the lateral femoral condyle. The fragment can be palpated blindly, grasped, and retrieved. The dissection then proceeds in the routine fashion.

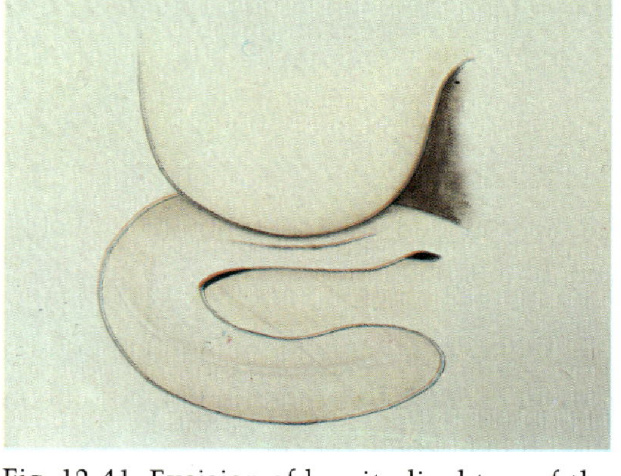

Fig. 12-41. Excision of longitudinal tear of the posterior third of the lateral meniscus.

Meniscal Flap Split From the Lateral Attachment

The knowledge gained at arthroscopy allows the patient's confusing symptoms

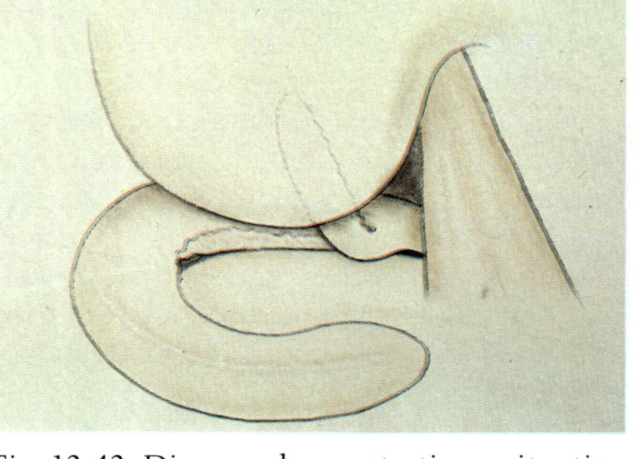

Fig. 12-42. Diagram demonstrating a situation that can occur if the lateral attachment of the longitudinal tear of the lateral meniscus is severed without retracting the body of the mobile fragment. The flap created by the surgical incision snaps beneath the lateral femoral condyle and disappears from view.

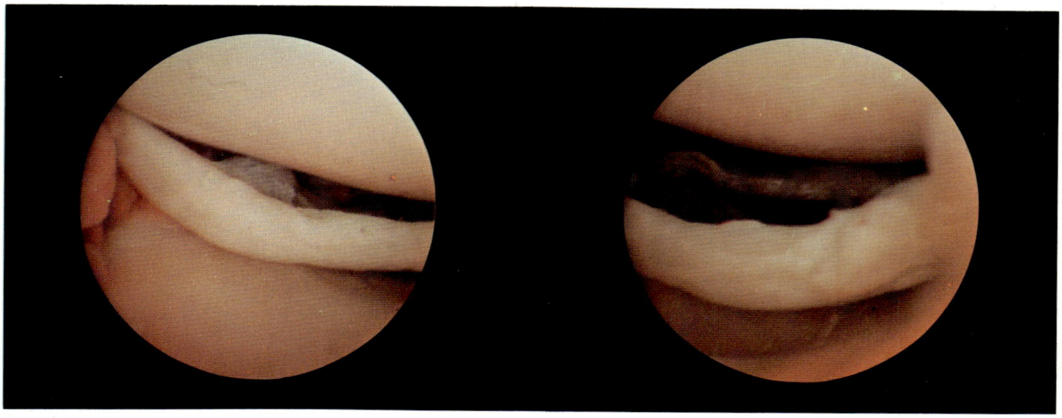

Fig. 12-43. (*Left*) A longitudinal tear of the left lateral meniscus has split from the peripheral rim laterally; it may rotate on its posterior attachment and be trapped in the medial joint line. (*Right*) The free end of the flap is seen behind a fold of synovium.

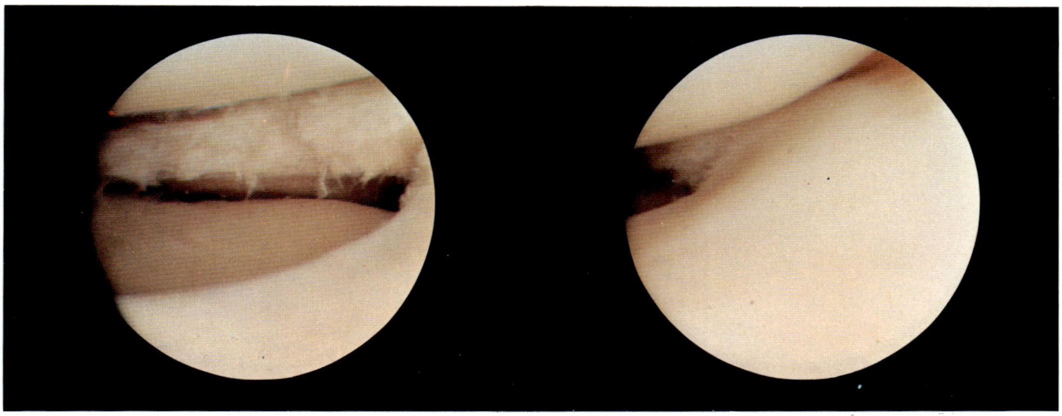

Fig. 12-44. The peripheral rim, following arthroscopic excision of this flap, is seen to be rounding off.

to be understood. A 30-year-old cowboy complained of intermittent pain (primarily of the medial joint line), and giving way. The medial joint line was found to be normal, but the anterior cruciate ligament was torn, compounding the problem and causing contralateral joint line symptoms (Fig. 12-43). In the lateral joint line of this knee (*left*), a flap of meniscus has split off from its lateral attachment, rotated on its posterior attachment, and, by virtue of the loss of the space-occupying anterior cruciate ligament, could be trapped in the medial joint line as well as the lateral joint line. The free end is seen behind the fold of synovium (*right*). Initial examination disclosed this fragment lying in the medial compartment. The meniscal fragment was simply severed at its posterior base.

In Fig. 12-44, the posterior and middle third of the lateral meniscus are rounding off. No further surgical attention was necessary.

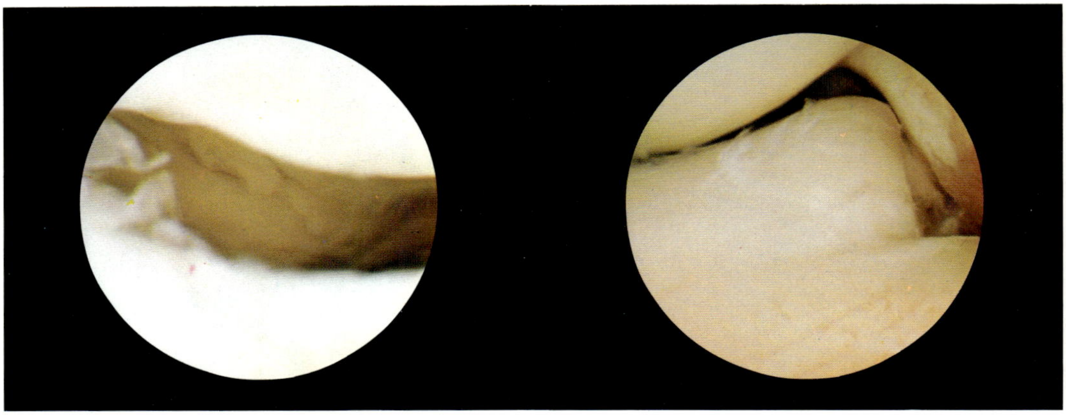

Fig. 12-45. Right knee. (*Left*) Tear of discoid lateral meniscus through the posterolateral corner. (*Right*) The rounded displaced body of the discoid meniscus.

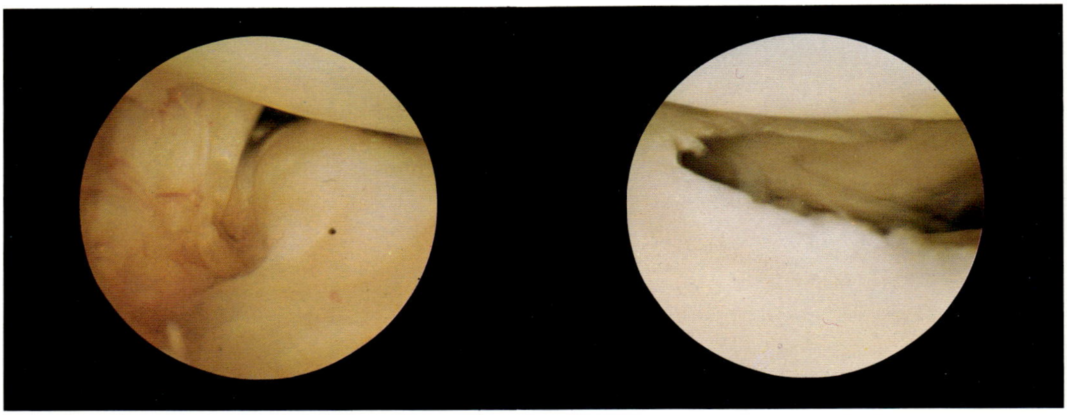

Fig. 12-46. An identical tear to the one in Fig. 12-45 is seen in this patient's left knee. (*Left*) Discoid meniscus is bulging centrally. (*Right*) The tear occurred posterolaterally. The popliteus tendon is seen in the background.

Identical Tears of Both Lateral Menisci

Occasionally unusual situations arise that require individual solutions. A 55-year-old sign painter was involved in an automobile accident injuring both knees. Arthrograms demonstrated identical tears in both lateral menisci. Arthroscopy disclosed a tear of the lateral meniscus (Fig. 12-45, *right*), torn at the peripheral posterolateral corner, (*left*) in a discoid lateral meniscus. The thickened inner rim of the discoid meniscus is seen centrally. Examination of the left knee demonstrated an identical tear (Fig. 12-46). The torn edge is better seen on the right view, and the outline of the popliteus tendon is seen in the background. Using the double puncture technique with the 5 mm. meniscal scissors and basket biopsy forceps, the central portions of the discoid meniscus were excised. The postoperative appearances of the joint lines are seen in Fig. 12-47 (right knee) and Fig. 12-48 (left knee).

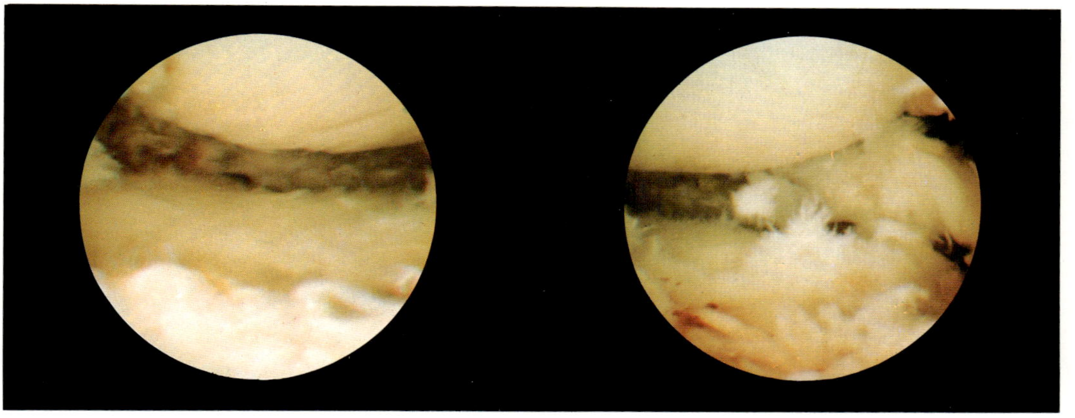

Fig. 12-47. The postoperative appearance of the right knee (see Fig. 12-45).

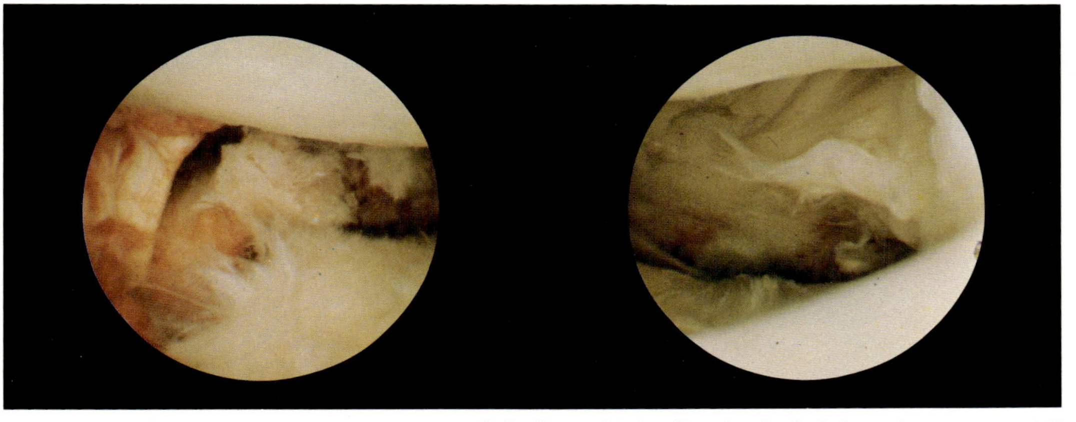

Fig. 12-48. The postoperative appearance of the lateral joint line in the left knee (see Fig. 12-46).

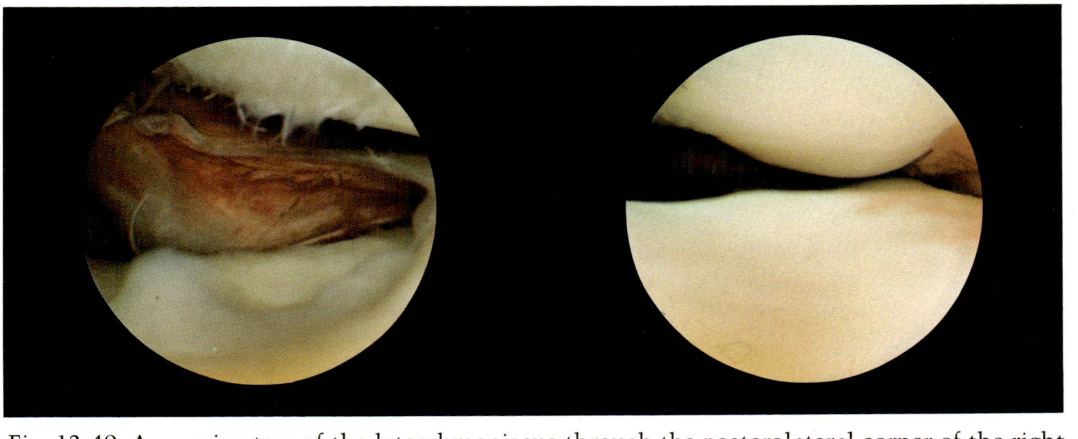

Fig. 12-49. A massive tear of the lateral meniscus through the posterolateral corner of the right knee. (*Left*) The popliteus tendon is demonstrated as well as the edge of the tear. (*Right*) The centrally displaced meniscus.

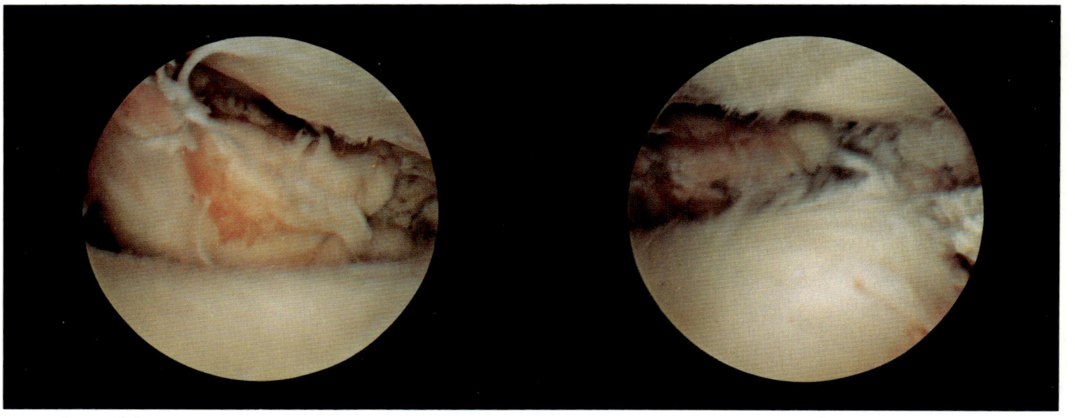

Fig. 12-50. The postoperative appearance of the right lateral joint line (see Fig. 12-49).

Massive Tear of Lateral Meniscus

Arthroscopic surgery may on occasion salvage a horrible result following meniscectomy. Eighteen months after a right medial meniscectomy, a 43-year-old female complained of severe knee discomfort and a severely limited range of motion. In spite of an attempted manipulation under anaesthesia, her range of motion actively measured only 15 to 50 degrees. The referring orthopaedist correctly suspected a lateral meniscal tear, but his clinical findings were not substantiated by arthrography.

A massive tear of the posterolateral peripheral margin of the lateral meniscus was found during arthroscopy (Fig. 12-49). On the left the popliteus tendon and the meniscus displaced anteriorly and centrally towards the intercondylar notch are visible. Under anaesthesia, the passive range of motion measured 8 to 80 degrees. Following excision of the meniscus using the double-puncture technique, and incision of the thickened synovium at the proximal quadriceps bursa, her passive range of motion measured 2 to 130 degrees. Arthrotomy and meniscal excision in this extreme situation undoubtedly would have conferred further disability on this woman. Figure 12-50 shows the postoperative appearance of the lateral joint line.

No serious complication, such as infection or vascular injury, has followed arthroscopic intra-articular surgery in this small series.

INDICATIONS FOR PARTIAL MENISCECTOMY (ARTHROSCOPICALLY PERFORMED)

As with any new technique or modification of an older technique, continued experience will more clearly define limitations and advantages. Based on over two years of surgical experience and follow-up (the results not included in this monograph), my opinion is biased in favor of arthroscopic partial meniscectomy. The short-term results are much more acceptable, allowing quick rehabilitation, shorter hospitalization, and speedy return to work. The important long-term results cannot be evaluated yet, but theoretically should show better results than total meniscectomy.

Obviously the surgeon should not embark on this type of procedure until he was a wide experience with diagnostic arthroscopy, can judge the extent of the tear, and can use the various portals of entry into the knee to obtain the proper cutting angle. A full set of tiny 3 mm. and 5 mm. instruments are necessary.

If scuffing of articular cartilage can be held to a minimum, the only disadvantage to attempted partial meniscectomy would be inadequacy of excision of the mobile meniscal tissue. This would require either repeat partial meniscectomy, or arthrotomy and subtotal meniscectomy. While this is more expensive to the patient, nothing has been done to jeopardize the results of arthrotomy and subtotal meniscectomy.

My brief experience with this technique can be summarized as follows:

Bucket handle tears of the medial or lateral meniscus are ideal tears for treatment by partial excision. If additional tears of the peripheral rim are encountered, these may be excised as well. Associated tears of the anterior cruciate ligament (suprisingly common) usually result in downgrading the final result due to the occurrence of late instability symptoms. Nevertheless, the short-term results appear better with partial than with subtotal meniscectomy.

Degenerative tears of the medial meniscus in the patient over 40 years of age are usually associated with hyaline cartilage degeneration of the medial femoral condyle, the patella, or the medial tibial plateau. Commonly, the tear pattern is either oblique or a flap. The response to partial excision in these patients is generally excellent. However, these flap tears may occur in patients in their second decade, whose functional demands are greater. The results of these cases have not been quite as salubrious. In fact, the majority of tears requiring revision have been those in the younger age group.

Degenerative tears of either meniscus in an older patient with gout or pseudogout that have had an associated effusion, are best treated by partial meniscectomy, if any surgery is to be performed. Arthrotomy in these patients may well result in a more prolonged convalescence than that in patients not afflicted with these metabolic conditions.

Tears confined to the posterior third of the medial and lateral meniscus are usually seen in the younger patient, and cause locking. Dealing with these tears arthroscopically is quite difficult, and I feel that, owing to the technical difficulties involved (especially of the medial meniscus), considerable arthroscopic surgical experience is necessary before these tears are attempted.

In the highly competitive athlete, partial meniscectomy may be indicated as a temporizing measure, allowing continuing activity until time is available for rehabilitation following arthrotomy.

A small flap tear in a meniscus that appears otherwise normal may allow at least several years of function. The small group of patients that could be included in this category have not yet needed arthrotomy.

ANALYSIS OF RESULTS OF PARTIAL MENISCECTOMY UNDER ARTHROSCOPIC CONTROL

One patient with a displaced bucket handle tear of the lateral meniscus, because of continuing clicking over the lateral joint line and tenderness over the popliteus tendon, was re-arthroscoped. A tear of the peripheral posterior segment of the lateral meniscus was noted (Fig. 12-51). The lateral femoral condyle and tibial plateau appeared normal, and photographs taken prior to partial meniscectomy and one year later showed no essential changes in the hyaline cartilage. He was treated by an excision of the peripheral rim without either subjective or objective improvement.

Two patients developed severe postoperative hermarthrosis, requiring aspirations. One was able to return to work after a month. He was treated by early aspiration of the effusion. The second pa-

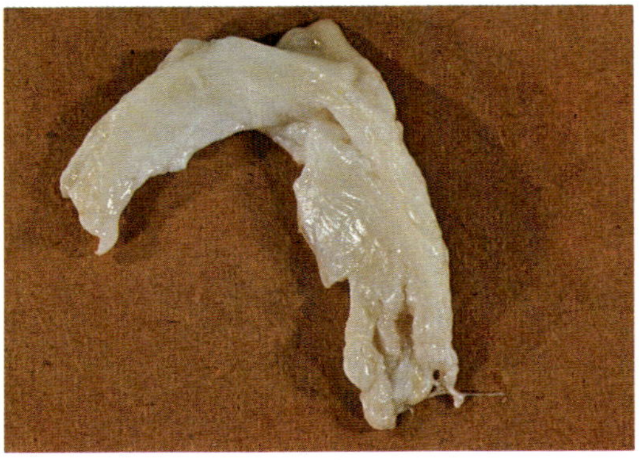

Fig. 12-51. Specimen of torn peripheral rim of lateral meniscus; one tear following arthroscopic excision of the displaced bucket handle. At repeat arthroscopy the articular cartilage appeared smooth. Despite a clean complete excision of the peripheral rim, the industrially injured patient still complained of lateral joint line pain, tenderness, and a click, and now has 1 inch of quadriceps atrophy.

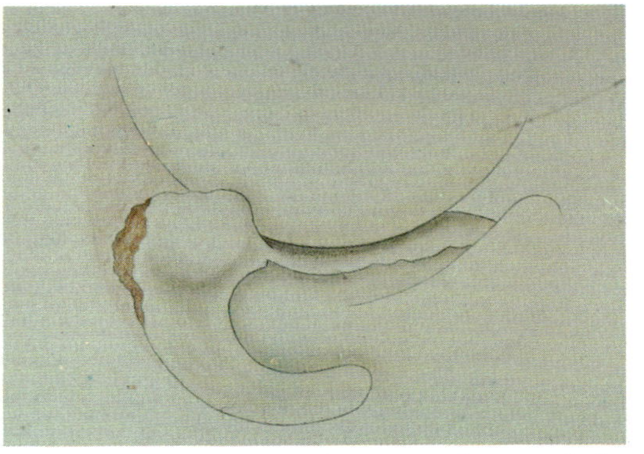

Fig. 12-52. A peripheral marginal tear of the left medial meniscus, seen through the medial portal is depicted in a quiescent rheumatoid patient.

tient could not return to work because of associated low-back difficulties.

One patient was released to lighter work only, owing to associated fracture of the lateral tibial plateau and severe chondromalacia of the patella. Another patient, age 52, with associated chondromalacia of the patella was not able to negotiate stairs or ladders, and was unable to return to work as a fireman. Still another patient, with 1½ inches of quadriceps atrophy following his industrial injury, was first seen 4 months following this injury, and quadriceps rehabilitation was difficult. After 3 months and a partial meniscectomy, it was discovered that this patient had a long history of litigated injuries, industrially incurred. He was successfully returned to work, however.

When the quadriceps was redeveloped, no patient failed to improve following partial meniscectomy, but the degree of improvement varied. Only one patient had continued buckling of his knee. No patient had continued locking of his knee. Two patients did have persistent tenderness over the posterior medial joint line, however. It has not been necessary to perform subtotal meniscectomy on any of these patients.

I am in complete agreement with Hughston[7] and others who recommend an intensive quadriceps development program, starting immediately after injury, inasmuch as quadriceps atrophy tends to delay recovery following partial meniscectomy, and it would be wise to build up the quadriceps prior to arthroscopy. Patients who failed to recover rapidly were usually industrial patients with considerable significant long-standing quadriceps atrophy. Perhaps arthroscopy should be delayed until the patient completely recovers his quadriceps tone and strength, particularly if this is an industrially incurred injury, as socioeconomic factors tend to obscure a good clinical result. However, I feel that a locked knee secondary to a displaced bucket handle tear should be handled aggressively, and arthroscopy performed immediately, in order to hasten recovery.

At the time of arthroscopy, an assessment of the synovium may well indicate a tendency for postoperative effusion. A vascular synovium will indicate a possible problem in the postoperative period. These patients are treated with high doses

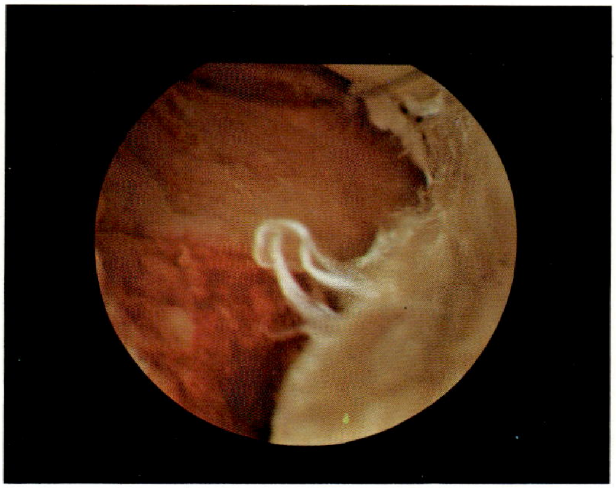

Fig. 12-53. Arthroscopic view of the meniscus separated from the capsule (medial portal).

of an anti-inflammatory agent immediately following surgery.

SUBTOTAL MENISCECTOMY UNDER ARTHROSCOPIC CONTROL

Ikeuchi has recently reported[8] four subtotal meniscectomies of the torn discoid lateral meniscus. The follow-up of the subtotal meniscectomy cases approached 5 years. He noted difficulty in the presence of a discoid lateral meniscus due to obstruction of view during the procedure and did not strongly advocate its use.

Subtotal Meniscectomy for a Displaced Anteromedial Peripheral Marginal Tear

A 58-year-old male in a remission of rheumatoid arthritis was employed as a machine mechanic. He gave a history of multiple episodes of giving way of his knee and occasional episodes of locking, but he had always been able to unlock the knee by manipulation of the leg. The evening preceding surgery, as he was ascending stairs, he felt his knee lock and was unable to unlock it. It was thought that the patient had a displaced bucket handle tear of the medial meniscus, and arthroscopy was performed in anticipation of partial meniscectomy of the displaced bucket handle portion. This was recommended by the patient's rheumatologist, who had previously treated him for rheumatoid arthritis with gold injections and who felt that he had been in a remission for approximately one year. A displaced anteromedial peripheral marginal tear was noted (Figs. 12-52, 53, 54) and subtotal meniscectomy was performed with a Kocker retractor inserted laterally and the arthroscope inserted medially, as well as a secondary quarter-inch stab wound beneath the telescope to accommodate the Smillie knives. The procedure required the use of a tourniquet, and the operating time was 1½ hours. The peripheral third of the meniscus was difficult to

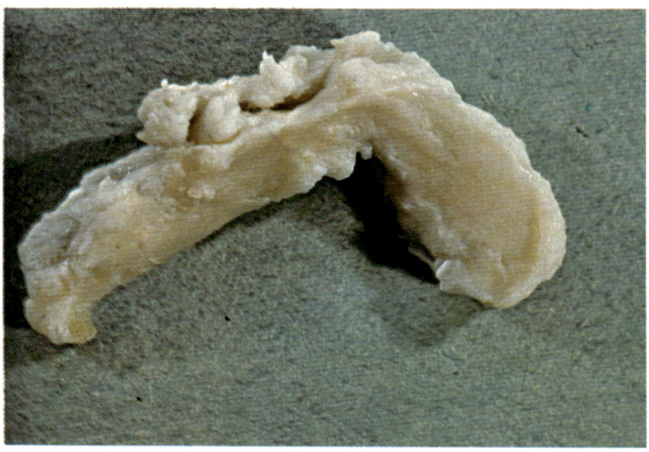

Fig. 12-54. The specimen attests to the difficulty of removing this meniscus. Interestingly, the patient developed no joint reaction to this surgery, but 5 months later manifested active rheumatoid involvement in the contralateral knee, both ankles, and, to a lesser extent, this knee.

dissect. It required the use of Smillie knives as well as arthroscopic scissors. The postoperative result was excellent and was obtained without activitation of his rheumatoid arthritis. The patient returned to full-time work in two weeks.

The gratifying surgical result, however, should not be interpreted as a reason to perform this routinely. Technically it is quite difficult, and, in the normal knee, undue cartilage (hyaline) damage may occur. Hopefully, with the proper instruments, in the future this procedure may hold some promise for the carefully selected patient.

REFERENCES

1. Cargill, A. O'R., and Jackson, J. P.: Bucket handle tear and the medial meniscus. J. Bone and Joint Surg., *58A:*248, 1976.
2. Cox, J. S. et al.: The degenerative effects of partial and total resection of the medial meniscus in dogs. Clin. Orthop., *109:*178, 1975.
3. Duthie, J. J. R., and Macleoad, J. G.: Meniscectomy on Soldiers, Review of Cases Discharged From an Army Convalescent Depot. British Medical Assoc., 1917.
4. Fairbank, D. J.: Knee joint changes after meniscectomy. J. Bone Joint Surg., *30B:* 664, 1948.
5. Gear, M. W. L.: Late results of meniscectomy after ten years; proceedings and reports. J. Bone Joint Surg., *47B:*270, 1965.
6. Huckell, J. R.: Is meniscectomy a benign procedure? A long term follow-up study. Can. J. Surg., *8:*254, 1965.
7. Hughston, J.: American Academy Instructional Course-Meniscal Injuries. Annual meeting. San Francisco, 1975.
8. Ikeuchi, H.: Meniscal excision under arthroscopic control. Second Congress, International Arthroscopy Association. Copenhagen, July, 1975.
9. Iseki, F.: The regenerated meniscus with special reference to functional anatomy. Second Congress, International Arthroscopy Association. Copenhagen, July, 1975.
10. Jackson, J. R.: Degenerative changes in the knee after meniscectomy. J. Bone Joint Surg., *49B:*584, 1967.
11. King, D.: The function of the semilunar cartilage. J. Bone Joint Surg., *18:*1069, 1936.
12. Love, R. J. M.: Prognosis after removal of semilunar cartilage. Br. Med. J., *2:*324, 1924.
13. MacConaill, M. A.: The function of intra-articular fibrocartilages, with special reference to the knee and inferior radiolunar joints. J. Anat., *66*:210, 1932.
14. O'Malley, A.: Clinical signs of torn menisci of the knee joint. Second Congress International Arthroscopy Association Meeting. Copenhagen, July, 1975.
15. Radin, E. L. and Bryan, R. S.: The effect of weight bearing on regrowth of the medial meniscus after meniscectomy. J. Trauma, *10*:169, 1970.
16. Tapper, E. H. and Hoover, N. W.: The late results of meniscectomy. J. Bone Joint Surg., *51A:*517, 1969.
17. Walker, P. S. and Erkman, M. J.: The role of the meniscus in force transmission across the knee. Clin. Ortho., *109*:184, 1975.
18. Watanabe, M., Takeda, S. and Ikeuchi, H.: Atlas of Arthroscopy. ed. 2. Tokyo, Igaku Shoin, 1969.

13 Correlation of Arthroscopy with Other Diagnostic Modalities

Many authorities, as I have pointed out, still question the utility of arthroscopy, despite continuing reports of its usefulness. Of the last 300 cases the author has examined arthroscopically, 42 cases (14%) presented confusing pictures that could only be resolved by arthroscopy. Twenty (6.6%) of these patients had conditions that could be specifically treated by intra-articular surgery, avoiding the postoperative morbidity associated with arthrotomy. (See Table 13-1.)

To demonstrate the advantage to the orthopaedist of assembling as much information as possible prior to arthrotomy, the aforementioned 300 cases of knee arthroscopy were analyzed. Those cases with marked discrepancies in the preoperative impression and the postoperative diagnosis were selected for tabulation. Of these patients, 58 per cent were referred by other orthopaedic surgeons, and several patients had been examined by as many as four orthopaedic surgeons. Often there was a discrepancy in compartmental localization between the clinical evidence and the arthrogram. In other cases, the original diagnosis was so bizarre that without arthroscopy a correct diagnosis could not be established. Given the multiplicity of previous examiners, the arthrograms were not all of excellent technical quality, and therefore the radiologists reports were used.

Not all intra-articular problems can be solved by the time-honored methods of history, physical examination and roentgenograms. Arthroscopy and arthrography complement these methods, resulting in more comprehensive diagnoses. With more surgeons mastering the technique of arthroscopy and thereby enhancing their diagnostic skills, microsurgical techniques that decrease postoperative morbidity may be developed. While the conventional restraints effective during all medical experimentation must be maintained for patient protection, a reasoned approach to microscopic intra-articular knee surgery by interested and talented surgeons will eventually lay down guidelines for treatment and improve the overall result. Hopefully this monograph will stimulate orthopaedists interested in arthroscopy, and partially free them from the shackles of conventional "wisdom" so that their minds may explore new avenues. Cassius noted in Shakespeare's *Julius Caesar* that "the fault, dear Brutus, is not in our stars but in ourselves." The future of the arthroscope is not preordained, but will only be realized through continued effort and thought.

Table 13-1. **Comparison of Knee Injuries Diagnosed With and Without Arthroscopy**

Preoperative Diagnosis	Arthroscopic Findings	Surgery Performed Arthroscopically
Torn medial meniscus (no arthrogram)	Localized pigmented villonodular synovitis Degenerative changes in medial compartment	Excision of localized pigmented villinodular synovitis
Changes following lateral meniscectomy (no arthrogram)	Adhesions in lateral compartment	Excision of soft tissue adhesions in the lateral compartment
Torn lateral meniscus (negative arthrogram)	Torn anterior cruciate ligament with overlying synovial chondromatosis	Excision of mass from anterior cruciate ligament
Tear lateral meniscus (2 negative arthrograms)	Lax medial capsule with healed medial capsular scar	
Torn medial meniscus (arthrogram negative for torn lateral meniscus)	Torn medial meniscus and extensive tear peripheral lateral meniscus	
Torn medial meniscus (arthrogram positive for torn medial meniscus and negative for torn lateral meniscus)	Torn medial meniscus and extensive tear lateral meniscus	
Torn lateral meniscus (no arthrogram)	Torn medial meniscus	Excision of small flap tear
Torn lateral meniscus (negative arthrogram)	Chondromalacia patella	
Torn medial meniscus (arthrogram negative for torn medial meniscus)	Hypertrophied medial inter-articular band	Excision of shelf
Torn medial meniscus (no arthrogram)	Tear of anteroperipheral margin of lateral meniscus, 2 chondral loose bodies	
Bucket handle tear of the medial meniscus (no arthrogram)	Synovial chondromatosis in the anterior cruciate ligament	Excision of 2 masses from anterior cruciate ligament
Torn lateral meniscus (2 negative arthrograms)	"Parrot-beak" tear of the medial meniscus, torn anterior cruciate ligament, anterior flap tear of the lateral meniscus	Excision of both tear arthroscopically and removal of multiple cartilaginous loose bodies
Torn medial meniscus (2 negative arthrograms)	Tear of the posterior third of the lateral meniscus	

Table 13-1. (Continued)

Preoperative Diagnosis	Arthroscopic Findings	Surgery Performed Arthroscopically
Chronic effusion after lateral meniscectomy (arthrogram negative)	Recent incomplete tear of the anterior cruciate ligament	Removal of a large necrotic sheet of synovium
Sequelae of medial meniscectomy (arthrogram negative)	Tear of the posterior third of the medial meniscus	
Torn lateral meniscus (arthrogram negative)	Chondromalacia patella	
Torn medial meniscus (arthrogram negative for torn medial meniscus)	Cartilaginous crater in the medial femoral condyle	
Displaced tear of the medial meniscus (arthrogram negative)	Hypertrophy and degeneration of band	Excision of medial interarticular band
Torn posterior medial meniscus (arthrogram positive for torn medial meniscus)	No meniscal tear	
Torn medial meniscus (arthrogram positive for torn medial meniscus; arthrogram negative for lateral meniscus)	Insignificant tear of the medial meniscus, large tear of the lateral meniscus	
Displaced bucket handle tear of the medial meniscus (arthrogram negative)	Arthroscopically normal knee	
Torn lateral meniscus (no arthrogram)	Torn medial meniscus	
Torn posterior medial meniscus (arthrogram negative for torn medial meniscus; arthrogram was correct but didn't show the pathology)	Cystic mass of the anterior cruciate ligament	Excision of cystic mass from the anterior cruciate ligament
Torn medial meniscus (arthrogram negative)	Incomplete tear of the anterior cruciate ligament	
Questionable tear of the lateral meniscus (no arthrogram)	Displaced bucket handle tear of the lateral meniscus	Excision of displaced bucket handle tear of the lateral meniscus

(*Table continues on page 150*)

Table 13-1. (Continued)

Preoperative Diagnosis	Arthroscopic Findings	Surgery Performed Arthroscopically
Displaced bucket handle tear of the medial meniscus (no arthrogram)	Complete tear of the anterior cruciate ligament	
Ligamentous instability to varus stress (normal arthrogram)	Transverse tear of the lateral meniscus	
Torn medial meniscus (negative arthrogram)	Torn lateral meniscus	
Cystic degeneration of the lateral meniscus (no arthrogram)	Displaced bucket handle tear of the lateral meniscus (ancient)	Excision of displaced bucket handle tear of the lateral meniscus
Torn medial meniscus (no arthrogram)	Multiple (hundreds) cartilaginous loose bodies	Irrigation removal of hundreds of cartilaginous loose bodies
Torn medial meniscus (arthrogram negative for torn medial meniscus)	Tear of posterior third of the lateral meniscus	Excision of inner torn fragment of the posterior third of the lateral meniscus
Unhappy triad (arthrogram positive for large tear of the medial capsule and normal for lateral meniscus)	Unhappy triad plus peripheral detachment lateral meniscus and tear of posterior half of the lateral meniscus	
Torn lateral meniscus (no arthrogram)	Depressed fracture of the tibial plateau, chondromalacia of patella	Excision of "parrot-beak" tear of the medial meniscus
Torn medial meniscus (arthrogram negative for torn medial meniscus and torn lateral meniscus)	Tear of the posterior lateral meniscus at tibial attachment, torn anterior cruciate ligament	Excision of stump of posterior lateral mensicus (in retrospect probably unnecessary)
Torn lateral meniscus (arthrogram negative for torn lateral meniscus; arthrogram shows only medial tear)	Torn medial and lateral meniscus	
Locked knee (arthrogram negative)	Arthroscopically normal knee	
Torn medial meniscus (arthrogram normal)	Transverse tear of the lateral meniscus	
Torn medial meniscus and lateral meniscus (arthrogram positive for torn medial and lateral meniscus)	Acute and chronic synovitis	Synovial biopsy

Table 13-1. (Continued)

Preoperative Diagnosis	Arthroscopic Findings	Surgery Performed Arthroscopically
Torn medial meniscus (arthrogram positive for torn medial meniscus)	Torn discoid lateral meniscus	
Torn medial meniscus (no arthrogram)	Avulsion (cartilaginous) lateral femoral condyle with interarticular loose body	Removal of large cartilaginous loose body
Torn medial meniscus (arthrogram positive for Bakers cyst)	Chondral fracture lateral tibial plateau with loose body	Removal of small cartilaginous loose bodies
Chondrolamacia of patella (arthrogram normal)	Torn posterior third of medial meniscus	Removal of cartilaginous loose body (Returned to referring orthopaedic surgeon)
Torn medial meniscus; torn anterior cruciate ligament (no arthrogram)	Isolated tear of ligamentum mucosum	

14 *Practical Suggestions and Possible Developments in Arthroscopy*

Robert C. Bechtol, M.D.

The natural desire of anyone starting in arthroscopy is to benefit from the experience of other arthroscopists. The newcomer is looking for suggestions that may make arthroscopy more informative, go along more smoothly, and present fewer hazards. At the same time, he has a desire to look ahead, to see what potential there is for some of the techniques that are being developed in the field.

A number of excellent techniques in arthroscopy are being used and taught. The suggestions given here are some that I have found helpful in my own work. The realization that arthroscopy can be an even more valuable diagnostic procedure in the future calls for the application of various scientific principles in its use and development.

PREPARATION FOR ARTHROSCOPY

Whatever the type or make of the arthroscope selected, some sort of protective box or enclosure is desirable (Fig. 14-1). This is to protect the instruments while they are in the preparation room

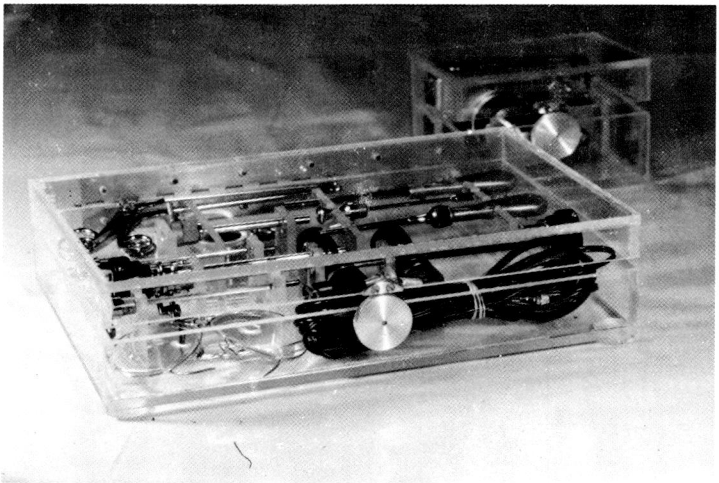

Fig. 14-1. Plastic boxes for gas sterilization of arthroscope, camera, and accessories.

and while they are being gas sterilized. Arthroscopes are fragile instruments and may be easily damaged if placed on a flat tray and wrapped for sterilization. If other instruments or trays are piled on top, the arthroscope is very likely to be bent. Cloth-lined, perforated metal trays or special plastic boxes are best, but certain types of plastic that adsorb ethylene oxide gas should be avoided.

It is well to have an extra telescope and light cable kept sterile for "back-up," in case of failure or contamination of instruments. In the case of tungsten bulb type instruments, a sterile light carrier with several extra bulbs should be available in addition. All other metallic parts can be quick-sterilized in the autoclave, so sterile spares are not necessary.

Whether the arthroscope is the fiberoptic type or the tungsten bulb type (Watanabe No. 21), in some instances neither the telescope nor the light cable can be steam sterilized in the autoclave. This may mean an undesirable interruption or even postponement of the arthroscopy procedure if contamination or breakage occurs. A few sterile standby parts can help avoid this embarrassing situation.

A special pair of glasses for arthroscopy is helpful for those who wear bifocals or trifocals. Ordinary bifocal or trifocal glasses require the operator to tip his head back at an uncomfortable angle, and they often produce half-blurred or double images. When the proper lens correction covers the entire glass, this annoying distortion of vision is avoided. The part of the lens that gives the best image definition can easily be found by actually looking through the arthroscope. With this information, any optician can make up a pair of glasses with the proper lens correction covering the entire glass. The lenses can be mounted in spectacle frames like those used in shooting glasses, which go above the operator's eyebrows. There should be no gas-adsorbing plastic on the frames if the glasses are to be gas sterilized. The operator's nose or face could be burned by the corrosive gas that might be retained by plastic parts.

Upon acquiring an arthroscope, the arthroscopist should become thoroughly familiar with all its parts. This is especially true of the more complicated or more fragile instruments. Practicing with the arthroscope before using it on a patient (for instance, using it to look inside the cupped hand, the mouth, the ear, or other familiar objects) develops facility in handling the arthroscope and aids in orientation. Practice in spatial orientation is particularly helpful in preparing to use a telescope with a field of view at or near a right angle to the instrument. Better still is practice with some of the realistic knee models that have recently been developed and used in arthroscopy training courses, or with fresh specimens if available. Photographing some of these objects helps to determine proper film exposure techniques. Practice ahead of time can save much time during the actual arthroscopy.

DOCUMENTATION

When a patient presents for arthroscopy, documentation begins with the recording of a complete history of the problem at hand and with a careful clinical examination. The extent of the prearthroscopy work-up will necessarily depend on the medical status of the individual patient at the time and the judgment of the physician. Even if the plan is to do arthroscopy only, under general anesthesia, it is well to have the patient's consent for both arthroscopy and possible arthrotomy. It should be explained to the patient that conceivably the arthroscope might fail in some way or an unexpected finding might arise and that either might necessitate an open operation to correct the problem. It is well, also, to have written records to show that the patient was informed of the objectives, advantages, limitations, and alternatives to arthroscopy, and that he or she was made aware of the possible complications of arthroscopy and of any open surgery that might follow.

For systematic photographic documentation of the arthroscopic examination, a modification of Watanabe's diagram of the knee, based on a frontal view of the right knee with the patella reflected distally, is helpful (Fig. 14-2). Various areas of the knee have been numbered and related to this diagram in a convenient order for arthroscopy. There are 21 areas, each of which is approximately the area encompassed by an average arthroscopic view. An attempt is made to photograph each area during examination. The ability to accomplish this will be commensurate with the arthroscopist's skill, and it will improve as he gains experience. The result is a series of pictures that can be kept as a permanent record, displaying the interior of the knee as seen through the arthroscope.

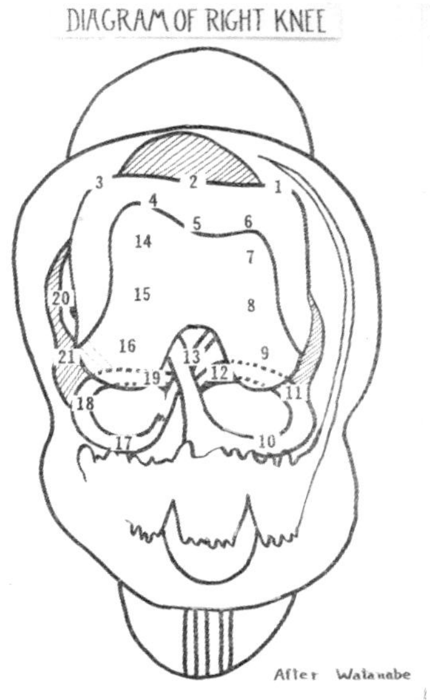

Fig. 14-2. This diagram of the right knee, after Watanabe, has areas numbered in convenient order for arthroscopy. (After Watanabe, M., Takeda, S., and Ikeuchi, H.: Atlas of Arthroscopy. ed. 2. Tokyo, Igaku Shoin, 1969.)

For visitors or those in training, a large diagram of the knee can be displayed in the operating room to show which area of the knee is under arthroscopic view at the moment. Simulation of the arthroscopic view through the eyepiece is achieved by a black cardboard ring on a pointer so placed on the diagram to encircle the area being studied (Fig. 14-3). Closed-circuit television for monitoring is superior, but it involves considerable expense and is not available at all hospitals.

A sterile work sheet with a similar printed diagram of the knee and a sterile marking pen are handy for sketching or making notes during the examination.

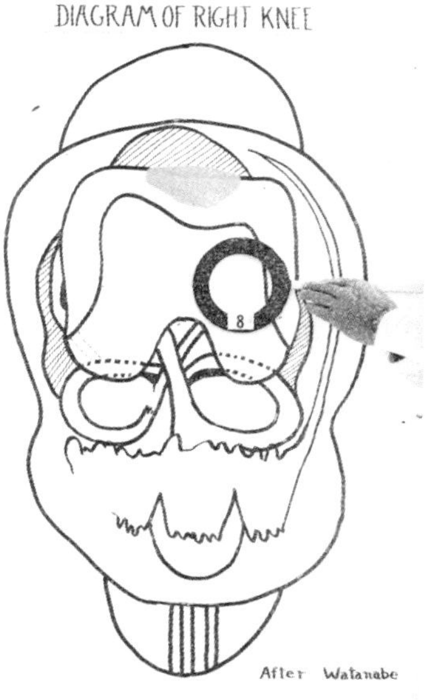

Fig. 14-3. For instruction, a pointer with a black ring is used to encircle the area being studied. (After Watanabe, M., Takeda, S., and Ikeuchi, H.: Atlas of Arthroscopy. ed. 2. Tokyo, Igaku Shoin, 1969.)

Photographic documentation, carried out systematically, is important for the following reasons: (1) for discipline, documentation develops a routine of orderly examination; (2) for learning, retrieval, projection, and labeling of the slides permits study and recognition of the normal and the abnormal; (3) for discov-

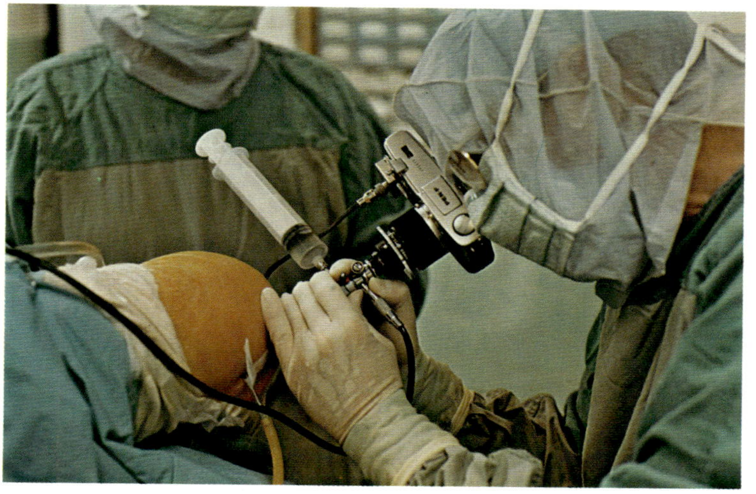

Fig. 14-4. Photographing through the arthroscope. A syringe for injecting saline is attached to the arthroscope sheath. The camera is held at right angles to the leg.

ery, study of the slides correlated with the clinical findings is an important avenue for coming upon new facts and relationships as well as for diagnosis; (4) for follow-up, a photographic record of the arthroscopic examination is just as important at subsequent examinations, as for example, a series of roentgenograms would be for follow-up; (5) for medicolegal use, photographs can be objective evidence. One is well advised to begin photographic documentation with the first case, if possible. After facility in use of the arthroscope and diagnostic skill have been developed, one may wish to document only the pathology.

Photography should be done with the camera always at right angles to the leg, in order to achieve proper and consistent orientation of photographs. It is helpful to have a 50-ml. syringe attached to the arthroscope sheath and to an overhead supply of sterile physiological saline by means of a three-way stopcock when one is taking photographs (Fig. 14-4). If the synovial fluid is cloudy, a bolus of physiological saline may be injected, and while the area is clear, a photograph can be taken. The same technique of injection allows inframeniscal views and differentiation of structures by observing their motion in the fluid stream.

INITIAL STEPS IN THE ARTHROSCOPIC EXAMINATION

When placing the patient on the table for arthroscopy of the knee, it is helpful to put a small pad, such as a folded towel, under the hip on the side to be examined. This prevents the lower extremity from rolling too far into external rotation. The arm on the side to be examined should be placed in abduction on a padded arm board rather than being pinioned at the patient's side (Fig. 14-5). If the arm and hand are held against the side, pressure is applied to the hand by the hip and upper thigh if the foot and leg on that side are dropped over the side of the table during examination. This may result in undesirable hand symptoms following the arthroscopic procedure, if general anesthesia is used. While the patient is relaxed, the knee is carefully examined clinically prior to being prepped. In this way further useful information can occasionally be gained by taking advantage of examination under anesthesia.

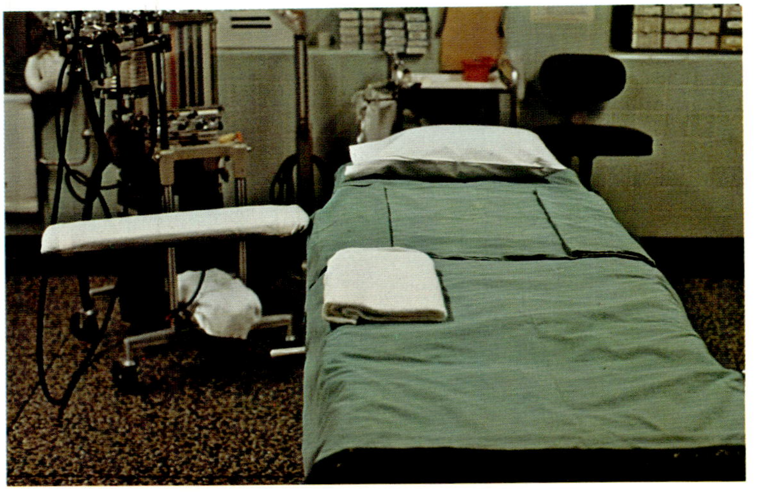

Fig. 14-5. Operating room table prepared for arthroscopy of the right knee. The padded arm board keeps the patient's arm away from his side and the folded towel at hip level prevents excess external rotation of the lower extremity.

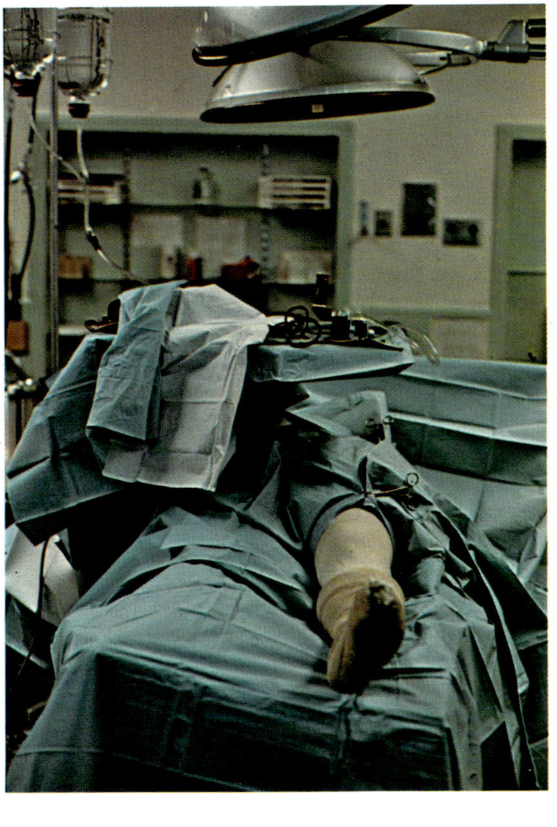

Fig. 14-6. The extremity draped for arthroscopy. Inflow system and Mayo stand with transformer are shown. Sterile photographic equipment is on the side opposite the knee to be arthroscoped. Arthroscopic instruments are on the back table, on the same side as the knee to be arthroscoped.

It is convenient to place all of the equipment—the stand holding the inflow system, the Mayo stand with sterile camera and attachments, and the light generator or transformer (Fig. 14-6)—on the side opposite that which is to be examined. The arthroscopic instruments may be placed on the back table, on the same side as the knee to be examined. The extremity is prepared and draped exactly as for an arthrotomy. Double stockinette is used below the knee, and below-knee wrap of Coban material helps to keep this area dry. A pneumatic tourniquet is applied to the upper thigh, but it is not inflated unless necessary.

The lateral suprapatellar pouch is entered with a large-caliber needle, and a sample of the synovial fluid is taken. The knee is washed out with approximately 150 ml. of sterile physiological saline at room temperature. If one is interested in studying the fluid for crystals under polarized light, great care should be used to avoid contaminating the sample of synovial fluid and the washings. Talc from gloves is a frequent contaminant, as is doubly refractile microscopic debris, which may be contained in hospital-washed syringes. Identification of calcium pyrophosphate dihydrate crystals can be difficult at times, and joints that may have been injected with crystalline corticosteroids within a month may contain residual crystals, which, because of their appearance under polarized light, can be confusing.

After the saline washings return clear, the needle in the suprapatellar pouch is removed, leaving a moderate amount of physiological saline in the knee to float the patella away from the femur. An arthroscope sheath with trocar point is then inserted into the lateral suprapatellar pouch and attached to the inflow system. This sheath can be used for placement of an arthroscope later, if desired. A second arthroscope sheath with trocar point is inserted in the usual manner at the lateral infrapatellar site and is connected to the outflow system. Normally, there is a voluminous flow of physiological saline from the suprapatellar pouch to the arthroscope sheath below. The direction of flow of the solution can be reversed easily at any time during the examination, if it appears advantageous to do so.

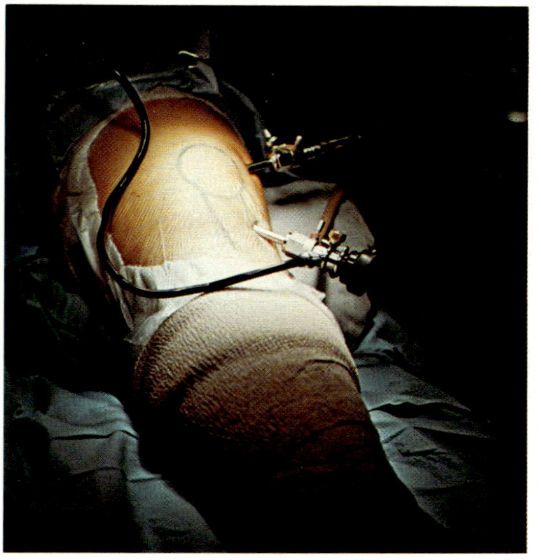

Fig. 14-7. The arthroscope in the knee at the lateral infrapatellar site. (Left knee) A second arthroscope sheath is in the lateral suprapatellar pouch, for irrigation and possible arthroscope portal.

After the arthroscope is inserted into the sheath at the infrapatellar site (Fig. 14-7), the operator and assistant don sterile glasses and hoods. If there is a good possibility that arthrotomy will also be performed, a sterile plastic face shield is also used. By careful aseptic technique in this manner, it is possible to remove the arthroscope after examination and, when indicated, proceed to arthrotomy with confidence. However, if arthroscopy is prolonged, the extremity should be completely re-prepared and re-draped. In this event, the operator should scrub again and be freshly gloved and gowned before arthrotomy is begun.

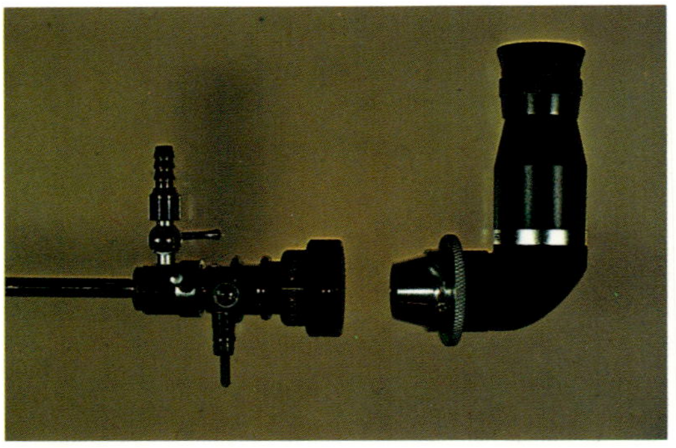

Fig. 14-8. A right-angle eyepiece for the arthroscope made from a right-angle camera finder.

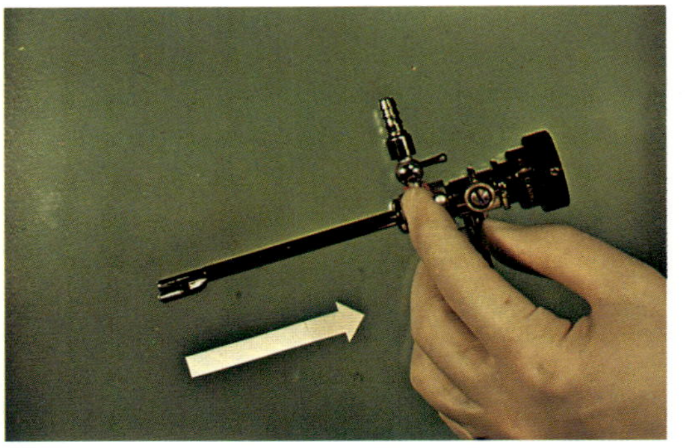

Fig. 14-9. The Watanabe No. 21 arthroscope is retracted by the sheath to prevent the telescope from sliding back and exposing the bulb to pressure.

The usual crouched position for examining the suprapatellar pouch is an uncomfortable one. At times the operator's head has to be almost against the patient's leg. Therefore, a right-angle eyepiece, made by modifying a right-angle finder from a camera to fit the eyepiece of the arthroscope, has been found to be of considerable value, both for comfort and for keeping the face and head away from the patient's leg (Fig. 14-8).

Before actually starting the examination, if one is using a Watanabe No. 21 arthroscope with a tungsten bulb, it is important to know that the arthroscope should be retracted by the sheath and advanced by the eyepiece. Any sliding motion of the arthroscope in the knee should be done toward the light bulb, to protect the light carrier from bending or breaking (Figs. 14-9–14-11).

Arthroscopes with glass-fiber light cables can also be used in open arthrotomy wounds because of the relatively cool fiber-optic light source. Occasionally this is helpful after meniscectomy for making sure there is no retained posterior meniscal segment. Although there is little danger of burning the tissues while using an arthroscope with a fiber-optic light source, the lighted end should nevertheless be tested to make sure no significant heat is being generated. Any arthroscope with an incandescent bulb at the

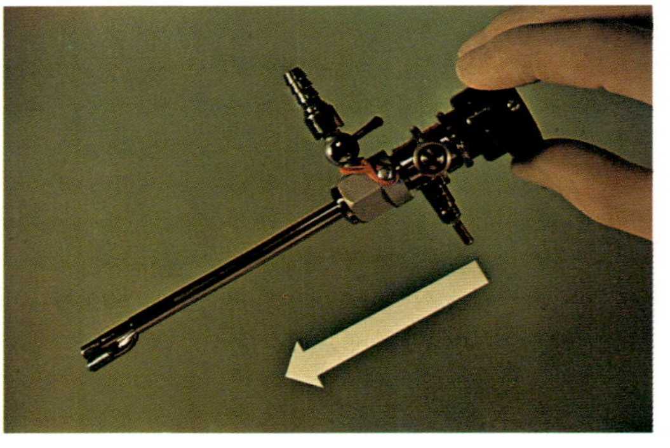

Fig. 14-10. The Watanabe No. 21 scope is advanced with the eyepiece. If the telescope slides back and then is advanced by the sheath, it may break the light carrier.

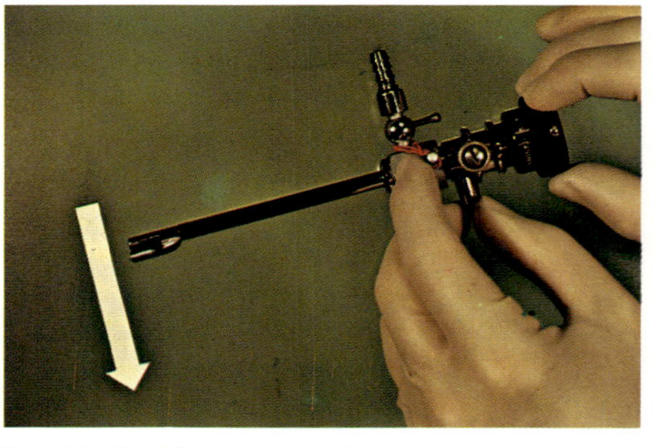

Fig. 14-11. The proper direction to slide the arthroscope is toward the bulb. This presses the bulb against the telescope and does not allow soft tissue to get between the bulb and the telescope.

end should be used within an irrigating solution for cooling and preferably should not be used "dry."

SPECIAL TECHNIQUES AND ADJUNCTS TO ARTHROSCOPY

In a field as relatively new as arthroscopy techniques are constantly being developed and improved. Some of these techniques are usable at the present time.

Transillumination

Articular cartilage and synovium may be viewed by transillumination. This can be done by using two arthroscopes in the knee. Usually one is used through a sheath in the suprapatellar pouch and the other at the lateral infrapatellar site. One instrument, with the light on, is moved about in the knee in such a way as to transilluminate the articular cartilage, while the other is used with the light off to view the cartilage by transillumination (Fig. 14-12). A single arthroscope and a fiberoptic light wand may be used in a similar manner. Transmission of light through articular cartilage can show fibrillation, fissures, cratering, and areas of osteochondritis dissecans, giving another visual dimension which may help in assessing the extent of pathology. Synovial villi can be viewed by transillumination, and magnified views of blood vessels can be obtained.

The light source for transillumination can be either intra-articular or extra-articular. In some instances, a fiber-optic light source can be used outside the knee to transilluminate the patella or be used inside the knee to transilluminate the medial femoral condyle to show the borders of an area of osteochondritis dissecans. This is sometimes helpful in accurately localizing an area for drilling or removal of the osteochondral fragment for replacement. The end of a fiber-optic light cable should not be used against the skin or soft tissue for transillumination if the cable is attached to a powerful photographic light source, because it may produce a burn. In any case, before use, the lighted end of the cord should be carefully tested against the operator's skin to be sure that no significant heat is being generated.

Measurements

The hallmark of meaningful, repeatable observation is measurement. During ini-

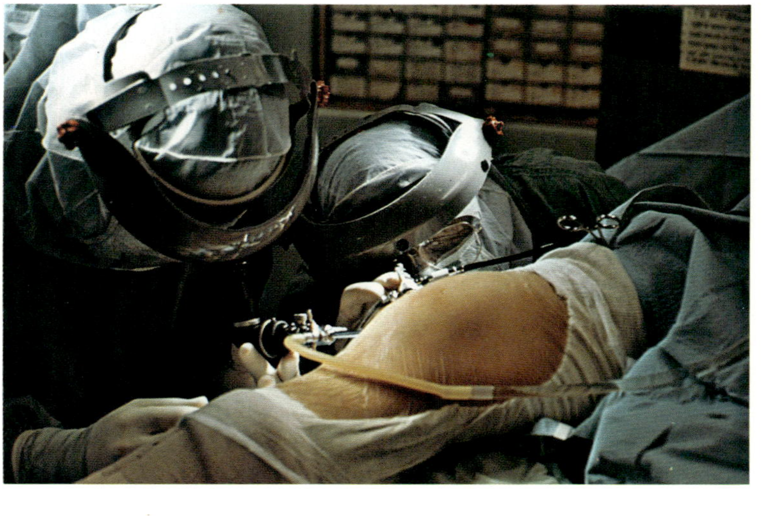

Fig. 14-12. Viewing by transillumination can be accomplished with two arthroscopes.

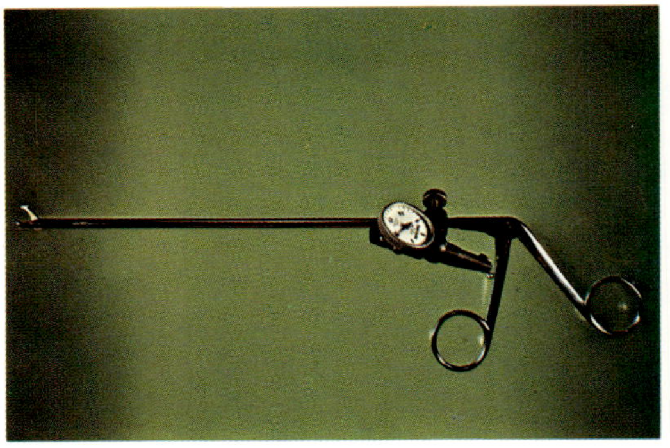

Fig. 14-13. Wolf scissors with a dial indicator attached to show distance between scissor points can be used as calipers up to 10 mm.

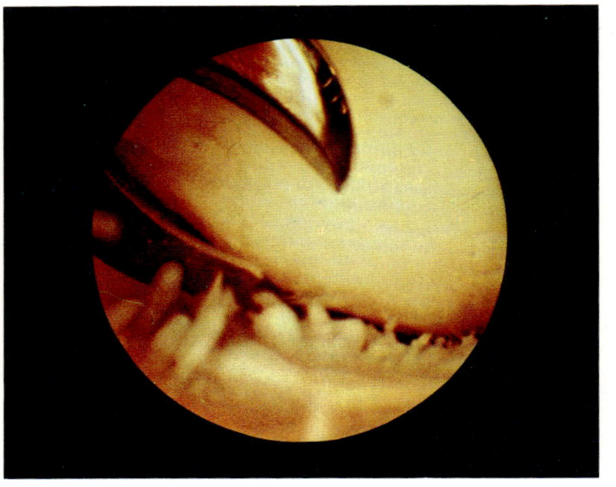

Fig. 14-14. This arthroscopic view of Wolf scissors in the knee shows how they can be used as calipers.

tial and follow-up examinations, it is useful to be able to measure lesions, such as areas of chondromalacia of the articular surfaces, or the size of the synovial villi, and to compare them. A change in measurements may give some quantitative idea of the progression or regression of a pathological state. Until eyepieces are built with reticles, one way of doing this is to attach a dial indicator to an instrument that can be used as a caliper (Figs. 14-13, 14-14). The hook-tipped scissors made by Wolf, Storz, and others are nicely shaped for this use. The scissors used, however, must have a minimum of backlash, in order to be accurate. A glance at the dial indicator outside the joint will give the exact distance between the scissor tips that are being observed inside the knee with the arthroscope. With this method, it is not necessary to have the same size field of view or even to use the same type arthroscope in order to obtain comparable measurements for different patients.

Measurements can also be made from serial photographs. When this is done, care must be exercised in order to obtain the same size field of view, relative to the knee, each time. Furthermore, a camera lens of the same focal length must be used on the same type arthroscope every time for the measurements to be comparable.

Intra-articular Dye

Instillation of innocuous dye into the knee can aid interpretation of the presence and extent of articular cartilage and meniscal lesions. Very small amounts of sterile methylene blue, introduced drop by drop while observing with the arthroscope, will stain and emphasize the borders of chondromalacia and tears or attritional lesions of the menisci. Abraded or softened areas of articular cartilage seem to have a greater affinity for the dye than the normal smooth cartilaginous surfaces.

Polarizing and Color Absorption Filters

A polarizing filter in the eyepiece of the arthroscope is sometimes useful in giving increased visual contrast when looking toward a light source that is being used to transilluminate articular cartilage. Rotation of the polarizer will often give better visual definition and contrast at one particular setting.

Color absorption filters can also be used to advantage at times. These can be fitted to the eyepiece for visual rather than photographic use (Fig. 14-15). Filters that transmit only the colors near the center of the visual spectrum (greens) most often

Fig. 14-15. A filter adapter can be used to mount filters for the eyepiece of the arthroscope. A polarizing filter is shown in the adapter.

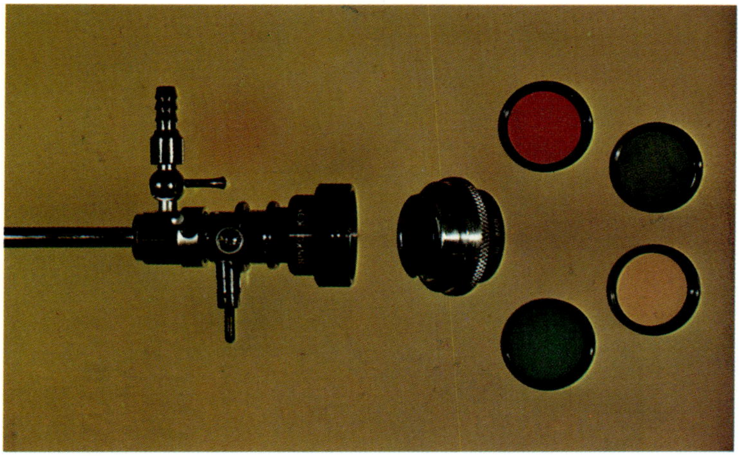

seem to give the best image definition through the arthroscope. This is, in part, an individual, subjective phenomenon and in part due to the fact that the extremes of the visual spectrum (red and blue) do not focus at the same point and are both absorbed by the green filter. When methylene blue dye is used in the knee, a yellow or red filter greatly darkens or emphasizes the stained areas, because both of these filters absorb blue light.

Projection

Projection enlargement of the photographs (slides) taken at the time of arthroscopic examination are often informative. With the magnification obtained by projection on a screen, lesions that were not seen or properly appreciated at the time of actual arthroscopy occasionally become apparent. On a smooth, completely matte screen the image will be sharper and more even in brightness than on any other surface. The relaxed atmosphere of the projection room often aids in thoughtful analysis of the photographic record and may result in a change of the treatment plan.

Another method of projection can give the arthroscopist a different perspective of a photograph taken at arthroscopy. The slide can be projected onto a rotatable screen whose axis of rotation is shown on the front of the screen by index marks (Fig. 14-16). If the index marks are aligned along the area on the projected image where magnification is desired and the screen is then tilted, the line on the projected image along the index marks will stay in focus. As the screen is tilted back and forth, a striking change in perspective

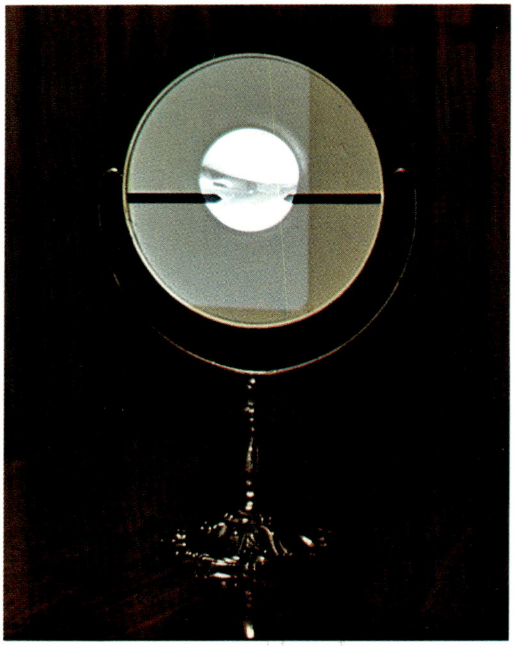

Fig. 14-16. The surface of the rotatable screen is smooth and matte. The index marks show the axis of rotation.

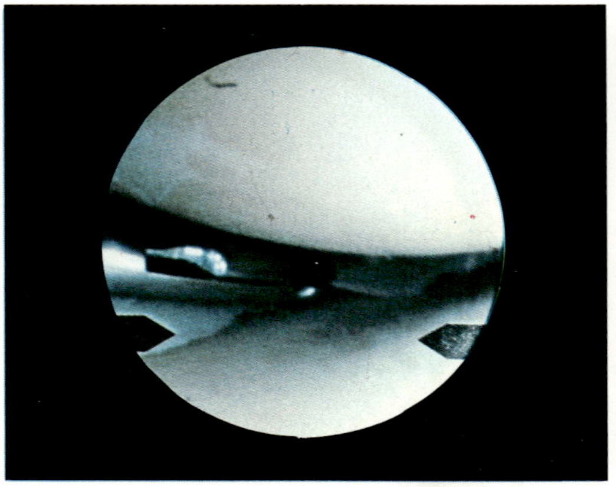

Fig. 14-17. A photographic slide is projected at right angles to the "tiltable" screen. Index marks show the axis of rotation of the screen. (See Fig. 14-18.)

is obtained (Figs. 14-17, 14-18). Horizontal lines (those parallel to the index marks) will be widened and vertical lines (those perpendicular to the index marks) will be lengthened. The obliquity of the screen results in both magnification and distortion over a selected area. If the index marks are placed along the joint line, when the screen is tilted it *appears* that the articular surfaces are pulled apart and more of the meniscus becomes visible. Small meniscal tears may thus be enlarged and made to stand out in contrast to the rest of the image (Figs. 14-19, 14-20).

POSSIBLE FUTURE DEVELOPMENTS IN ARTHROSCOPY

Infrared Photography

Visible light is a very small band of wavelengths ranging from approximately 400 to 700 nm. in the electromagnetic spectrum. One way to "see more" with the arthroscope is by breaking visible light up into monochromatic bands by the use of adsorption filters (see p. 160). Another way is to widen the small crack that we look through when we use visible light; this is done by going beyond the visible spectrum into the infrared band (700–900 nm.; Fig. 14-21).

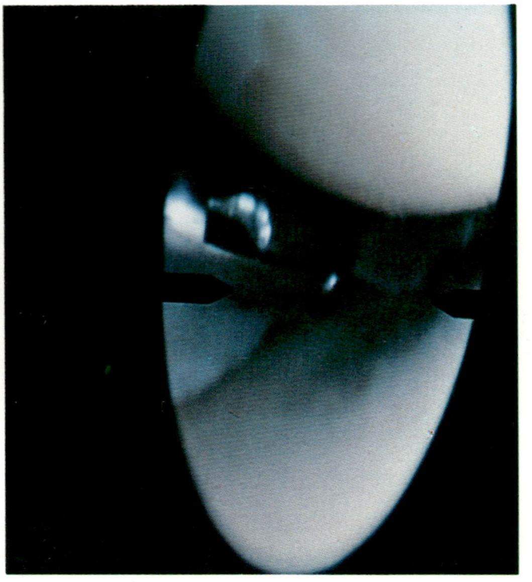

Fig. 14-18. Compare this projection on the screen rotated 40 degrees with the same slide in Figure 14-17. Forceps are grasping the posterior segment of the medial meniscus.

The rationale for the use of infrared is that it has already been found to penetrate the skin to a depth of several millimeters,

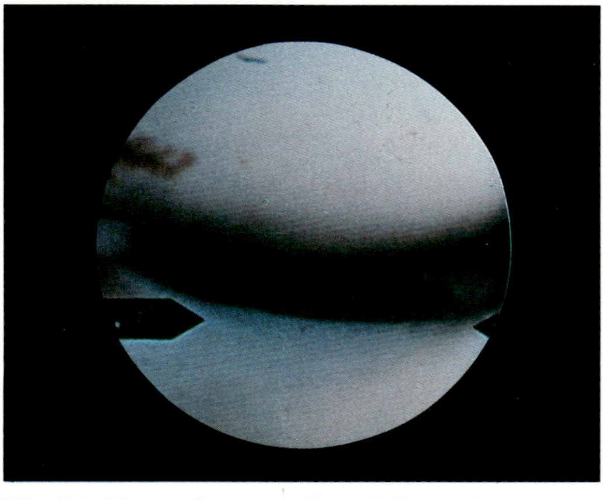

Fig. 14-19. A photographic slide of the lateral meniscus is projected at right angles to the screen. (See Fig. 14-20.)

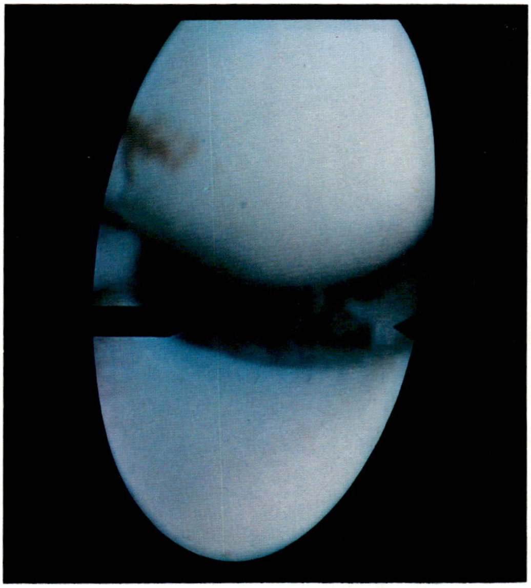

Fig. 14-20. When the slide shown in Figure 14-19 is projected onto the screen rotated 40 degrees, irregular tears of the meniscus become more obvious. Note the index marks.

and it will penetrate an opaque cornea to reveal the iris. Tests show it will also penetrate articular cartilage to reveal reflections or absorptions from a deeper layer than would be the case with visible light (Figs. 14-22, 14-23). Because infrared light goes through ordinary glass, it calls for no special lenses for photography.

Kodak Ektachrome Infrared film is used in this type of photography. The films should be kept refrigerated at 13 degrees C (55° F) until about 2 hours prior to use, in order to avoid loss of infrared sensitivity and to avoid a color balance shift. Although the camera need not be loaded in a darkroom, it should be loaded in subdued light, as there is a tendency for infrared to penetrate the slot in the film cassette. A Wratten No. 12 filter is used, either in the eyepiece of the arthroscope or in the camera. When a tungsten light source is used, a color-correcting filter is desirable. The Watanabe No. 21 arthroscope has been the model used most for infrared color photography because of the high output of infrared from its white-hot tungsten filament in close proximity to the area being photographed.

Some of the initial infrared photographs made through the arthroscope suggest that infrared not only accentuates articular cartilage lesions but also seem to show changes in the articular cartilage beyond the lesions seen with visible light. Lines of healing of osteochondral fractures also seem to show nearby loss of the homogeneous appearance of the articular cartilage. The interpretation of infrared findings in arthroscopy is not sufficiently settled at this time to warrant conclusions. Rather, more investigation needs to

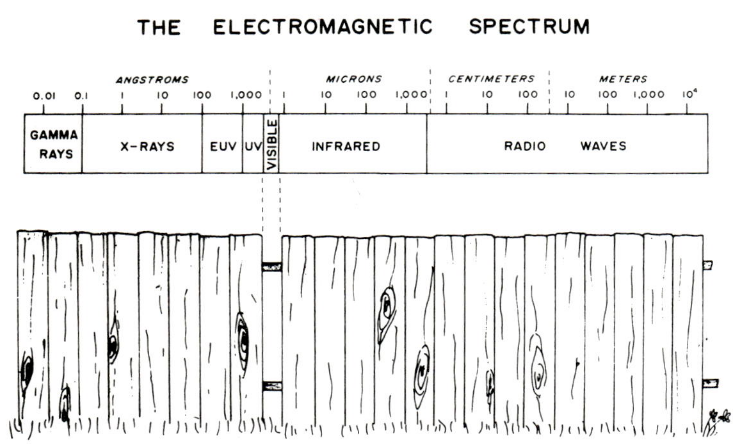

Fig. 14-21. A diagram of the electromagnetic spectrum shows the narrow band of visible light. The spectrum may be compared to a board fence. The object of infrared photography is to pull another board out of the fence, in order to "see" more. (Top of diagram showing spectrum is reproduced by permission from *Sky and Telescope*.)

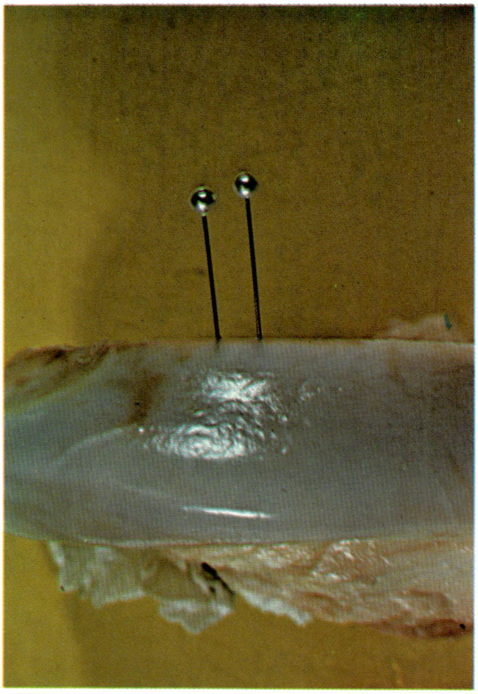

Fig. 14-22. A photo of a beef joint made with conventional color film. Two common pins have been inserted under the articular cartilage. Slight shadows of the pins can be seen near the points of entry. (Compare Fig. 14-23.)

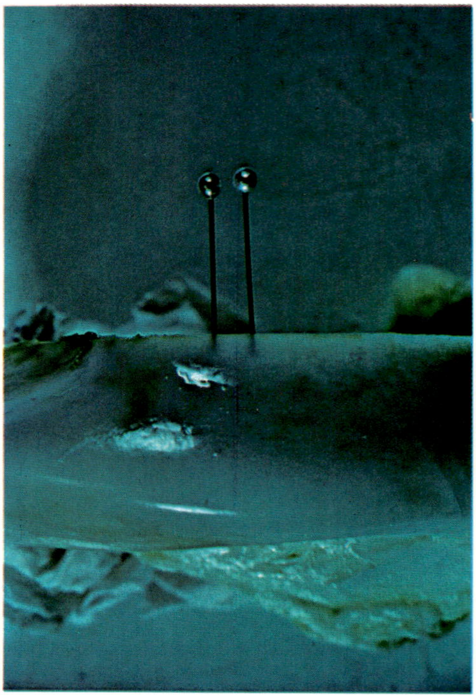

Fig. 14-23. The joint shown in Figure 14-22 was photographed with infrared color film (filtration: Wratten No. 12; CC 50C-2). The shadows of the pins are much sharper and visible out to the ends of the pins. Note the "false" color rendition.

be done along these lines before infrared can be recommended as a routine diagnostic or prognostic aid.

Intra-articular Roentgenograms

An intra-articular roentgenogram is defined here as a roentgenogram taken with the film inside the knee joint. Recent gas sterilization techniques have made it safe to place sterilized film inside the knee joint. It is considered possible to introduce a film into the knee, expose the film, and remove it under arthroscopic control. The limiting factor to date has been lack of dimensionally stable film thin enough to be rolled into a cartridge of 4 or 5 mm. diameter. The advantage to be gained by placing the film under the patella for an anteroposterior view of this bone is that the shadows show a strikingly high degree of detail. This could be useful clinically, for example, in showing undisplaced linear fractures and retinacular avulsions which are not well visualized on the conventional views. Furthermore, the detailed internal architecture of the bone thus revealed may hold some keys to understanding the function or malfunction of the patella. Similarly, by placing the film up against an area of osteochondritis dissecans in the medial femoral condyle, it may be possible to show the earliest stage of fatigue fracture in the lesion which might not show on a film taken in the standard way. Roentgenograms made with gas sterilized film placed within the knee at arthrotomy are shown as examples of the detailed obtainable (Figs. 14-24, 14-25).

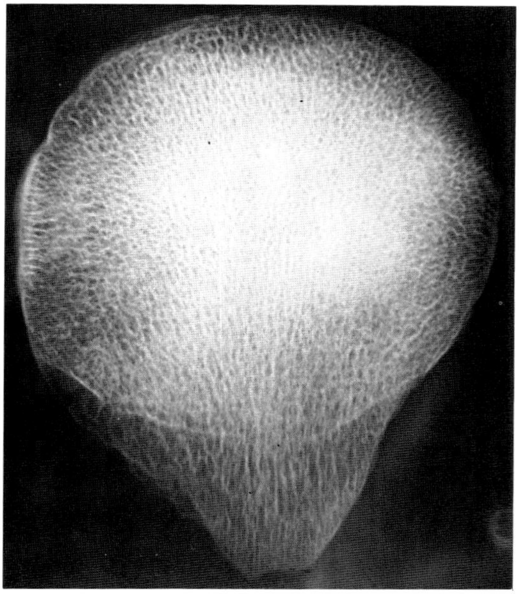

Fig. 14-24. Note high order of trabecular detail on this intra-articular roentgenogram of a normal adult patella made at arthrotomy.

Improvements in Surgical Instrumentation and Procedures

Not only will improved instruments and techniques lead to easier and more accurate diagnosis, but the increasing sophistication of operating instruments will be even more spectacular. Indeed, some of the intra-articular surgery (partial meniscectomy) being done through the arthroscope or under arthroscopic control, even at this time, has converted some rather major knee surgery to nothing more than an overnight stay in the hospital followed by immediate ambulation. This promises to be a great boon, particularly to the middle-aged patient who may not be in the best physical condition and cannot afford to miss much work.

Surgical help can be offered in this way where previously the magnitude of the procedure, from the patient's standpoint, often seemed prohibitive. This is not to say that the procedure is a minor one from the operator's standpoint or is easily performed. On the contrary, at present it requires much practice and impressive skill.

At present, of course, only certain conditions are amenable to intra-articular surgery with the arthroscope, and the long-term results are not known. However, the increasing accumulation of observational data correlated with treated clinical conditions and the results, will indicate in what cases these measures can best be used.

The future may see further electronic developments in the arthroscope, possibly the use of cutting currents and light-emitting diodes. Even the use of

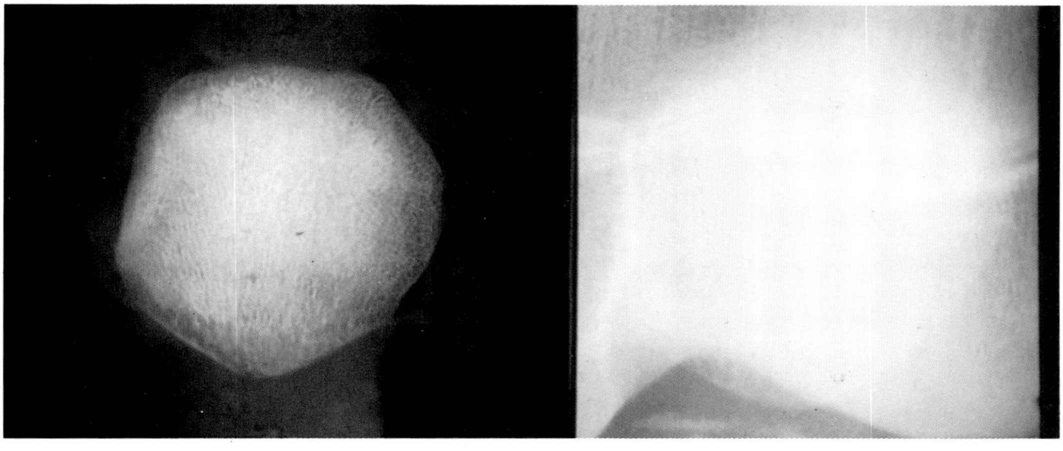

Fig. 14-25. Compare the intra-articular roentgenogram of the patella of a 12-year-old girl made at arthrotomy (*left*) with the conventional roentgenogram (*right*).

fluorescent, non-toxic irrigating solutions for lighting is envisioned. Perhaps the use of laser beams in partial meniscectomies or in removal of areas of chondromalacia may be developed sufficiently to be practical.

Arthroscopy in Research

The arthroscope is an amazing tool of discovery, because it fuses comfortably with so many physical modalities that can be used with it without affecting or harming the patient. Arthroscopy under local anesthesia will permit the mapping out of sensitive areas in the knee and locations of pain spread or radiation when various structures are stimulated in the course of a routine diagnostic examination. For example, how common is postero*medial* pain in the knee when the posterior segment of the *lateral* meniscus is the site of pathology? Or, does point pressure on articular cartilage cause pain? What areas are sensitive, if any, and what type of discomfort or pain is produced? The answers to these questions and many more will come through use of the arthroscope and will greatly improve clinical diagnosis in the future.

The use of low-level sound and ultrasound energy during arthroscopy may lead to interesting discoveries. Would standing waves develop on the meniscus or in other structures in the knee? Would there be a detectable difference between wave forms on an intact meniscus or articular cartilage and wave forms on torn, damaged, or degenerated areas? Perhaps the use of this type of low-level energy combined with simultaneous stroboscopic observation could lead to findings of practical value in the future.

By increasing the energy and decreasing the area subjected to ultrasound, emulsification of meniscal tissue may be possible with a technique similar to that being used in certain cataract operations. Perhaps meniscectomy by this technique will be feasible in the future.

Combined with the use of dyes, an arthroscope with a high-power lens to view the transilluminated synovium might make microscopic study of vascularity and pathological lesions of the synovium an arthroscopic procedure. Use of polarized light in this situation could add even more information, especially in regard to crystal deposition.

Eyepieces that convert infrared or ultraviolet to visible light may be developed and used as part of a routine arthroscopic examination. Such phenomena as infrared transmission during transillumination of structures, and infrared and ultraviolet fluorescence are incidental properties that may be found useful in diagnosis and prognosis.

Photometric measurements of visible light reflection from normal and abnormal articular cartilage may give an indication of changes too early to recognize by other means, the reflection or absorption of narrow light bands (reflection spectrography) possibly indicating specific changes in the cartilage or synovium. A recent development is laser resonance Raman spectroscopy, which can probe specific structural changes in complex molecules without interference from surrounding structures.

Holograms, three-dimensional "photographs," of at least part of the knee may become possible in the future by introduction of coherent light through the arthroscope or through a supplementary light wand. If so, this will be almost like plucking the knee out through the arthroscope for examination.

It may be possible to implant minute sensors into the knee by means of the arthroscope. The sensors, whether pressure, ballistic, chemical, or other types, might be left in place long enough to gather information into a computer tie-in, and might then be arthroscopically removed later with very little inconvenience or disability to the patient. Such computerized information then could influence the type of surgery proposed or possibly even anticipate when and what kind of medication would be necessary to prevent acute episodes of inflammatory or metabolic conditions in the joint. Detection of abnormal shock or distribution of weight on the bearing surfaces by this means may make long-range prognosis of osteoarthrosis possible and prevention practical.

REFERENCES

1. Eilert, R. E.: American Academy of Orthopedic Surgeons, Course on Arthroscopy and Arthrography of the Knee. Laboratory Demonstrations. Chicago, Ill., November 21–22, 1975.
2. Guten, G.: Staining articular cartilage with methylene blue during arthroscopy. Read before The International Arthroscopy Association. Copenhagen, Denmark, July 10, 1975.
3. Ikeuchi, H.: Surgery under arthroscopic control. "R" Rev. Internat. Rhumatol., *33:*57, 1976.
4. Jackson, R. W., and Abe, I.: The role of arthroscopy in the management of disorders of the knee. J. Bone Joint Surg., *54B:*310, 1972.
5. Kahn, C. B., Hollander, J. L., and Schumacher, H. R.: Corticosteroid crystals in synovial fluid. J.A.M.A., *211:*807, 1970.
6. Kodak Publication No. N-1: Applied Infrared Photography. Ed. 3. 1973.
7. Kodak Publication No. M-28: Medical Infrared Photography. 1972 Edition.
8. McGinty, J. B.: Closed circuit television in arthroscopy. "R" Rev. Internat. Rhumatol., *33:*45, 1976.
9. O'Connor, R. L.: The arthroscope in the management of crystal-induced synovitis of the knee. J. Bone Joint Surg., *55A:* 1443, 1973.
10. Phelps, P., Steele, A. D., and McCarty, D. J., Jr.: Compensated polarized light microscopy. Identification of crystals in synovial fluids from gout and pseudogout. J.A.M.A., *203:*166, 1968.
11. Research News: Laser spectroscopy: probing biomolecular functions. Science, *188:*1002, 1975.
12. Watanabe, J., Takeda, S., and Ikeuchi, H.: Atlas of Arthroscopy. ed. 2. p. 53. Tokyo, Igaku Shoin, 1969.

Index

Numbers in *italics* indicate a figure; "t" following a page number indicates a table.